Keys to EMR/EHR Success

Selecting and Implementing an Electronic Medical Record

SECOND EDITION

Ronald B. Sterling, CPA, MBA

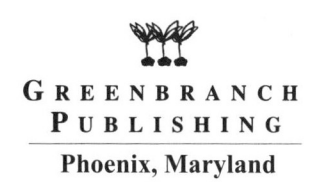

GREENBRANCH PUBLISHING
Phoenix, Maryland

Keys to EMR/EHR Success: Selecting and Implementing an Electronic Medical Record

Copyright © 2010 by Greenbranch Publishing, LLC

ISBN: 978-0-9827055-0-6

Published by Greenbranch Publishing, LLC
PO Box 208
Phoenix, MD 21131
Phone: (800) 933-3711
Fax: (410) 329-1510
Email: info@greenbranch.com
Website: www.greenbranch.com, www.soundpractice.net, www.codapedia.com

All rights reserved. No part of this publication may be reproduced or transmitted in any form, by any means, without prior written permission of Green branch Publishing, LLC. Routine photocopying or electronic distribution to others is a copyright violation. Please notify us immediately at (800) 933-3711 if you have received any unauthorized editorial from this book.

Requests for permission, information on our multi-copy pricing program, or other information should be addressed to the Permissions Department, Greenbranch Publishing, LLC. (800) 933-3711 or info@greenbranch.com

This publication is designed to provide general medical practice management information and is sold with the understanding that neither the author nor the publisher is engaged in rendering legal, accounting, ethical, or clinical advice. If legal, technological or other expert advice is required, the services of a competent professional person should be sought.

Screen shots of EMR/EHR products reprinted with permission from industry representatives.

CPT® is a registered trademark of the American Medical Association.

Printed in the United States of America by United Book Press, Inc.

PUBLISHER
Nancy Collins

EDITORIAL ASSISTANT
Jennifer Weiss

BOOK DESIGNER
Carter Publishing Studio

COPYEDITING AND INDEX
Hearthside Publishing Services

TABLE OF CONTENTS

Introduction v

Author's Note, Second Edition vii

Author's Note, First Edition ix

About the Author x

Acknowledgments xi

Chapter 1: Should I Invest in an EHR? 1

Chapter 2: Evaluating an EHR Investment 15

Chapter 3: Your Practice Management System and an EHR 37

Chapter 4: Compiling a Practice Focused Evaluation List 53

Chapter 5: EHR and Malpractice Risk 85

Chapter 6: Selecting Products to Review 99

Chapter 7: Reviewing Products for Your Practice 113

Chapter 8: Making a Final Decision 133

Chapter 9: Negotiating a Contract 149

Chapter 10: Implementing an EHR 177

Chapter 11: Activating an EHR 249

Chapter 12: Supporting an EHR 259

Appendix: List of EHR vendors 269

Index 283

Glossary 292

Dedication

To my wife Janis, and my parents,
Kenneth and Hannah.

INTRODUCTION

The lack of effective medical record tools is dangerous for patients and intolerable for doctors and their practices. Without computerized support for patient services and practice operations, your must contend with inefficient operations and obstacles for doctors, staff, and even patients. In the final analysis, staff, doctors and patients are frustrated with the delays in patient service. Doctors and staff must sift through ever-growing mountains of paper to find the essential information and/or treatment plans for patients.

Unfortunately, few practices understand the challenges and demands of selecting and implementing an EHR. In too many cases, EHR decisions are made for the wrong reasons. In other cases, implementation is undertaken with too few resources and even less internal support. The result can be expensive ventures that leave members of the practice frustrated, maybe even angry.

Keys to EMR/EHR Success guides you through the demanding and challenging process of selecting and implementing an EHR. The book is filled with hundreds of tips, ideas, and advisories to help you avoid problems and achieve success.

From figuring out what you to need, to selecting an EHR and negotiating a contract, **Keys to EMR/EHR Success** will help you realistically focus on the key issues to consider and help you develop a balanced relationship with your vendor. After completing your contract, **Keys to EMR/EHR Success** will help you structure and manage implementation in a realistic and constructive manner. **Keys to EMR/EHR Success** presents strategies to preserve your EHR investment and insure that the EHR, and its use in your practice, evolves with your needs, and remains relevant to your colleagues.

There is no question that the selection and implementation of an EHR is a "bet-the-practice" proposition. If you fail, you end up with more costs and greater frustration. On the other hand, few practices will be able to avoid implementing EHRs as these tools become necessary to meet patient expectations, payer quality requirements and pay-for-performance demands. The Healthcare Information Technology (HITECH) Stimulus Program, that will pay up to $44,000 for each eligible provider that participates with Medicare and even more for Medicaid participating eligible providers, has triggered an unprecedented level of interest and plans to implement EHRs. Indeed, the sheer force of the HITECH stimulus program will generate enough EHR use that practices without EHRs could be at a disadvantage serving patients and interacting with other healthcare providers. Understanding and accommodating the all-encompassing changes that EHRs produce will help you properly implement and effectively capitalize on these ultimately critical tools for your practice.

Properly implemented EHRs can provide a wide range of benefits to a practice and its patients. However, the implementation of an EHR is not an easy proposition. An EHR clearly demands a strategic vision and tactical focus. Attention to managing change and proactively working to keep the EHR relevant to your practice will help you more effectively serve patients and make better use of staff and doctors.

Keys to EMR/EHR Success: Selecting and Implementing an Electronic Medical Record was written by Ron Sterling, President, Sterling Solutions, Ltd., Silver Spring, Md. Ron, a nationally recognized expert, has guided a variety of primary care and specialty practices in over 30 states in the selection and implementation of electronic health record and practice management systems. He has authored four books on practice-based computer tools. Mr. Sterling has reviewed electronic health record and practice management systems from over 150 vendors. He can be reached via *info@sterling-solutions.com* or 301-681-4247.

AUTHOR'S NOTE
Second Edition

Nancy Collins and I attended the Healthcare Information and Management Systems Society (HIMSS) awards ceremony at the 2009 HIMSS (Healthcare Information Management and Systems Society) conference in Chicago. The awards ceremony recognized the groundbreaking accomplishments and service to the Electronic Healthcare Record industry. A variety of awards are presented for service to the industry as well as the innovative use of technology to serve patients and improve results. And the first edition of the book in your hand was awarded the HIMSS Book of the Year Award. The citation stated:

> *Keys to EMR Success: Selecting and Implementing an Electronic Medical Record*
> By: Ronald Sterling, CPA, MBA
>
> "*Keys to EMR Success: Selecting and Implementing an Electronic Medical Record* was selected because it comprehensively covers the selection and implementation of electronic medical records for the physician practice. The book contains solid advice, worklists, and other tools to help physicians and office managers succeed in leveraging EMRs to improve patient services and practice performance. The book presents a guide for sorting out myriad options for the practice, including the vendor choice, contracting, and establishing a framework in the practice to ensure a successful implementation. Topics include defining requirements; using a weighting score to make a final decision on product selection; negotiating contracts to avoid tricky situations with warranties, termination clauses, upfront fees, etc; and staff training and motivation."

I really appreciate recognition of the book and its content from the EHR industry. I also appreciate the many people who purchased the book as a result of the award and the uniquely comprehensive and practical advice contained in *Keys to EMR Success*.

So, the problem was how could I improve upon a book that is widely recognized as "best in class." Fortunately, the answer came from Congress.

In June 2008, the first edition of *Keys to EMR Success* was published by Greenbranch Publishing. Within a year, the term EMR has been superseded by Electronic Healthcare Records (EHR) through the Healthcare Information

Technology (HITECH) aspects of the "Stimulus Package." There were a couple of ironies that resulted from this situation:

> EHR, the new abbreviation, sounds a lot like "Error" when you try to pronounce it. I thought that for $17 Billion they could have afforded a pronounceable acronym, or at least one that Microsoft Word would not try to "correct" every time your type it.

> Significant commercial activity was triggered by all of the "old" EMR vendors who had to rename and rebrand their products as EHRs.

And following the lead of the EMR industry, I thought that we could rename the book *Keys to EMR/EHR Success* and voila Second Edition. I thought that would make Nancy Collins happy. In reality it is a lot of work since we had to change all references to EMR while Microsoft Word pushes back every time you type HER. But industry events overtook us.

In order to meet the evolving issues of the suddenly overactive EHR interest of practices and other healthcare organizations, I wanted to add more useful tables and coverage in areas that are just not on the radar screen of enough people when trying to meet the demands of selecting and implementing an EM...EHR.

An entire chapter has been added on EHR and malpractice risk and coverage of conversion issues for practices that have an old EHR was added to the chapter on implementation. Several new worksheets have been included as well as a number of new advisories and notes.

These improvements will help you more effectively organize, track and manage the significant amount of work that you face to succeed in taking advantage of these critical patient care and clinical tools.

Thank you,

Ron Sterling

Ron Sterling

AUTHOR'S NOTE
First Edition

Doctors, medical practices and their patients suffer from the limitations of paper-based medical record systems and processes. Even with the best clinical and interpersonal skills, the limitations of paper records undermine effective interactions with patients. From taking a message instead of answering a question, to office visit delays in locating the expected test results (or even documenting if the test was done), patients are subjected to diversions from the quality of care provided by the vast majority of medical practices.

I have personally experienced practices losing requests for information about a family member in the hospital, and even the complete disappearance of a medical record with 20 years of information. I have waited for practices to find "missing charts," and witnessed doctor and staff frustration with the time needed to get their hands on important patient information. I have been given incorrect information on a medical situation, because the doctor could not effectively gather the complete information from the mass of paper that is my own medical record. Are these unusual situations? Am I the exception?

Based on my extensive work with doctors and staff in practices from 30 states, I know that the doctors, nurses and staff that serve patients are as frustrated, if not more frustrated, with the limitations of paper medical records. Fortunately, there are viable solutions to the problem. There are a number of practical EHR products, and the hardware prices have dropped. In the final analysis, practices need to value their own time and focus on improvements that can address the paper chase. Once you have achieved this conclusion, you must approach EHR selection and implementation with a serious commitment and clear understanding of the strategies and demands to assure success.

I would like to thank Beth Matosko for her help with the book.

Thank you,

Ron Sterling

ABOUT THE AUTHOR

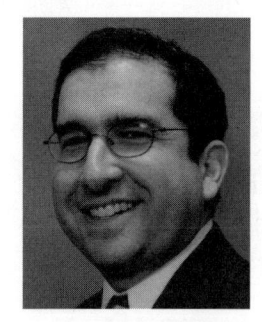

Ronald B. Sterling, CPA, MBA, President of Sterling Solutions, Ltd. (www.sterling-solutions.com), helps physician practices and other healthcare organizations capitalize on technology to improve patient service, clinical operations and financial results. Sterling Solutions provides project leadership and guidance to achieve tangible results and benefits from an EHR investment.

Ron is a nationally recognized expert on the selection and implementation of electronic healthcare record (also known as electronic medical records) and practice management systems. He offers a full range of services to achieve success backed up by an extensive background in technology, physician practices and project management. He has reviewed software products from over 150 vendors.

With more than 30 years experience using technology and information as a competitive weapon, he has managed transitions to new computer tools for health care organizations in 30 states. He has served a wide range of primary care and specialty groups including some of the premier ambulatory organizations in the country.

Ron manages the transition to EHRs from conception to selection to implementation and deployment. He is vendor neutral, and focuses on the interests of the medical practice. He continually monitors product and vendor developments in this rapidly evolving and diverse software market.

He is a frequent speaker on EMRs to a variety of provider and industry groups including MGMA, American Association of Orthopaedic Executives and Hospitals. He has contributed to a wide range of publications including the widely used *Marketing Your Clinical Practice*, 4th Edition, by Neil Baum, MD. He has also written "How to Select and Install Medical Practice Software" and the "Guide to Medical Practice Software."

Ron earned a B.S. in Information Systems from the University of Maryland and an MBA in International Business from George Washington University. He is a member of the AICPA and Maryland Association of CPAs.

ACKNOWLEDGMENTS

Writing *Keys to EMR/EHR Success* was actually cathartic and fun. *Keys to EMR/EHR Success* is based on real life EHR selection and implementation projects. The cathartic part was coming back from a particularly difficult situation and writing a book section about how to avoid and deal with the problem. The fun part was the open ended creativity that a book allows. Based on that origin, I am most thankful to the many practices that I have been privileged to serve and work with. I also appreciate those readers who took the time to contact me and share their own problems which resulted in additional guidance in the Second Edition.

I would also like to thank Beth Matosko of Sterling Solutions for her continuing help with the second edition, editing the book, and maintaining the list of EHR companies. Between mergers, and new products, as well as my obsession with certain aspects of the book, Beth has toughed it out with me in putting the book together.

Writing the original first edition was one thing, but finding an appropriate channel and avenue for it is another. Maureen McCarthy, CPA of Snyder Cohn Collyer and Hamilton was kind enough to take a look at the book, and refer me to Nancy Collins of Greenbranch Publishing. Nancy and her team were enthusiastic about this book, improved the manuscript, and implemented their creative and comprehensive approach to publishing and distributing the book in your hand. The most amazing part was the speed and responsiveness that they demonstrated. Thank you to Greenbranch Publishing for freeing me up to work with my clients while they focus on the book.

For the second edition, I want to thank Nancy Collins for her insights and enthusiasm about the book as well as her input on additions to make the book more useful and helpful. In dealing with a topic that is in hyperdrive, Nancy has been invaluable helping me determine the more important aspects of the avalanche of information and changes to the EHR industry. I also appreciate the speed with which Nancy and her team got the Second Edition to print that almost matched the hyperdrive speed that has taken over in the EHR industry.

Should I Invest in an EHR?

Even today, most medical practices don't have an electronic health record (EHR.) And many practices that have an EHR have not generated the savings or efficiencies they expected. So, why should you make a major investment in an EHR?

Medical practices and physicians underutilize computer systems. Few, if any, other industries have so many key individuals going through their standard workday without any support or interaction with computers to support customer/client/patient service and their business purpose.

For example, car dealers and service stations have extensive recall campaigns for oil changes while the average medical practice does not have the tools to track or manage patient recalls for life threatening health issues. Some retailers are using radio frequency identification to track the location of a $50 case of paper goods, but medical practices cannot track the disposition of a battery of diagnostic tests costing hundreds of dollars. A service company can review every service call on your equipment for the past 5 years, but many practices cannot access a reliable list of prescriptions that the doctor has issued for the patient or quickly determine the pending immunizations for a child.

Physicians, clinicians and administrative employees are competing for access to and possession of the vital paper medical record. Without the paper medical record, the patient waits and the doctor is less efficient.

As you prepare to consider EHR, you need to contemplate the key differences between this effort and anything you have done. Before getting too caught up in the technological wonders of the EHR, let's take a reality check into the challenges that lie ahead:

Organizational—To take advantage of an EHR, your practice will need to rethink the way it works. From interactions with patients to the working relationship between the physicians and staff, the EHR will become a critical repository of historic and operational information that everyone will use. You need to redesign interactions with patients, other practices, payers and other outside parties. EHRs change the speed of information flow within the practice as well as the availability of information. Since the medical record is available immediately to any authorized user, the practice needs to determine the best processes to capitalize on and accommodate this dramatic change.

Management—Many EHR vendors like to portray system flexibility by offering that each doctor could use the EHR as he/she sees fit. In theory, your practice could pay several times to solve the same problem, and have to live with the consequences. The problems with inconsistent paper-based documentation do not go away with inconsistent EHR documentation. EHRs can offer a wide range of benefits to almost every practice but these benefits must be driven by practice policies that establish a structure to meet practice organization and patient care objectives. For example, each practice should carefully consider how their EHR is set up to insure that the collection of patient information will meet your care and documentation needs. Each practice needs to assure that patient information will be practically accessible to the wide array of doctors and staff involved in patient care. These strategies need the backing of the practice management team to insure that the EHR is used in a manner that most effectively helps the practice meet care and management objectives.

Procedure—EHRs will become an integral part of the practice's procedures and workflow. Indeed, you will have to account for the effect of the EHR on how you work as well as what every employee and doctor will do. EHRs will become the point of focus for every process and activity. Your practice will not be able to manage patient issues without the EHR, and you will have a vested interest in the ability of your staff to manage patient flow through the EHR. In essence, the EHR becomes the repository of patient information as well as the facilitator of patient movement, care items and messages. Practices that fail to recognize the pervasive effect of EHRs may fail to look for the correct features, and/or implement the EHR with fewer resources than required.

Technology—EHRs will dramatically increase the use of and reliance on computers for your practice and doctors. Arguably, you could walk over to your current practice management system (PMS), pull the plug out of the wall, and you will still see patients today. If you have an EHR, your tolerance for any disruptions will be limited since the lack of EHR access will prevent you from serving patients. You may go to great lengths to work around your current PMS because it may not be set up the way you want or need, or you may have outgrown the system. Unfortunately, you could end up in a bad situation working around the inadequacies of an EHR that is not effective. For example, you cannot view the outstanding orders for a patient, if the orders were dictated into a note that is stored in the EHR, but not entered into the patient order feature of the EHR. As important, you will need to invest money to mitigate the chance that you could lose access to your EHR. Practices may invest in redundant hardware and communication lines as well as extra workstations and tablets.

Staff—Most of the doctors and people in your practice do not rely on your current computer systems to do their job. With an EHR, everyone relies on the computers throughout their working day. As such, staff and doctors need adequate training, support on day-to-day use and a mechanism that insures that the EHR is available and relevant to patient care and practice operations. In some cases, this requires remedial training for staff and doctors who may have little experience using computers at all, let alone relying on computers for their activities throughout the day.

Regulatory—The interest in the use of computers by healthcare organizations has shifted from the compliance and support of the Health Insurance Portability and Accessibility Act (HIPAA) to the American Recovery and Reinvestment Act (ARRA.) ARRA included over $19 Billion to stimulate the use of EHRs and other technology tools to attack the increasing cost of healthcare. ARRA includes specific timelines, incentives and penalties to apply computers to frustrating and costly operational problems in the healthcare system. HIPAA defined mechanisms to exchange information through the HIPAA transaction set, as well as standards for privacy and security. However, HIPAA did not require the replacement of existing systems in physician practices or the use of EHR. ARRA affects the deployment of new systems by offering incentive monies to those practices that buy, AND use EHR tools. Indeed, ARRA established a mechanism to certify which products would meet and accommodate the EHR vision. Practices that are considering EHR investments must focus on those products that will meet ARRA standards as well as the process needed to fully utilize the EHR to support the forthcoming revolution in healthcare technology triggered by the ARRA Healthcare Information Technology Incentives.

EHRs dramatically differ from the traditional use of computers in physician practices. Indeed, one would have to go back prior to the use of a computerized billing system to get a feel for the changes that lie ahead. EHRs are particularly challenging due to the following:

EHR Product Changes—Shifting from one EHR to another is much more complicated than making changes to your diagnostic equipment, PMS or other computer systems. EHR products significantly differ in how they track issues, store information and present patient charts. EHRs also differ in the support of clinical workflow. (See the section on EHR conversion in Chapter 10—Implementing an EHR.) For example, some EHRs have special prescription refill management features. Buying an EHR to try it out, or buying a different EHR for various departments in the practice is a waste of your time and money. Ultimately, you could put your patients and practice in a risky situation. For example, having prescriptions on one software system, images on a second, and other patient information in a third could result in patients being given advice using less than all of the information that the practice may have. You should buy an EHR to achieve and support your patient service, operational and management objectives for the foreseeable future.

> **TIP:** Another important issue about EHR changes is the fact that you need to maintain the patient record for years. If you change EHRs, you may not be able to get all of the information that you need converted over to the new EHR and may have to maintain access to the old EHR for years after you finish using it. Therefore, pick the EHR that meets your needs and has the staying power as a product and company to avoid problems.

EHR Starting Point—Most practices have little to no existing computer-based clinical information and/or content to convert to the EHR. In most practices, clinical staff do not use computers to work with and serve patients. So you must formulate a variety of structures, strategies and procedures that are completely new to the practice. The practice needs access to the EHR from locations that may have no current workstations or equipment. For example, many practices have few computers in the clinical area since all of the patient information is in the paper chart. Additionally, most practices must train a number of users on how to integrate the EHR into their patient service style. Nurses will need to reference the EHR to know that patients are waiting for the doctor and/or the doctor has ordered a procedure or test.

Service Coverage—An EHR should support the variety of services, as well as support the workflow, between the clinical departments. These processes will facilitate patient services between departments, and support collaboration among doctors and staff. For example, doctors and nurses would issue lab orders to the internal lab through the EHR. The ability to call on staff and stay informed on patient issues instantaneously changes the working environment and time management of physicians and staff.

Strategic and Tactical Effect—The implementation of an EHR will have a dramatic effect on your practice and operations. An EHR will speed the flow of information in your practice, but you must redesign your practice to capitalize on these improvements. Many practices have failed to see results due to a lack of guidance and experience with these tools. To facilitate such a transformation, you need effective project leadership and management of the implementation process.

Looking at these significant challenges and effects, many practices have yet to pursue an EHR strategy.

EHRs AND THE HEALTHCARE INDUSTRY

Let's look at the healthcare industry and how you fit in. Today, you mostly exchange paper with a wide variety of players, including hospitals, insurers and other doctors.

Typically, you send them your paper and they send you theirs.

Many practices work with healthcare organizations that have their own computers but produce few benefits for the practice. For example, some laboratories provide computer systems for practices to enter orders and print results that are placed in the patient's paper chart. Other organizations are providing onsite printers that print their reports at the practice. In other cases, hospitals provide workstations for physician order entry and printing of hospital information. More recently, the push to deploy electronic prescriptions has added an additional task to physician practices that provides substantial benefits to pharmacies and PBMs, but has mostly resulted in additional costs to many practices. Indeed, a number of practices support electronic prescriptions by pulling the paper prescription at the checkout/clinical desk and having an employee enter the prescription into a prescription service website. In the final analysis, the practice may do the data entry for those organizations with computer systems, but these schemes produce few benefits for the practice. Indeed, the doctor may still need to record the orders, and, in some cases the results, in the patient paper chart.

This avalanche of paper includes a number of gems and important issues as well as a lot of "snow" that does not have a bearing on the patient's health and your business. Indeed, finding the important information in the paper blizzard consumes valuable doctor and staff time. In many practices, clinical staff "prepare charts" for patient visits by pulling important notes and pages to the front of the chart. At the end of the visit, someone must refile these pages in the appropriate place.

To get anything done, you have to co-locate the message or problem, the patient's medical chart and the doctor or clinician who will decide on the next steps. Typically co-location involves faxing information among your offices or passing charts around the office in search of the doctor. In fact, most of the faxing in many practices is to pass patient information among offices to get patient information to the doctor and/or, in some cases, maintain multiple charts for the same patient. In some cases, a staff person will read information to the doctor over the phone. In many cases, the issues must wait until the doctor has time to work through the stack of patient files on his desk. To serve patients, the doctor must wade through a variety of pages and notes to find important information. Doctors may note information or use dictation to record the patient visit.

Looking forward, the employer and government buyers of healthcare services are keenly interested in producing industry wide efficiencies through EHRs and the electronic exchange of information among healthcare organizations. Rising health care costs and an aging population fuel this interest.

Payers, and healthcare organizations that you do business with, want to eliminate the cost and inefficiency of paper charts and paper exchanges with electronic solutions. Whether a key payer starts requiring electronic information or patients come to expect a more timely response to their questions and problems, EHRs will become a required tool for physician practices to meet patient expectations and work with payers and other providers. In short, you may not have a choice whether to invest in an EHR.

Current industry issues that may affect your EHR thinking include:

American Recovery and Reinvestment Act (ARRA)—ARRA places EHR on the critical issues agenda of every practice. The key issue facing practices is that ARRA will force many practices to implement an EHR. Practices that do not implement EHR could be at a disadvantage as well as give up the incentives offered under ARRA.

ARRA includes a $17 Billion payout to physician practices that implement and achieve "Meaningful Use" of an EHR. Practices that meet the meaningful use standard could receive up to $44,000 from Medicare or $63,750 from Medicaid. Simply purchasing an EHR or partially using one is not sufficient to receive the incentive payments. As important, the meaningful use standard includes 25 individual items such as electronic prescriptions, patient order entry, and interacting with patients over a patient portal. Practices will be expected to meet these standards through stages that will be clarified in June 2010. Be on the lookout for additional details on meaningful use from the Office of the National Coordinator for Healthcare Information Technology (healthit.hhs.gov).

Physician practices have no choice but to use tools that are necessary to be an active player in the healthcare industry, and, more importantly, effectively serve patients. Patients are interested in interacting with their doctors over the Internet. Indeed, the ARRA inspired Meaningful Use standards include availing patients of information over the Internet as well as the percentage of your patients that take advantage of that option. CAUTION: If other practices and healthcare organizations are serving patients through Internet connects, how will practices that keep patients waiting on hold, or leave cryptic HIPAA compliant phone messages be perceived?

A significant aspect of ARRA is the support of "interoperability." Interoperability is the electronic exchange of information among various healthcare providers. Indeed, most practices support some form of interoperability today, but these exchanges are mostly limited to administrative information.

ARRA encourages the installation of EHR infrastructures that would enable practices to exchange clinical data with other healthcare organizations. If your practice does not have the support infrastructure, you may be at a disadvantage. For example, Doctor A has an EHR and produces a note that includes complete information about the patient service and exam. Doctor B does not have an EHR and receives a paper copy of the complete report that many doctors consider excessive. The length of the paper report is daunting and the important information is difficult to identify. Doctor A also transmits an electronic version of the report to Doctor C who uses an EHR. Doctor C can view the Doctor A report in their EHR and accept the prescriptions, conditions, and selected information into the Doctor C EHR based patient record. Doctors A and C will be able to share their patient information with others and immediately access their patient information. Doctor B will continue thrashing through pages of patient charts to find pertinent information. Why should a patient wait for an hour in an emergency room bed for Doctor B's staff to accumulate the list of drugs and fax them to the hospital when Doctor A and C can send over the patient's prescriptions through their EHR on demand at any time?

The same lack of EHR and interoperability support for patients could inhibit the ability of a practice to receive referrals, manage patient treatment orders and even communicate with other providers in the local referral network. For example, if other orthopedic doctors in your physician network have the ability to receive referrals from primary care providers, download patient prescriptions prescribed by other doctors, and receive and send clinical reports electronically, which orthopedic practices will be easier to work with from the primary care practice's perspective?

Pay for Performance—A number of insurance carriers and Medicare/Medicaid are looking into pay for performance options that tie some compensation to support for quality measures. Quality measures can range from use of clinical treatment protocols to proactive management of patient care.

Medicare's 2010 Physician Quality Reporting Initiative (PQRI) includes 129 quality measures that are reported through the standard claims submission process. The PQRI program started in 2006 with less than 20 measures. One of the more interesting aspects of the PQRI standard is that the reporting mechanism may cover a look back period for the condition. Included in the current PQRI measures are some quality measures that report on up to a 12 month look back window. Medicare is offering 2% of total allowed charges as a financial incentive through 2010. Regardless of your view of PQRI, an increase in measures as well as incentives (both financial and perception) is not beyond the realm of possibility. Keeping track of and reporting on these measures is difficult at least without an EHR. For example, the current coping "tools" consist of papers that are used to record the quality measures. But paper reporting tools do not help your practice determine if reports were submitted for appropriate patients, and how your practice is performing. More insurance companies could follow Medicare PQRI strategies.

Highmark BCBS in Pennsylvania awards pay for performance points for practices that have implemented an EHR (See page 7–6-43 at https://www.highmark.com/health/manual/Chp7-Unit6–1-06.pdf.) Many physicians expect additional pay for performance items that are based on having an EHR. For example, verifying clinical protocols, or following patient treatment plans are not practical without an EHR.

EHRs can help practices monitor compliance with practice level and industry level protocols while insuring that all doctors and staff can easily access patient care issues and outstanding treatment orders. For example, an EHR can identify outstanding patient care issues and orders for a particular patient when you access the patient medical record as well as in response to a general query for overdue services. Similar analysis of paper records would require an expensive and time consuming review of the paper charts for all patients. Such a review is not practical for many practices.

ARRA Meaningful Use measures include listing patients by specific condition for quality improvement and accompanying measures for compliance such as colorectal screenings for patients over 50, and eligible patients who receive flu vaccine. Such reporting and collecting the underlying information requires the use of EHR tools.

Common Care Standards—Medicare focuses on "prevention and early detection" and may raise patient expectations of care management and risk tracking. Your practice will want to be able to capitalize on such initiatives to improve patient service and management. For example, an EHR could help identify at-risk patients who have not been in for follow-up visits. Incidental patient contacts could be used to check up on patient compliance with clinical pathways and treatment standards. Examples of common care standards include

> Bright Futures—A health care standard for children from birth through the age of 21 (available at http://brightfutures.aap.org/web/) and
>
> Bridges to Excellence—Establishes strategies to improve care for targeted diseases (available at http://www.bridgestoexcellence.org/bte/)

Disease Management Initiatives—Many payers are interested in improving the management of patients based on clinical standards and guidelines. Indeed, a number of PQRI standards include disease management program reporting. An EHR can support better management of patients with continuing care requirements and issues. For example, future services and testing can be entered and tracked as pending orders in some EHRs. EHRs can also present typical treatment orders for patients based on a particular problem or condition. Practices that can support disease management initiatives have more to offer patients, employers and payers.

Electronic Interfaces/Interoperability—The ability to exchange information among health care organizations is a key objective of the healthcare industry and a significant aspect of the ARRA standards for a certified EHR. Current electronic exchanges of claim and payment information between payers and practices are a small fraction of the exchanges that are done with paper. Additional electronic transactions will insure that healthcare organizations are better informed about patient issues through electronic exchanges including:

> The HIPAA Transaction Set (CMS Transactions and Code Sets Regulations, available at http://www.cms.hhs.gov/TransactionCodeSetsStands/) includes a transaction that allows providers to request specific patient information (Ex. Office Note, Blood Pressure) as well as a transaction that electronically returns the requested data. An electronic transaction

that supports a full set of exchanges with pharmacies is included in the HIPAA Transaction Set.

The Continuity of Care ("CCR") record supports sending patient information to a referred provider from a provider that is currently treating the patient. The Continuity of Care Record is available at http://www.centerforhit.org/PreBuilt/chit_ccrnyc.pdf

These transactions will allow practices and other healthcare organizations to more effectively collaborate on patient care and services. Providers without an EHR will not be able to capitalize on these exchanges and the resulting efficiency for the healthcare system as well as the practice.

Given that the healthcare industry is seeking to implement these changes, your practice faces a decision: you can establish a practice-based infrastructure to support these exchanges or you can print paper copies of information received and enter information from your paper records into a tool that will formulate the electronic transaction instead of an EHR. For example, some practices are entering prescriptions over the Internet to a service that formulates the electronic prescription. However, this strategy does not improve practice operations and may add another step in your prescription procedure: route the prescription to the front desk to enter the prescription into the prescription Internet site. EHRs help you take advantage of the vast amount of clinical information that you collect but cannot practically access in a paper medical record.

EHRs AND YOUR PRACTICE

The reality for many practices is that an EHR will become an operational necessity and a cost of doing business in the next few years. Computers have dramatically increased efficiency and changed every other industry, and now the focus is moving to your practice. Nonetheless, you need to consider the specific needs of your practice including:

Size—Many physicians are frustrated with the lack of economies of scale as the practice grows. Expecting to see a variety of benefits from added size, many practices find that their existing procedures and policies do not produce a comparable benefit to the physicians or patients. A close look at these practices will reveal that many problems are caused by the larger number of people chasing after the paper medical record. Indeed, some employees will keep their own copies of various medical record documents to act as a back up. For example, many surgical schedulers, lab technicians, and triage nurses maintain a "shadow" patient record to keep track of their patient issues. In some cases, multi-office practices will keep duplicate charts for a single patient in order to serve the patient from multiple locations. Unfortunately, not all copies contain the same information. Working with outdated information can lead to problems. For example, a surgical scheduling form that does not have current payer information could lead to a rejected claim. In other situations, the cancellation of a procedure may be recorded on only one of the many different copies of the surgical scheduling form. Other employees and staff may not be aware of the change.

Quality of Service—In many cases, patient services and management are not provided as effectively and at the same level of quality as the clinical services. Patients may call in several times for information and are frequently put off until the practice can retrieve the medical record. With the paper chart, finding the appropriate information can take time. An EHR changes the patient service dynamic by providing instantaneous access to the patient medical chart and/or specific information in the chart. More importantly, the patient chart can be viewed in a variety of ways and the EHR can highlight important issues. For example, EHRs may allow you to view patient information by date of service, episode of care, or type of information (e.g., prescription list, outstanding orders). EHRs may flag pending orders and incomplete treatment plans.

Electronic Exchanges—To fully appreciate the current state of electronic exchanges of clinical information, let's look back to the early days of electronic claims. A number of insurance companies would actually give away PCs with their "key to disk" software that allowed your staff to enter the information into a computer and transmit the claim to the payer. The benefit to your practice was that the electronic claim was more quickly paid. The benefit to the payer was that you were doing their keypunching for them: the payers could eliminate rooms full of data-entry employees in the claims department.

Similarly, you may already be entering lab orders into the reference lab systems and reviewing the electronic results. Typically, the results are printed and moved around your office with other paper information. With the advent of clinical electronic transactions, you will be sending and receiving clinical information electronically. Lab interfaces are available with a number of EHR products. You enter and track tests on your EHR and results are loaded into your EHR. You may be able to review results on a flow-sheet and graph lab tests over time. You will be able to exchange clinical information and information on patient care issues through evolving transaction standards. These exchanges will become as common as electronic claims and electronic credit card transactions.

Electronic interfaces or interoperability is a major component of the ARRA driven meaningful use standard. Backed up with the ARRA incentives, many practices will be installing practice based tools that will support such exchanges in time to receive the promised ARRA incentives.

This book helps you work through the selection and implementation of an EHR. Following your analysis of the business case for an EHR (Chapter 2—Evaluating an EHR Investment,) the book examines your current computer situation (Chapter 3—Your Practice Management System and an EHR).

Proceeding through the selection process, the book will review compiling an evaluation list (Chapter 4), present malpractice issues associated with EHRs (Chapter 5), selecting products to review (Chapter 6) and actually reviewing the EHR products (Chapter 7). The book covers compiling your findings and making a final decision (Chapter 8), as well as negotiating a workable agreement with your chosen EHR vendor (Chapter 9). Succeeding chapters cover your implementation effort (Chapter 10), and the activation of the EHR (Chapter 11). Your continuing support efforts are itemized in the last chapter.

A checklist to guide you through the entire selection and implementation process is included at the end of this chapter.

NOT BUYING AN EHR

Some practices will choose to wait to implement an EHR for a variety of administrative, political, management and financial reasons. Nonetheless, such practices should consider the following strategies to facilitate the implementation of an EHR in the future:

Paper Chart Preparations—Scanning of paper charts into an EHR is a monumental task. Unfortunately, practices do not design their paper charts to be scanned. Preparing a paper record for scanning is a major barrier to activating an EHR and takes 5–30 minutes per paper chart. To prepare charts for a future EHR, you may evaluate your paper charts and undertake a chart cleanup/reorganization process. The cleanup process may focus on eliminating old paperwork, unnecessary documents and duplicate documents. You may also seek to group chart documents that will ease a future scanning process. For example, if you decide that you will scan the last two years' worth of documents when you move to an EHR, you may want to organize your charts to support this plan.

Accumulating Key Information—The first time a patient is seen using the EHR, the EHR typically contains little to no information. Depending on the type of practice and implementation strategy, the practice may choose to enter key historic information. Immunizations for pediatricians, previous surgeries for a surgical practice and last colonoscopy date for a GI practice are examples of key information that may be needed to start a patient record. However, if this key information is not easily and clearly discerned from the patient chart, the cost of initial information entry could be exorbitant. If the information to be entered is not easily available, the practice may want to consider creating a new face sheet and start a campaign to get accurate information for initial entry into a future EHR.

Diagnostic Equipment Interfaces—When the practice purchases new diagnostic equipment, make sure that the new equipment will support an interface with a future EHR. You should get information on how you can interface with an EHR and include an option to buy the interface, if necessary, in the future. You can look for HL7 (Health Level 7 is an industry standard that supports the electronic exchange of information among healthcare systems and other devices) interfaces as well as a list of EHRs that the diagnostic equipment is interfaced with. Note whether the interface includes the study order from the EHR as well as returning the results to the EHR. These interfaces may be included in your future EHR evaluation list.

Transcription Capture—The vast majority of practices fail to capitalize on their investment in transcription. Typically, practices maintain word-processing files with the transcription, but do not store the files in a protected environment or with information to facilitate future loading in an EHR. To support future conversion to an EHR, your transcription files should include only one report for one patient per file. Some practices place all notes for a day in the same word processing file. Most EHR vendors would not be able to accept such a file into their EHR. Your transcription files should be protected from changes and editing, and include sufficient identifying information for the patient. For example, the patient's name, date of birth, gender and account number should be in the same exact place in each transcription file.

PMS Features—Several PMS products include workflow tools that support administrative based to-do's, and, in some cases, an imaging or basic EHR capability. Basic EHR capabilities could include a patient note capability and messaging feature. If you have such a product, seriously consider implementing the features that will let you capture key electronic data in a controlled structure. Potential options include an imaging capability to store images needed by many staff members as well as maintaining transcription documents. For example, you may scan in copies of the patient insurance card, and referral paperwork. Using these capabilities may help your practice in the interim. However, you need to preserve the integrity of your complete medical record in the paper chart.

Technology Strategy—Your practice should insure that any additional investments in technology will support the implementation of a future EHR. For example, replacing your PMS should include an option to choose your future EHR. Some PMS vendors have exclusive relationships with an EHR that may not meet your needs. Similarly, you may want to insure that additional workstations and communication upgrades can be easily used or upgraded to accommodate a future EHR.

Deciding to put off the implementation of an EHR may be the best decision for your practice. However, you should position your practice to more easily segue to an EHR in the future.

EHR CHECKLIST

Checklist Item	Assigned	Due	Comment
General Project Approval			
1. Initial Approval—Present EHR concept to management committee for approval to proceed.			
2. Select Selection Committee—Select representative doctors, clinicians and administrative staff to serve on the selection committee.			
3. Create Timeline—Establish a timeline for the selection process.			
Select EHR Product			
4. Review Current Operations—Review current paper record and clinical processes to support the creation of the Evaluation Criteria.			
5. Compile Evaluation Criteria—Compile evaluation criteria to measure potential EHR solutions.			
6. Develop a List of Potential EHR Products—Contact similar practices and local clinics to identify potential EHR products to consider.			
7. Review EHR Products—Review viable products in detail using the evaluation criteria.			
8. Focus Selection on a Limited Number of EHR Products—Based on the review of EHR products, select a limited number of products for a demonstration.			
9. Compile Demonstration Script—Develop a demonstration script that reflects the needs of the practice.			
10. Conduct Scripted Demonstration—For appropriate doctors and staff, conduct a scripted demo for a limited number of products.			
11. Compile a Budget—Compile an EHR Budget for products being considered.			
12. Select Final Product(s)—Based on the scripted demonstration, select a final one or two products to consider as the final selection.			
13. Conduct Reference Checks—Contact similar practices that are using the EHR product to check on the issues and practical use of the product in a similar environment.			
14. Visit an EHR User—Send a team to visit a practice and view the EHR in a live environment.			
Make Final Decision			
15. Compile Results of Selection Activities—Create a document summarizing the results of the selection activities.			

— Continued

Continued from previous page

Checklist Item	Assigned	Due	Comment
16. Make a Final Decision—The Selection Committee makes a final recommendation to management.			
17. Approve EHR Decision—Practice management should approve the EHR decision and empower the EHR Implementation Team and Process.			
Negotiate Contract			
18. Negotiate Business Agreement—Reach an agreement with the vendor on the business terms of the agreement including pricing, services and products.			
19. Negotiate Contract Terms—Work out contract issues to create a balanced agreement with the vendor that can support the EHR going forward.			
20. Approve Contract—Management approves and signs off on the contract.			
Implement EHR			
21. Detailed EHR Plan—Create a Detailed Practice Implementation Plan.			
22. Assign Resources—Create an implementation committee with doctors, clinicians and other staff.			
23. Establish Supporting Policies—Create a management structure to support the implementation process.			
24. Design EHR Workflow—Develop a workflow model for the practice that takes advantage of the EHR.			
25. Establish Technology Infrastructure—Build out the technology and communications base needed to support and protect the EHR.			
26. Setup EHR Software—Set up the various master files needed to support the use of the EHR.			
27. Verify and Enhance Clinical Content—Work with the clinical content to optimize the use of the EHR within the practice.			
28. Data Conversion—Convert or preload information into the EHR to support patient service and meet retention requirements.			
29. Train—Train doctors and other staff on the use of the EHR and the practice procedures.			
30. Activate the EHR—Transition to full use and deployment of the EHR.			
Continuing Support			
31. Transition to Support—Work with the vendor and practice staff to transition from implementation to continuing use.			

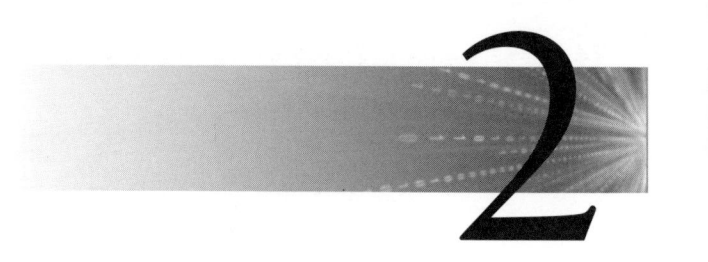

Evaluating an EHR Investment

EHRs can produce cost and revenue benefits. However, the expected benefits are not realized by many practices. The main barriers to realizing economic benefits are:

Insufficient Investment—For the vast majority of practices, an EHR will be the largest technology expense and project ever undertaken. Indeed, the EHR investment will significantly exceed the investment in your PMS. The costs can be justified by the fact that the EHR will have to serve a larger number of employees, and the critical nature of the EHR. However, some practices establish an unrealistic cost expectation. In order to meet the budget, some practices cut EHR hardware, training, and support. For example, practices that buy too little hardware will not allow for access to the EHR by all clinical staff. In frustration, some staff may start printing, and saving information from the EHR to get their jobs done. Other practices do not invest in hardware that can sustain hardware failures on a cost-benefit basis. For example, "hot swap" redundant disk drives can help the practice avoid lost data in the event of a disk crash.

Buying the Wrong Product—EHRs can vary widely in capabilities and features. Some EHR vendors will state that their product is not designed to support a paperless office, while other vendors offer their EHR by module. In the final analysis, your practice should prepare to fully implement an EHR to avoid paying for both EHR and paper charts. Otherwise, you may be better off not pursuing an EHR strategy. Some practices purchase the wrong product. The product may lack sophistication, clinical content (Ex. Charting tools for your specialty or area of medicine) or sufficient stability to be practically used. Practices may be lured into buying the product with the expectation that the vendor will make enhancements, and changes to address product deficiencies. For example, one practice waited three years for promised enhancements to address problems that prevent clinical charting with the EHR. Unless you want to expend time and resources to support the development of the EHR, you should make sure the product substantially satisfies your needs today.

Implementing a Less Than Complete EHR—Other practices stop in the middle of an EHR implementation. For example, some practices have bought all of the equipment, but only use the EHR to post charges and print prescriptions. In many cases, they end up with many EHR costs, but few of the benefits. The implementation of an EHR is certainly a challenge, but ultimately, the EHR is a strategic move that must be carried through to completion. Otherwise, the practice can end up worst off. For example, some practices have patient information split between the EHR and the paper record. The split complicates patient service, creates discrepancies, and risks problems with the designated record set, a HIPAA requirement.

Failure to Change Processes—Some practices use an EHR within their original paper-based workflow. The implementation of an EHR changes the information velocity and accessibility. For example, continued dictation may prevent updating the EHR list of medications and prescriptions to ease refill management. Similarly, an EHR cannot highlight incomplete tests when the test orders are in the dictated note, and not in the EHR order module. Some practices go to a lot of effort to make the EHR look and act like the paper system. For example, one practice would print the patient's record stored in the EHR when the patient presented for service. The printing of the patient record created a line at the front desk and kept the doctors waiting for patients.

Failure to Deploy Sufficient Hardware—Some practices fail to invest the money in the hardware to fully support the EHR. The basic challenge is to allow the doctor, nurses and staff to get access to the EHR from where they would have been normally working with the paper chart. For example, a stationary workstation in an exam room may prevent the doctor from maintaining eye contact with the patient during the exam. In other cases, practices do not provide EHR access to all of the people involved in clinical services. To save money, some practices limit tablets to the doctors. For example, one practice had nurses record intake information on forms that were entered by the doctors on their tablets before the doctor could work with the patient. In the final analysis, an employee without access to the EHR is analogous to preventing an employee from looking for information in your current paper chart.

The failures of many EHR projects can be found in the original scope, and planning for the project. To avoid these problems, establish a realistic expectation of the hard and soft costs for an EHR. Then you've set a strategic mandate to see the EHR project through to completion. In the final analysis, the strategic mandate will allow the practice to balance between the benefits of an EHR and realistic costs.

DETERMINING THE BENEFITS

An EHR will produce a variety of benefits for the practice. Some of the benefits impact revenue; others expenses. A number of EHR benefits improve services and productivity, but may be difficult to quantify financially:

Support Patient Collaboration—If serving a patient involves a variety of staff, technicians, or mid-level providers, an EHR will enhance collaboration on patient services and issues. By providing immediate access to information in the chart as well as outstanding patient issues, practice staff and doctors will be able to make better use of their time and avoid interruptions to track missing information. For example, immediate access to patient information may allow doctors to defer certain types of services to nurses and clinical support staff. Immediate access to the patient record may allow doctors and staff to address incoming patient calls when the patient calls and not later when they gain access to the paper chart.

Improve Documentation—EHRs enable practices to produce documentation on a more timely and consistent basis. For example, instead of the nurse recording information on a piece of paper that the doctor will dictate into their note, the nurse enters information directly into the EHR: the doctor only has to enter the new information or findings. Optionally, some EHRs combine dictated notes with information entered by the doctor or staff. Charting at time of service produces documentation when the doctor signs the note. More consistent documentation is enabled through use of a common set of clinical documentation tools as well as retrospective analysis of documentation for previous visits. For example, some EHRs allow the user to cite forward information from previous visits. More consistent documentation mitigates the risk of a patient service error, and enables all doctors and staff to quickly locate the appropriate clinical information. For example, doctors and staff will not have to adjust to the documentation styles, level of detail and placement of information (e.g., prescriptions and outstanding orders) for each person in the practice.

Improve Access to Information—EHRs allow doctors and staff to instantaneously access patient records. EHRs improve access to medical records by allowing doctors and staff to review patient information through a number of views. EHR records can be organized by date of service, type of document (*examples*: note, prescription, order), doctor, diagnosis and other criteria. Key information can be separately reviewed. For example, the user can see a list of medications, allergies, procedures and visits.

As important, EHR users can dig down into related documents by merely selecting the criteria and looking at the associated documents. Immediate access to patient records can cut the time needed to serve a patient as well as allow for immediate servicing of patient issues. With paper records, action on patient issues must be deferred until the paper medical record, and issue can be presented to the doctor.

More effective access to information is a significant benefit that can dramatically affect efficiency and productivity. Thrashing through paper records consumes valuable time for all doctors and staff. Paper thrashing steals time in increments that are difficult to measure and track. For example, an extra 15 seconds needed to locate the last prescription in a pile of patient prescriptions is virtually eliminated with an EHR. Add to that multiple 5 to 45 second delays thrashing for other patient information during each patient visit or the time staff spends re-organizing the patient chart before and after every patient visit. Eliminating paper thrashing will have a significant effect on how doctors and staff spend their time as well as how the practice is perceived by the patient.

Improve Patient Services—Patient service is inhibited by the inherent limitations of the paper record. Only one person can practically use the paper record at a time, and several pages may have to be reviewed to locate the appropriate information. For example, the nurse needs to access the previous note and reconcile the doctor's plan with other received documents (Ex. Lab results, MRI studies) to verify whether the information needed to serve the patient is available.

Patient messages and notes are circulating in the practice, but staff cannot easily determine the status and resolution of particular issues. Indeed, frustrated patients may call several times for the same issue and generate several notes that need to be matched up with a single paper medical record. Online access to patient issues and to dos as well as the medical record empowers staff and doctors to more effectively and quickly respond to patient queries. EHRs clinical orders, patient issues, and pending procedures can be accessed and reviewed by managers to track patient service issues and avoid lapses in care. As important, management will know with certainty the status and disposition of the various patient issues that the practice must manage.

Eliminate Lost Files—In many practices, lost files cause frequent interruptions to the staff and patients. Indeed, some practices have designated staff members who do nothing but look for lost files. Other practices return all files every day to the medical records department or employ someone at night to record information on the current location of patient files in the medical office. EHRs eliminate lost files and the associated disruption to the patient service process. All patient files are accessible through the EHR.

Even though the service and productivity improvements are substantial, you need to have a high level of assurance that the economic benefits of the EHR will offset the costs. The key economic benefits usually are:

Transcription

Practices that use transcription can spend from $1,000 to $2,000 per month per provider. An EHR can eliminate transcription expense if the physician charts patient information at the time of service. Unlike transcription, EHR charting can occur as the physician is seeing a patient. The physician enters the information into the EHR throughout the encounter. At the end of the encounter, the documentation is completed and transcription is eliminated. For doctors that dictate during the day, charting at time of service may allow for more patients. For doctors that dictate at night, charting at time of service will produce lifestyle benefits.

Numerous physicians are wary of charting at the time of service due to the impact on patient interaction, navigating through the computer screens, and being unable to change the record after signoff. However, the key issue is charting at time of patient service is a massive change to their patient service style. If the results improve the ability of the physician and staff to serve patients, then the change to charting will be worth the cost.

If the practice chooses to not chart at the time of service then don't expect transcription savings at the practice level. In the final analysis, charting at time of service is a physician decision. Some physicians may choose to chart all patients at time of service while other doctors may decide to continue using dictation. In any case, prepare for an extended transition period for the doctors and the practice. In general, concerns with charting at time of service can be addressed through appropriate clinical content, effective training, responsive support and the ability to amend the medical record as needed.

Medical Records

Medical record expenses include the costs of the medical record staffs, folders and materials, storage, printing and space. Hidden medical record costs include interruptions and delays due to lost medical records or the difficulty of finding information. In multiple office practices, faxing medical record information to the doctor can be a disruptive and expensive process. Practices with several offices may use up to 80% of their faxing to send clinical documents to another office or the billing department. A major productivity problem with paper charts is that many practice employees and doctors are competing for access to the same medical record.

EHRs eliminate the actual medical record expenses and allow everyone instantaneous access to the patient medical record. However, the practice will still need EHR support staff as well as staff to manage the exchange of paper records with other healthcare organizations. The initial transition to the EHR may include a scanning effort that will keep the medical record staff and additional resources completely absorbed for several months after the EHR is activated. Due to the EHR transition costs, the actual EHR costs should not be expected to go down for 6 to 12 months depending on your patient service cycle.

After the initial transition period, medical record expenses may drop by up to 50%. EHR patient file folder and paper expenses will dramatically decrease. A significant number of dedicated paper medical record staff will no longer be needed to pull, file, prepare and update paper charts. However, these resources will be initially dedicated to the EHR transition. The remaining medical record expenses will be needed to support the EHR operations.

EHRs may not produce any cost savings in offices that do not have medical record employees. For example, a satellite or small office, where several employees split preparing and processing medical records, will not necessarily see a decrease in expenses. That is you will continue to need someone at the front desk to greet patients and answer the phones, even if you do not need them to work with your paper charts.

E&M Coding Levels

Many physicians code office visits at a lower level than the services provided. Physicians may adjust coding due to concerns with the documentation quality or the belief that down-coding protects the practice from other problems. Unfortunately, down-coding prevents the physician from being fairly compensated for the services provided.

Some EHR products address this problem by calculating the E&M code at the time of service based on physician and staff charting. As the physician enters patient information, the EHR tracks the level of service. In many cases the additional revenue from more accurate E&M coding can pay for the EHR as well as mitigate the risk of a coding compliance problem in the future. Note that some EHR products do not calculate the level of service based on the information entered but on the factors selected by the doctor. For example, the product may display a worksheet that accepts the complexity and other coding factors from the user to calculate the E&M code.

Revenue enhancement from improved coding will vary widely depending on the coding accuracy of the physician. In some cases, the practice will see no improvement. In other cases, physicians may see $3,000 or more in additional revenue per month per physician for the same patient services.

> **CAUTION:** Some EHR products correctly calculate the E&M code for primary care visits but not necessarily for specialty visits.

> **TIP:** To estimate the effect of improved E&M coding, produce a report of the E&M code distribution for all of the doctors in the practice. Based on analysis of current coding distributions from sources such as CMS and subspecialty groups, project the effect of a more accurate coding on revenue. Review current distributions to identify providers that are not using appropriate codes. For example, some providers may always use Level 2 codes when the patients may really have deserved Level 3 or Level 4 codes, which pay higher. Comparing the expected distribution with the current E&M coding pattern will produce an estimate of the marginal revenue potential. For example, a doctor with only level 3 codes compared with a more evenly distributed provider may indicate that a certain percentage of the current level 3 visits should be level 2s and level 4s. By calculating the expected payment for the redistributed codes, you can calculate the potential marginal revenue.

ARRA Healthcare Information Technology Incentives

America Recovery and Reinvestment Act (ARRA) allows up to $44,000 per provider from MEDICARE or $63,750 per provider from MEDICAID for the "meaningful use" of electronic healthcare records (EHR) These incentives are only available to practices that implement EHR products and maintain meaningful use of the EHR by 2014. Therefore, practices that expect to implement EHRs should seriously consider taking advantage of this one time incentive. See the discussion on ARRA in Chapter 1.

Pay for Performance (P4P)

Pay for Performance programs cover a variety of issues and practices. For example, some pay for performance programs pay a certain amount of money to practices that have and use electronic prescriptions, and/or an EHR. Other pay for performance programs are based on managing patient care items that require patient management strategies that are only possible with an EHR. For example, monitoring diabetic patients or patients with a heart condition requires automated tools to track last patient visits and diagnostic tests as well as effectively insuring that the patient comes in for the next recommended visit. In the future, pay for performance programs could depend on your ability to quickly identify and contact at risk patients and promote the management of their care.

> **TIP:** Pay for Performance programs are a moving target that you need to monitor. For example, the pay for performance factor that requires electronic prescriptions could be enhanced to require periodic patient visits for selected drugs. Be sure that you understand the strategic implications of pay for performance for you practice.

> **TIP:** Medicare's Physician Quality Reporting Initiative (PQRI) includes 129 Quality Measures. Individual practices choose the appropriate measures to report and track. PQRI Measures include reporting treatment activities, as well as reporting events over a look back period of up to 12 months. EHRs can help the practice determine if PQRI reporting was performed when required as well as help the provider find the relevant information for those measures with a look back period.

Charge Capture

Many practices miss charges due to communication and process errors. Several studies have shown many providers miss several charges per day. Practices may miss charges due to recording problems in the office, lack of coding knowledge, and quick add-ons to patient services. Indeed, many practices dedicate complex procedures and staffing resources to minimize lost charges. For example, some practices use nurses to review all charts for lost charges on a daily basis.

In an EHR, all services and doctor orders are entered in the clinical chart to record the order and establish the framework to track the order through completion. For example, you may be able to identify outstanding or overdue services. That order information notifies other departments (e.g., lab, radiology) of services and pending patients. At the end of the patient visit, the doctor is presented with the list of services that were ordered and can initiate the posting of the services for billing.

EHRs also provide powerful research tools for coding staff. Patient medical records can be accessed on demand to review the actual record, billed charge information from the EHR and clinical documents to verify specific coding issues. Immediate access to the patient record will improve productivity of coding staff and increase coding accuracy. With a paper chart, the billing office may need to send a request to the clinic and the clinical staff may copy the relevant materials for transmission to the billing office.

To estimate the potential marginal revenue, the practice could audit a sample of clinical records for a selected day to estimate the missing office charges. Project the missing charges for a year to calculate the estimated revenue from missing charges.

Volume

Although most doctors have more than enough to do already, selected physicians have seen more patients daily with an EHR. The increase in volume is due to making better use of office time, support staff and facilities as well as the particular working strategy of the physician.

Physicians may be able to save time by having immediate access to patient issues and medical records through the EHR. Immediate access to relevant EHR information eliminates the all too common interruptions to leaf through the medical chart throughout the visit to locate the last note, test information or historical patient care issues. Additional time may result from elimination of dictation and more effective handling of messages and patient issues.

In some practices, doctors perform record keeping and transcription during the workday. For example, some doctors spend up to one and a half hours each clinical day on transcription. Charting at the time of service freed up dictation time to see other patients. For doctors who dictate after hours, charting at time of service will improve their quality of life.

These benefits will be realized after a physician is using the EHR effectively. In some cases, physicians may take a few weeks and in other cases physician may need several months to use an EHR efficiently.

Improved Collections

EHRs can improve collections by allowing the insurance collectors more effective access to clinical documentation on patient services. Instantaneous access to charts and E&M coding documentation empowers the biller to succinctly present the key information to the payer. For example, in the course of discussing a collection issue with a payer, an employee could call-up the relevant office note, and fax the note to the payer—more effectively and efficiently providing supporting information for claims.

More effective access to supporting information will help your practice avoid or eliminate denied claims that are not appealed. Nationally, 15% of denied claims are not appealed.

In many cases, the practice has provided the service, but lacks the supporting documentation that can withstand the scrutiny of an insurance company or support the dispute. In other cases, getting the information to challenge the denial is so difficult or costly, that the billing department bypasses collecting the money that is due the practice.

The practice should see an improvement in collections and virtually eliminate late-claim filling.

The worksheet below organizes your estimated cost and benefits for the EHR:

TABLE 2.1

Cost Reduction and Revenue Benefits Worksheet	Strategy/ Rationale	Current Expense	Projected Expense	Projected Savings/ Revenue
Cost Reductions				
Transcription Costs	Eliminate transcription expense for doctors who chart at time of service.			
Medical Record	Eliminate medical chart folder costs through the EHR.			
	Eliminate medical chart paper and copying costs through the EHR. Costs may include additional copiers that would no longer be necessary with EHR.			
	Cut medical record staff by half due to elimination of chart movement. This benefit will be phased in 9 to 12 months after EHR Go Live.			
Revenue Benefits				
E&M Coding Improvement	Calculate expected marginal revenue from a more accurate E&M coding method.			
Pay for Performance	Some payers are now offering pay for performance incentives based on a variety of factors. Calculate the pay for performance revenues that require an EHR.			
Charge Capture	Extrapolate the total lost charges from the sample charge review survey.			
Volume	On a physician-by-physician basis, determine the additional time available to physicians with the charting at time of service. Project the change in number of patients and apply the average revenue per patient.			
Improved Collections	Calculate late submissions that lead to untimely filing over the past year.			
ARRA Stimulus Incentives	Calculate the potential ARRA Stimulus monies. Be sure to allow for sufficient time to attain Meaningful Use.			
ANNUAL POTENTIAL BENEFIT				

The total potential benefit will be compared with the estimated EHR cost below.

DETERMINING THE HARD COSTS

To save you time and money, a working budget of the EHR cost should be established early on in your process. Of course, the exact cost will be subject to final negotiations, but a working budget should be set up as soon as possible. The working budget establishes a benchmark for the practice as well as a reference point for your return-on-investment (ROI). As important, the practice owners need to understand the EHR scope and financial commitment. *Beware*: Most practices significantly underestimate the cost of moving to an EHR.

The understated cost estimates are based on experience with practice management systems, vendor cost estimates and optimistic scenarios. Practice management comparisons are inaccurate since more people need EHR access than the PMS users. PMSs are used by administrative staff, but the EHR must be accessible to every single clinical staff member and doctor as well as a number of administrative users. As important, EHR use is intense throughout the workday; sharing workstations is not practical. For example, nursing staff may share a workstation to review the PMS schedule, but, with an EHR, each nurse may need to access a different patient chart at the same time. Similarly, the EHR's list of messages and to-dos may be specific to each nurse.

Practices also invest money on a cost-effective basis in equipment and services that will minimize the risk of EHR loss, but may not be highlighted by the EHR vendor. For example, you may invest in redundant main systems, and spare workstations to insure that you can continue to access your EHR even if a particular item is out of service. Some practices also maintain backup communication facilities with remote sites.

Vendor cost estimates frequently exclude key costs. Vendor software costs do not include training, support, hardware and other items. In some cases, vendors may not include system software costs which are needed to run their system, but is not included in their EHR software license cost. Optimistic scenarios are based on what the practice perceives as a reasonable cost. However, many of these estimates are based on historic computer expenditures which are low for healthcare in general and certainly not designed to handle a major change to the practice's technology base.

Initially, you should determine what you consider a cost of the EHR, and what is not considered a cost of the EHR. A variety of items may be required to move to the EHR but it is your decision to require a comparable ROI or consider this the cost of doing business. This determination is not an issue of semantics since some of these investments may be needed by the practice whether or not they go to an EHR:

>**Workstation Upgrades**—Practices that are using a character-based system with basic terminals or have old PC workstations will probably need to upgrade their current workstations. EHRs frequently require more computing power to support the imaging data and other EHR capabilities. Additionally, EHRs may necessitate more workstations due to the constant need for most staff to have access to the EHR. For example, a workstation may be needed at the nursing station. In

situations where a workstation may be shared by two or more check-in desk staff, the practice will need a separate workstation for each staff member.

Network Upgrades—Data moves between the workstation and the server over an internal communication network and/or phone/high-speed lines. Your current system probably does not require the line speed needed by EHRs. EHRs require additional line speed due to the use of imaging in the EHR as well as the initial scanning of the current paper medical records. Upgrades to the internal network speed may be needed. Communication lines to your remote facilities may need similar improvement. Ironically, a number of practices have seen their interoffice communication costs drop when moving to higher speed connections. For example, an old connection used for PMS workstations was upgraded to a faster connection for EHRs at one half the cost of the slower connection since the practice had never renegotiated the contract for the old connection.

PMS Upgrades—PMS upgrades may involve upgrading your current PMS to the latest version. An upgrade could require installing a new PMS as well as training, and even data conversion. In some cases, the new PMS version may require a new server and even new workstations. In other situations, practices may replace the PMS as part of the move to an EHR. PMS upgrades are clearly the cost of doing business for a medical practice. However, the cost of integrating the PMS with the EHR product could be considered an EHR cost.

Compiling an initial budget can be complex and frustrating. However, the purpose of creating an initial budget is to set expectations and avoid future problems. For example, a practice established a budget of $20,000 for a 4-doctor practice. Another practice of 10 doctors wanted to implement an EHR for under $100,000. Given that a tablet device costs $2,000 to $3,000 and an EHR user license costs $2,000 to $4,000, the 4-doctor practice was looking at a minimum of $16,000 for the doctor setups without any money for other staff hardware, training, EHR server and other EHR essentials. Similarly, the 10-doctor practice needed $45,000 to meet the basic needs of the doctors without allowing for any other EHR costs.

You can compile an initial budget based on three strategies: **Basic EHR Estimate**, **Quick EHR Working Budget** and/or **Comprehensive Working Budget**. All three budget strategies are based on a 5-year amortization of the original costs of the EHR. Note that all three methods may not correspond to any quotes you have received since the budget may include items not in the vendor quotes, and the vendor quotes may have items that are not in the budget. For example, the working budgets do not include PDA applications for the doctors. The current vendor quote may not include a server with selected redundancies to cut the risk of a failure that could limit or prevent access to your electronic health records. (The table on the page 27 will help you calculate a Quick EHR Working Estimate).

The **Basic EHR Estimate** is a monthly EHR cost of $1,000 to $2,000 per provider per month or $12,000 to $24,000 per provider per year. Communication expenses, mid-level employees, locations and a wide range of other factors can significantly impact this estimate. The basic estimate is based on general costs for a tablet, licenses, a low level server, basic training, implementation fees, and other costs. You can validate that estimate by completing a more detailed working estimate.

The **Quick EHR Working Estimate** does not include the details in the Comprehensive Working Budget, but does present a reasonable estimate of the EHR costs for the small to mid-size practice. The Quick EHR Working Estimate bundles a number of items that are detailed in the Comprehensive Working Budget (pages 27 and 28).

The Comprehensive Working Budget details the various items needed to implement an EHR. At a minimum, the Comprehensive Working Budget allows you check that you have included the various components needed to activate your EHR. The estimated costs column in the Comprehensive Working Budget can vary based on additional factors. For example, a very large practice could invest over $100,000 in their EHR server. The Comprehensive Working Budget Worksheet is at the end of the chapter.

CONSIDERING SOFT COSTS

In addition to the hard costs, EHRs require the expenditure of time and effort that are hidden and/or difficult to quantify:

> **Initial Productivity Losses**—Most physicians are concerned about dramatic losses in their productivity as well as increased staff time. The implementation of an EHR is a massive change, but the impact to productivity varies widely by physician. Some physicians report dramatic improvements after a few weeks while others never get up on the EHR. The key strategy to minimize losses is to insure that you have one or more physician champions who can lead the way and demonstrate the results and benefits of the EHR.
>
>> **TIP:** Each physician should carefully phase in use of the EHR according to the particular nature of their practice and services. For example, a primary care physician should start out using the EHR to document a single patient with a selected condition (Ex. Upper Respiratory Infection) on a selected day. The physician can add additional URI patients in succeeding days and then add additional clinical conditions. Thereby, the doctor is not risking problems throughout the day and with every patient.
>
> **Provider Time to Start Medical Records**—Any EHR will require physician time to support the initial startup effort. Physicians must validate the clinical content for the practice as well as train and start use of the EHR to serve patients. Physicians must review the clinical content, establish the vision of how the EHR should work in the practice, and support the initial efforts to "Go Live" with the EHR. One or more physicians must lead the way for the rest during the implementation effort. Note that delegating the responsibility solely to nurses and other clinical staff will not build the physician skills or support that will be needed to deploy and use the EHR in the practice.

TABLE 2.2

Quick EHR Working Budget	Quantity	Unit Cost	EHR Total	Comment
Servers				
EHR Application Server		$15,000–$50,000		1 per practice to run the EHR, but you should buy 2 if you want redundancy for the EHR Server.
Imaging Server		$10,000–$25,000		1 per practice but some EHRs store images in the EHR Application Server.
Large File System		$20,000–$100,000		Larger Practices may need a large storage device to improve performance and security.
Backup Hardware		$4,000–$25,000		1 per practice
FAX Facilities Equipment				
Multi-Line FAX Server		$4,000–$10,000		1 per practice
System Software		$250/device		For each workstation and tablet
Printers		$1,000/printer		To upgrade old printers
Scanners				
Front Desk Sets		$300–$600/scanner		1 for each front desk station. To scan a few pages from patients at the front desk.
Production Scanner		$2,000–$6,000/scanner		At least 1 per medical record location to support Medical Record Scanning
User Devices				
Workstations		$1,000–$2,000 per workstation		Staff that share PMS workstations or have no access today may need an individual workstation.
Tablets		$2,000–$3,500 per Tablet		One tablet per doctor, nurse and clinical staff person
Application Software				
Electronic Health Record (EHR)		$2,500–$4,000 per user		1 license per doctor, nurse clinical staff and others who access the current paper record.
Imaging Software		$500–$1,000/user		1 license per user
Installation		10%–30% of hardware costs		Varies widely based on number of servers, current hardware and a variety of factors.

— *Continued*

Continued from previous page

Quick EHR Working Budget	Quantity	Unit Cost	EHR Total	Comment
Training		40% to 60% of EHR Application Costs		Varies widely based on training strategy, location, and staff sophistication.
TOTALS				
Hardware Contingency				Allows for unexpected upgrades to hardware.
Other Contingency				Covers other potential costs that are not covered elsewhere.
Services Contingency				Supports additional training and implementation services for practices with complex situations.
TOTAL WITH CONTINGENCY				

Staff Time to Start Medical Records—An EHR necessitates a complete change to the way the staff works and manages patient care. The change to workflow will require a significant amount of time to develop, and deploy the changes as well as train and support staff. The transition of patient paper charts to the EHR is a massive undertaking for any practice. Transition activities may include scanning paper charts, back loading information into the EHR from the charts and/or setting up an existing patient on their first EHR visit. For example, you may have to load in previous procedures into the EHR and existing problems to take advantage of the EHR Patient Summary Screen. The startup efforts will absorb all of your current staff time and then some from the time you select your EHR until at least 6 months after the EHR is activated.

Unexpected Upgrades to Current Computers and Communications— In many practices, some current workstations and communications must be upgraded to support the EHR. Additionally, current versions of key software may not be the most current version required by the EHR. For example, you may need to upgrade your practice management system, and purchase an interface for the EHR to exchange data with the PMS. The communications network designed for the PMS may not be sufficient for EHR volumes and images. Note that communications changes could affect intra-office and inter-office communications. For example, a slow router may require replacement to increase the speed of the network in the office, while a slow direct dial-up or DSL connection must be upgraded to a faster T1 connection.

> **TIP:** Unfortunately, these communications upgrades can have an extended lead time for installation and activation. For example, a new communication service between your office and a satellite may take 30 to 90 days to deploy. Make sure that you time your communications orders to avoid delays to the rest of the project.

Additional Security and Network Protection—EHRs significantly raise the security and network protection requirements for a practice. Internet access without controls, unprotected workstations and lax system security policies will cost a practice a lot of time, effort and money. For example, a practice had a serious problem with a software virus that was introduced from software that was loaded on their system by accident. The practice must evaluate security vulnerabilities and address those issues for the initial implementation as well as establish procedures to monitor security. For example, changing passwords on a periodic basis is an important security procedure.

Continuing Staff and Provider Support—The practice must establish a continuing process to support staff and manage changes to the EHR. Ad hoc changes to EHR standards and procedures expose the practice to a variety of risks and undermine the EHR investment.

> *TIP:* You should establish a continuing process to assure all users are properly trained in the use of the EHR as well as how the EHR is used at the practice. For example, a standard training and mentoring strategy for new clinical employees will help maintain the appropriate level of expertise and standards for the EHR.

The working EHR budget will go through several iterations as the project moves forward. The working budget format can be used to compare products, as well as manage the budget.

INVESTMENT ANALYSIS

After calculating the cost and the projected benefits, you can now analyze your EHR investment. In general, larger practices will develop a more compelling financial reason to implement an EHR. The relation between size and benefits is directly related to the number of people who access the paper chart. In smaller practices, the competition for patient information is not as fierce since patient service involves fewer people. If your practice has more than one person working on care for a particular patient, then your practice is well positioned to capitalize on an EHR. If your practice has been frustrated with the lack of economies of scale even as you have grown, then the EHR may help you generate these benefits.

But a financial return on EHRs will make the decision easier. The worksheet on page 30 helps you calculate a return on investment based on the information you gathered above. Note the worksheet spreads the initial costs (A) over a 5-year period.

Note that the EHR Return on Investment does not include interest expenses, soft costs or the phase-in of benefits noted above. However, the worksheet does present the magnitude of the project and potential benefits.

If the benefits and marginal revenues present a compelling return on your EHR investment, that is great. However, the lack of a compelling ROI may not necessarily free you from the ARRA influenced need to implement an EHR. You need to consider the com-

TABLE 2.3

EHR Return on Investment	Amount	Comment
A. Cost Estimate		Cost estimate from one of the three strategies listed above.
B. Five Year Annualized Cost		Divide A. by 5 to calculate the annual cost over the first 5 years (For Basic EHR Estimate, multiply monthly cost by 12)
C. Annual EHR Software Support		Add Annual Software Support of 18% to 33% of the original software cost (0 for Basic EHR Estimate)
D. Annual EHR Hardware Support		Add Annual Hardware Support of 12% of the Hardware Cost (0 for Basic EHR Estimate)
Total Annual Costs		**Sum of B, C, and D.**
E. Annual Potential Benefit		From Cost Reduction and Revenue Benefits Worksheet Above.
F. Annual Potential Profit or Loss on EHR Investment		Subtract Total Expected Costs (D) from Annual Potential Benefit (E)

petitive issues, patient expectations and the general movement of the healthcare industry to insure that you maintain a responsive and viable practice. Otherwise, you may be left at a disadvantage. For example, practices that can interact with patients over the Internet provide an alternative to waiting on hold to schedule an appointment or request a refill.

TABLE 2.4

Comprehensive Working Budget	Item	Purpose	Key Issues	Estimated Costs
Hardware	EHR Server	EHR servers contain the medical record information and the EHR application. In most cases, the EHR operates on a different server than the PMS application.	Various levels of protection from server failure can be purchased. A cluster server includes two or more servers sharing the same data repository. Cluster servers can continue to provide service in the event of a serious problem with one of the servers in a cluster.	$15,000–$250,000
	Image Server	Many EHR products store images on a separate server. The server contains the images that are accessed through the EHR. EHRs that use a single server for both the EHR and imaging do not require a dedicated Image Server.	Image volume can be very substantial. Scanning of current paper records as well as storing new incoming documents and images may require very large storage capacity.	$10,000–$30,000
	Storage System	EHRs may store massive amounts of information and images. A Storage Area Network (SAN) allows you to accommodate large amounts of data and images in a fast and secure environment. Not all practices need a SAN.	Larger practices may need the SAN to handle the amount of information as well as provide a viable way to backup all of the data.	$20,000–$150,000
	Backup System	EHRs contain much more data than you collect with a PMS system. The backup system may be attached to one of the main servers (e.g., EHR Server).	A dedicated backup server may allow for greater flexibility by downloading the information to the backup server storage, and backing up the storage to tape. PMS backup devices are mostly too slow to handle EHR backups.	$4,000–$35,000
	Interface Server	In the event that your EHR will be interfacing with a PMS, PACS, or other systems, you may need an interface server. In some cases, EHRs exchange information without an interface server. Without an interface server, the information is sent as a transaction between the PMS and EHR.	The interface between the EHR and the PMS may conflict with each other and require additional equipment or testing.	$4,000–$10,000
	FAX Server	Incoming faxes will be immediately entered into the EHR in paperless environments. Otherwise, you would need to scan the fax into the EHR and store the image in the EHR. Fax servers accept the image of the Fax, and track incoming faxes. The fax server bypasses the print and scanning process to add the image to the EHR.	Many EHR vendors do not offer fax servers. An alternative to fax servers are Internet-based services that deliver your incoming fax as an email with an image attachment.	$5,000–$10,000

— *Continued*

Continued from previous page

Comprehensive Working Budget	Item	Purpose	Key Issues	Estimated Costs
	Other System Servers	To support a computer network, you may need additional servers to manage overhead issues. Overhead issues include email (Mail Server), printer management (Print Server), and network traffic management (Domain Server and Active Directory Server.)	If you currently have a network, you may still need to upgrade the additional servers for additional capacity, and/or backup the key servers.	$4,000–$8,000 per server.
	Remote Workstation Server	Remote workstation servers allow you to improve the support for wireless devices and decrease the communications needed for remote offices. Basically, remote workstation servers act as a local proxy for a remote user (like *PC Anywhere*). All of the information that is typically exchanged between the workstation and the EHR server is done locally in your computer room; only the screen information is transmitted to the remote user. The remote EHR uses fewer communication resources than without the remote workstation server. Some EHRs are based on technologies that eliminate the need for remote workstation servers. Note that ASPs typically provide the remote workstation facilities for practices using their service.	Remote servers also help mitigate lost data due to communication problems or interruptions in contact with the remote user. Remote workstation servers improve and simplify management of the system since you can affect many users through working with the remote workstation sever. Costs of Remote Workstation Servers can vary widely and is impacted by the number of users.	$10,000–$40,000.
	Network Infrastructure	A wireless network will be needed to support the EHR at each location. A variety of options exist. The wireless network should be considered with any other improvements to the communication infrastructure.	Locations may need multiple access points based on size, interference and other factors.	$700–$3,000 per location
System Software	Network Access Licenses	Workstations and Tablets on a network require licenses to access the servers. Licenses may also be needed to access applications, such as email.	A variety of network licenses may be needed including access, virus protection and other facilities. These requirements vary widely by vendor and can be impacted by your own installed systems. For example, you may need a special terminal emulation program to access the current PMS application from the new EHR workstations.	$40–$200 per workstations/tablet.

— Continued

Continued from previous page

Comprehensive Working Budget	Item	Purpose	Key Issues	Estimated Costs
	Database Access Licenses	Most EHRs are built on a database system. Many database vendors require each user or each workstation/tablet to have a database license.	In some cases, the EHR vendors include the database license in the EHR costs.	$100–$250 per workstation/use
Tablets and Workstations	Additional Workstations	Additional workstations may be needed to support users who will need EHR access but do not have current access to a workstation. Additional users may be found in the clinical and administrative area. For example, procedure schedulers and insurance collectors will need access to the EHR. With workflow features, virtually every employee and doctor needs EHR access.	Workstations may be needed for staff who share workstations with other employees as well as staff who use the medical chart, but have no workstations today. Additional workstations may be allocated for nursing stations, doctor offices and other locations, as needed.	$1,000–$1,500 per workstation.
	Tablets	Virtually every doctor, nurse and clinical worker will need access to the EHR. If the person in question moves around to serve patients, he may need a tablet instead of a workstation. Tablets communicate with the EHR over radio frequency connections and allow the user to maintain contact with the system as they move around the facility. Tablets also simplify HIPAA Privacy and Security compliance. For example, if a workstation was in each exam room, the screen would have to be secured each time the user left the room.	The practice needs a strategy to accommodate doctors and staff who move between facilities. Tablets may be shared by part-time employees. Each location needs tablets for peak staffing. Each location may need a spare tablet.	$2,000–$3,500 per tablet.
Printers	Color Printers	Color printers can print patient education information from the EHR and other sources.	Some practices do not use color printers since they are more expensive and slower than other printers.	$500–$3,000 per printer
	Other Printers	Additional printers may be needed to support the EHR.	The practice may replace old PMS printers to improve print quality for EHR products.	$300–$2,500 per printer

Continued from previous page

Comprehensive Working Budget	Item	Purpose	Key Issues	Estimated Costs
Scanners	Front Desk Scanners	Front desks will receive miscellaneous forms, reports and information from presenting patients. Typically, the patient only has a few pages. Due to space constraints at most front desks, a small hand-fed scanner has been successful in a number of practices.	Small scanners may be needed by other staff that may receive a few pages from patients. Nurses and surgery schedulers may need small scanners.	$200–$600 per sheet-scanner.
	High Volume Scanners	To maintain the designated record set, some practices scan the existing paper records into the EHR. Scanning old paper charts requires a faster, heavy duty scanner that can handle the initial workload.	Incoming mail will be scanned into the EHR and routed to the appropriate doctor, nurse or staff. After the first 6–12 months, the paper chart scanning volume may drop to a level that requires fewer scanning devices.	$1,000–$10,000 per high volume scanner
Software	EHR Application	EHR application licenses allow access to a set number of users based on the actual user count or provider count. The EHR application licenses may be for full access or partial access depending on the vendor. License fees vary widely based on the target market for the EHR and staffing composition. For example, some EHRs are licensed by a provider, but only allow a certain number of users for each provider.	Licensing fee strategies vary widely by vendor. Definition of a provider license can dramatically impact the cost. Some EHRs are sold by module with discounts given for packages.	$2,500–$4,000 per user
	Scanner Software	Some EHR vendors include the scanning software in the base EHR price. Many vendors charge extra for scanning software.	Scanning software may be licensed differently from the EHR application.	$500–$1,000 per user
	PMS Interface	A separate interface may be required for the demographic information, appointment schedule and charge interfaces between the PMS and EHR systems.	The interface between the EHR and PMS may require a separate server. In addition to EHR interface costs, the practice may have to pay for PMS interface modules.	$3,000–$10,000 per interface per system.
	Equipment Interface	The practice may have diagnostic equipment that could be interfaced with the EHR. The equipment interfaces may transmit an order from the EHR to the diagnostic equipment and download the results.	May require upgrades to the diagnostic equipment and/or an interface module from the diagnostic equipment vendor.	$3,000–$5,000 per diagnostic device with an interface.

Continued from previous page

Comprehensive Working Budget	Item	Purpose	Key Issues	Estimated Costs
Third Party Licenses		EHRs may require other software from third parties. In addition to system software, the practice may need to buy word processing, and other items.	In a document management EHR, the practice may have to purchase a variety of software products to produce the files for storage in the EHR.	0–$300 per workstation and tablet.
Services	Installation	Installation services include the installation of hardware and software as well as the setup of access to your workstations.	Installation services include hardware setup, software setup and connecting the EHR system to your network. Each workstation, tablet, scanner and other device will require a certain level of setup.	10%–30% of Hardware Costs
	Customization	Customization of the EHR may be required for certain vendors while other vendors may include customization in the sales price. Do not mistake customization for setting up user preferences. Ultimately, the practice is better off if each user knows how to maintain his specific setups and preferences (e.g., medications).	The scope of changes varies widely. The more clinical content that is already in the system, the less customization will be necessary. Some vendors will train the practice but leave customization to practice resources and third parties.	Varies Widely
	Training	EHR training includes computer-based training, classes at the vendor offices, practice office training and web-based training. Some vendors have structured training programs.	Many vendors train a small group of users who then train other practice staff. Training services typically vary in price.	40%–60% of EHR Application Costs
TOTAL EHR COSTS				
Contingency Costs	Communication Upgrades	Allow for upgrades to inter-office and intra-office communications to support the EHR.	Depending on the current level of communications and the last upgrade.	Varies Widely
	Workstation Upgrades	Allows for upgrades to workstations that are questionable in light of the EHR requirements.	May be easily determined by surveying the existing workstations.	$1,000–$1,500 per workstation
	Services	Implementation and training services are typically based on time. In many cases, you may want to include a contingency fee to allow for additional training and EHR customization.	This contingency fee allows the practice to allow for additional help in this demanding project. The estimate can be refined as the vendor proposal and practice requirements get more specific.	10%–20% of estimated services
TOTAL EHR COSTS WITH CONTINGENCY COSTS				

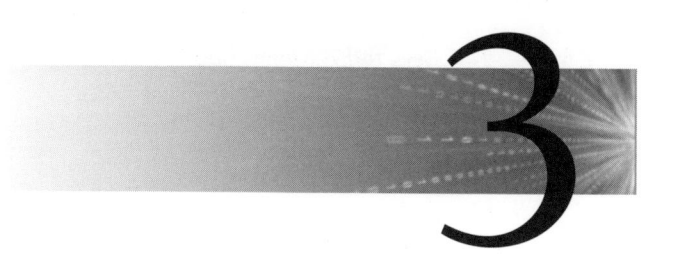

Your Practice Management System and an EHR

An EHR does not exist in a technological or organizational vacuum. EHR usefulness will be affected by your processes, staff and your practice management system (PMS). Your PMS can help or hinder your EHR and vice versa. The key issue is where you draw the border between what you expect from your EHR as well as how you will use your EHR in conjunction with your PMS. If you are not careful, you could end up duplicating efforts, and undermining both your clinical and billing operations.

HOW EHRS WORK WITH PMSs

Most EHR systems were designed as stand alone products that work with a variety of PMS systems. As such, many EHRs have their own demographic files, procedure codes, and—in some cases—full feature appointment schedule modules: information that is also maintained in the PMS.

As the EHR industry has progressed, many PMS vendors and EHR vendors have developed relationships to offer a complete package of software to your practice. Other vendors have developed a completely integrated EHR/PMS combination where the EHR and PMS components are inseparable.

With more than 1,000 PMS options and over 400 EHR products, a wide range of relationships exist between EHR and PMS systems. The following chart shows two technology relationships (Integrated and Interfaced Products) as well as business relationships between EHR and PMS products.

TABLE 3.1

	Description	Strengths and Limitations	Examples
Integrated Products (See Diagram 3.2)	Integrated products were designed as a single product from a single vendor. The products share information from the same database.	+ Supports reports including PMS and EHR data. + Costs may be lower since only one technology base is needed. + One set of master files is shared by PMS and EHR. − EHR or PMS product may not be best of breed.	eClnincalWorks Electronic Health Systems Intergy Med-Informatics
Interfaced Products (See Diagram 3.1)	Interfaced products exchange information between the EHR and PMS. Basic exchanges are demographics, and appointments from the PMS to the EHR. Charges are passed from the EHR to the PMS. In many cases, the interfaces are based on an industry standard called HL7 (Health Level 7). However, HL7 allows for a wide range of options. Interfaces should be tested to insure that the PMS and EHR are properly exchanging information. Interfaced products may be from one or more vendors.	+ Mostly allows for multiple EHR options for a PMS. + Interface is standard product. − User look and feel may differ between PMS and EHR. − PMS and EHR products may have overlapping features that requires careful analysis during implementation. − May obscure audit trails for charges from the EHR to the PMS. − May require separate entry of master file data (Ex. CPT/ICD9 codes) in EHR and PMS. − Software upgrades could cause interface problems. − May require additional licenses and costs for products based on different technologies. − An interface server may be needed to pass information between the PMS and EHR.	Centricity PM and several EHR Products
Companion Products	Companion EHR and PMS products are interfaced by a single vendor and sold as a pair.	+ One vendor responsible for the PMS and EHR. − Vendor may not be open to other EHR options. − User look and feel may differ between PMS and EHR.	Horizon Ambulatory Care and Horizon Practice Solutions Healthport EHR and PM Micro MD and PM

— Continued

Continued from previous page

	Description	**Strengths and Limitations**	**Examples**
Joint Marketing	A PMS vendor and an EHR vendor have a preferred product relationship. Their separate products work together through an interface between the PMS and EHR.	+ The practice may get preferred pricing. + Interface is used by other clients. − User look and feel differs between PMS and EHR.	MARS and Several EHR products.
Open EHR Options	Some PMS vendors do not have a relationship with an EHR vendor. The PMS vendor offers to develop an interface with any EHR chosen by the practice.	+ Supports "Best of Breed" selection. − Interface may be costly and used by few practices. − Practice may be on its own when dealing with the PMS and EHR interface. − Upgrades to one of the products may cause interface problems.	Many smaller vendors.

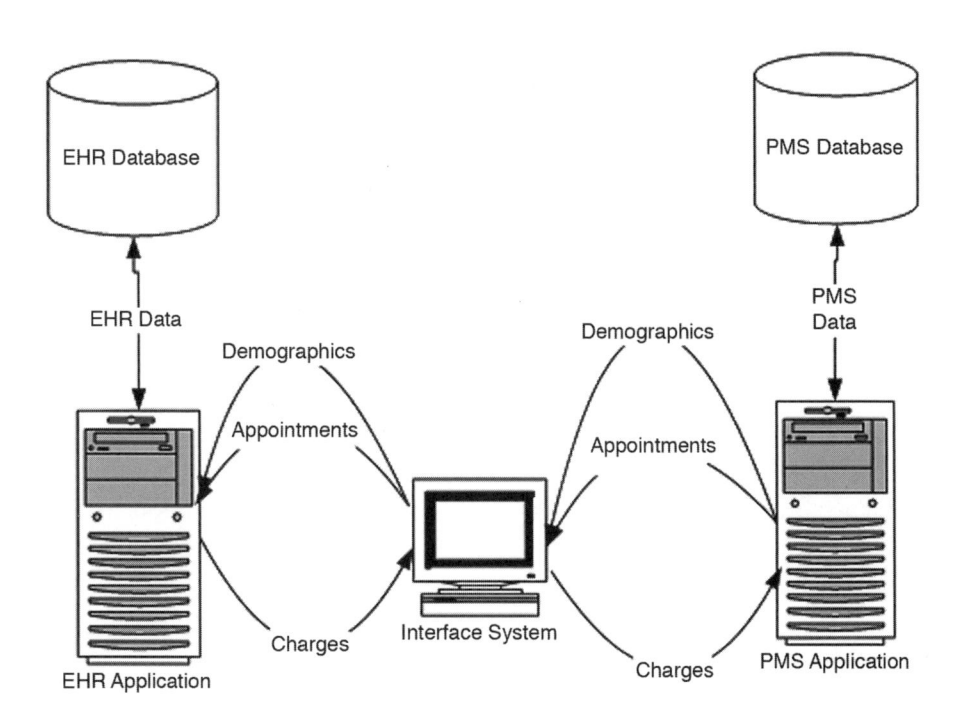

DIAGRAM 3.1—*Interfaced EHR and PMS*

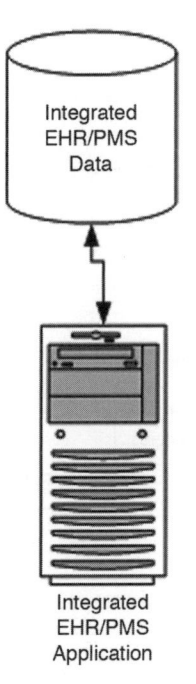

DIAGRAM 3.2—*Integrated EHR and PMS*

All things being equal, you would rather buy a single product and deal with one vendor rather than deal with two separate products, vendors and their interfaces. However, not all products are equal. In some cases, you select an EHR that meets your need, but may not have a companion PMS offering. Some integrated products and interfaced EHR/PMS offerings have significant disparities between the sophistication and capabilities of their PMS product compared with other PMS products, and their EHR product compared to other EHR products.

EXAMPLE: You may encounter a PMS product that can handle multiple locations, but the companion EHR product does not manage audit trails and appointment activities by location. Similarly, the PMS product may not have computer assisted collection tools to manage your A/R. In other cases, the PMS may be targeted to a variety of practices, but the EHR may only have clinical content for a primary care practice.

INFORMATION EXCHANGES BETWEEN EHRs AND PMSs

Several logistical issues must be considered when you are considering an interfaced EHR. In most cases, interfaces are limited to receiving patient demographics and appointment schedules from the PMS and sending charges to the PMS. However, the practice will need a number of other data exchanges to allow PMS and EHR users to serve patients effectively and manage the practice.

The chart on pages 41 through 43 illustrates these types of information exchanges a practice would expect between an EHR system and its PMS, along with limitations to be aware of.

Some practices use EHR and PMS products that are not interfaced at all. Practices will work without an interface due to the lack of a working relationship between the two vendors/products or the costs of such interfaces. **EXAMPLE:** Some PMS vendors may not support an EHR interface with your desired EHR product. Some interfaces require substantial investments for PMS interface software, EHR interface software and a separate system to manage the interface. Be aware some PMS vendors do not accept electronic charge transactions from an EHR.

> **CAUTION:** Separate entry of patient demographics can lead to account numbering discrepancies between the PMS and EHR systems. For example, some systems attach prefixes or suffixes onto the patient number for a variety of reasons, while other systems use internal aliases to track related patient records.

TABLE 3.2

Information Type	Primary Source	Needed To	Status
Master Files	PMS	Master files include CPT codes, ICD9 codes, appointment types and other data used in the EHR and PMS systems. Some of the files are fairly standard, but other files may significantly differ between the two systems. For example, PMS products may include pricing and payer reimbursement information while the EHR merely tracks the basic CPT code and description. EHRs may maintain formulary information that must be associated with your PMS payer file. EHRs also have a number of master files that are not in a PMS including drugs, clinical database, orders, and allergies.	Some EHR vendors will load selected PMS master file data into the EHR at installation, but updates are manually entered.
Patient Demographics	PMS	Demographic information establishes the identity of patients in the EHR. Most EHR products store the PMS patient ID in the EHR demographic information. *TIP:* Although many EHRs allow you to set up demographics, you should fully evaluate how the demographic information is coordinated with the PMS. Note that not all interfaces support bi-directional demographic exchanges: the PMS may send demographic information to the EHR, but the EHR does not send demographic updates back to the PMS. A demographic link allows you to maintain consistent information between the two systems and coordinate information. Otherwise, you will be adding patient demographic information to both PMS and EHR separately.	Most EHR systems can accept demographic information from a PMS, but few PMS systems will accept demographic information from an EHR.
Appointment Information	PMS	EHRs use appointment information to track patient visits and progress. In most cases, patients are scheduled for appointments in the PMS. The appointment schedule is sent to the EHR to track the status of patients. Appointments for the day are typically displayed on the main EHR workflow screen with tasks, and to do's, patient visits and progress. Some PMSs allow patients to be checked in to flag patient appointments awaiting charges. PMSs typically do not track patient service progress (room, status) or the completion of the appointment process. PMS systems recognize a completed appointment when the charge is posted. Some EHRs track the patient throughout the visit. Medical staff determines that patients are waiting, and doctors can see which patients have been placed in a room. Internal labs, nurses, and technicians can see which patients are waiting for a service ordered by the doctor. The PMS system would only show that the patient has checked in.	Many interfaces send appointment information to the EHR, but very few PMS products accept appointment information from EHRs.

— Continued

Continued from previous page

Information Type	Primary Source	Needed To	Status
Payer Information	PMS	In the course of treatment, physicians and clinical staff need payer information to correctly guide patients through treatment options, locations and processes. For example, some payers may prohibit use of an internal lab or require procedures at a designated ASC. The payer information for a patient is typically included in the EHR demographic record. However, many EHRs do not necessarily maintain coverage details that may affect care options. Payer information may be used to determine prescription formularies and/or referral requirements in the EHR. Physicians may also reference insurance information to determine coverage or authorization requirements for in-office procedures. *CAUTION:* In many cases, the PMS payer codes have to be translated into a different code for the EHR. Otherwise, the EHR may not properly handle the payer specific issues and formulary.	Typically sent over to the EHR with demographic information.
Recall Information	EHR	Recall triggers are generated through clinical visits. Some EHRs allow you to generate recall notices and letters as well as track the completion of recall items through office visits. However, recall information in the EHR is not available through the PMS to assist appointment schedulers. Many PMS products have recall features to allow appointment scheduling to track recall issues. However, few interfaced EHR products send recall information to the PMS. *CAUTION:* PMS appointments will not necessarily reconcile EHR recalls or orders. Similarly, EHR plan items and orders will not be reflected in the PMS recall or appointment modules.	Typically, practice staff must separately enter the recall in the PMS. Scheduling staff may need access to the EHR to track recalls.
Clinical Orders	EHR	Clinical orders are entered by physicians/practitioners in the treatment plan for a patient. Additional orders based on disease driven protocols may be automatically generated by the EHR. Examples of orders include lab tests, procedures and other studies. Orders are needed by appointment scheduling to confirm that the patient has completed necessary testing or to schedule the patient for the appropriate type of visit in the PMS. PMS products do not typically allow for clinical order information.	Scheduling staff needs access to the EHR to track orders.

— Continued

Continued from previous page

Information Type	Primary Source	Needed To	Status
Surgery Scheduling	EHR	Surgery requests are communicated to the clinical support team by the doctor. The clinical support staff manages a variety of administrative, insurance authorization, testing, and facility coordination tasks to support surgery scheduling. Surgical procedures may be entered in the PMS appointment schedule, but the actual status of the various tasks associated with the appointment is normally documented in the EHR.	Scheduling staff needs access to the EHR to track surgery scheduling status. Clinical staff may need access to the PMS to manage surgery scheduling.
Charge Information	EHR	Many EHRs collect the charge information during the patient visit. Charge information is gathered when procedure and test orders are entered as well as the calculation of the E&M code at the completion of the visit. When approved by the doctor, the charges are sent to the PMS. In many interfaced PMSs, the PMS user accesses the charges from the EHR and posts the charges collected during patient service to the patient account. The PMS uses the charge information to produce patient statements and claims. In many cases, the PMS audit trail will show the charge posting person and not the clinical staff who approved the charge in the EHR. Note that many PMS products allow the user to change the posted information without creating any flag or notice that the posted charge differs from the information sent by the EHR.	The interfaces are available, but audit trails may not be clear. In most interfaces, the PMS user can edit the charge from the EHR. Some PMS vendors do not allow for charge interfaces with EHRs.
Incoming Referral Information	PMS	Incoming referral information is entered in the PMS to support claim submission. However, the doctor may need to see the referral information to determine the allowed services during the patient visit. Lacking the referral information, the EHR user will not be able to determine the specific treatment requirements. The PMS referral order will not be electronically sent to the EHR.	Doctors and clinical staff will need access to the PMS for incoming referral information.
Internal Referral Information	EHR	Doctors record internal referral information in the EHR at the time of service. Internal referrals may include a payer communication or may be directly authorized by the doctor. Internal referral information is needed in the PMS to manage appointments, file claims, and insure that you do not provide services beyond the referral.	The referral information is manually transferred to the PMS. Administrative staff may need access to the EHR system to review the original referral information.
Clinical Notes	EHR	EHRs contain the clinical record for the patient. Anyone who accesses dictation, prescription information or any other clinical information will need access to the EHR. As a practical matter this may cover a large number of your clinical and administrative staff. For example, • Payer-collection staff uses clinical notes to justify insurance claims. • Surgery schedulers need information on procedures.	Many administrative staff members will need access to the EHR.

Practices that do not use interfaced or integrated products must separately enter the basic information needed by the PMS and EHR. Typically, the practice will enter the demographic information in both systems, and enter appointments for the next day into the EHR from the appointment schedule printed from the PMS. Charges are posted into the PMS from a fee slip that is used by physicians around the EHR. The fee slip is printed from the PMS, and the charge information recorded on the fee slip during the patient visit. *Warning*: This workaround may lead to discrepancies between the EHR charge information and the PMS charge posting. For example, the doctor may record a certain level of service on the fee ticket before completing the clinical chart note and calculating the level of service in the EHR

> *TIP:* Do not sign the contract to purchase the PMS until you fully understand how your EHR will work with your practice management system and vice versa.

REVIEW YOUR PMS BEFORE OPTING FOR AN EHR

Take a close look at your current PMS in light of your EHR plans. Your PMS can affect the EHR options that can be practically implemented. Before beginning your search, assess your current situation. Carefully consider:

Are you Satisfied with the PMS?

Many practices are not happy with their existing PMS due to a variety of issues. The practice may have outgrown the product, or the PMS vendor may have not kept the product up to date. Unfortunately, EHRs will not necessarily improve your PMS. If your practice is not content with the PMS, then you should not attach too much significance to the current PMS in your EHR selection process. For example, you may be dissatisfied with the PMS appointment scheduler and seek a better appointment scheduler in the EHR, but a future PMS may actually be the tool used for appointment scheduling.

If you are not happy with your PMS, you should consider replacing the PMS in conjunction with the EHR implementation. Thereby, you won't compromise your final EHR selection with a PMS base that is not right for you. Additionally, you may more seriously value the integration with a PMS replacement and not limit your practice to EHR options with interfaces to your current PMS.

Does the PMS have a Preferred or Exclusive Relationship with an EHR product?

Many PMS products have preferred or joint agreements with one or more EHR vendors. Some PMS products have exclusive agreements with EHR products. If you do not choose a vendor-endorsed EHR, you may be on your own to get the PMS and EHR to interface.

> *TIP*: However, don't unnecessarily settle for the EHRs offered by your PMS vendor.

If the PMS's EHR does not include a workflow tool, or lacks features needed by your specialty, you should determine (and get the vendor commitment) when the PMS's EHR partner will address your preferences. Otherwise, you should select a more appropriate EHR product and work out the relationship needed with your PMS vendor. You do not want to compromise your EHR project to make the PMS vendor happy. You may have some leverage, since the PMS vendor would prefer to have you as a PMS customer rather than risk losing you because it forced you to go with an EHR product that is not appropriate for your practice.

Does the PMS Support EHR Interfaces?

Initially, you need to determine if the PMS product supports interfaces with EHR products. Some PMS vendors support open interfaces for any EHR vendors using industry standard transaction structures. Other PMS vendors develop custom interfaces that are used for each EHR situation. Of course, you can always create your own interface between your PMS and the selected EHR. Some interface strategies even allow you to interface two products without the assistance of either the PMS or EHR vendor.

> **CAUTION**: Do not undertake a custom interface effort without fully understanding the implication including potential changes with future versions of the EHR or PMS, and the fact that you may be among the few (or only) practices using the combination of products.

Does the PMS Vendor Lack an EHR Strategy?

Surprisingly, a number of PMS vendors still lack an EHR strategy. These PMS vendors claim to be customer-driven and will offer to create an interface with products selected by their customers. However, some of these vendors have never interfaced their products with an EHR. Other PMS vendors have developed interfaces with a variety of EHR options, but the PMS vendor does not have extensive expertise with a particular EHR. In these cases, the costs of maintaining the interface may be spread over a few practices and be more expensive that an interface that is used by a large number of practices.

If your practice ends up developing a new PMS interface, or an interface with an EHR that the PMS vendor is not interfaced with, you will have to coordinate the work of the PMS and EHR vendors to implement the interface. The interface development effort may include designing the mechanism and strategy, as well as the specific information that will be exchanged and the sources and destinations of the interfaced data.

Interface design requires attention to a number of technical details including what triggers sending a demographic and appointment update to the EHR and the amount of time it takes to post changes to the EHR. For example, you may need the patient check-in from the PMS to update the EHR within a minute to insure that the clinical staff is adequately informed about patient flow issues.

You will not be able to benefit from the work of other practices, and you will have to coordinate changes to allow for upgrades to either the PMS, EHR or the interface. For example, a change to the PMS product appointment scheduler may change the information that is going to the EHR. You would have to test the PMS/EHR interfaces anytime you upgrade either the PMS or EHR.

Will the PMS Technology Base Support an EHR?

Most EHR products are based on a graphical user interface (GUI), such as Windows or Linux, and a database structure, such as Microsoft SQL Server, Oracle and Informix. Many older PMS products are based on old technologies and a character interface that may not easily work with your EHR selection. Similarly, you may be using "dumb" terminals that would not work with an EHR. Even if you have PCs, your PCs may not be powerful enough to support an EHR.

Upgrading your existing technology base to support an EHR could also require additional investments in the PMS infrastructure. For example, you may have to buy software to make your new PC workstations appear as dumb terminals to your existing PMS product—creating a new interface between the EHR and PMS. In some cases, you may need to pay additional money to move to a new version of the PMS, or even the next generation product of your existing PMS product.

Are Additional User Licenses Needed?

If doctors, nurses and clinical staff have access to the EHR, they may also need access to the PMS. Such access may require additional licenses fees and maybe even new PMS hardware. For example, the additional users may exceed the number of users that your current PMS hardware can manage.

The table on page 47 and 48 reveals several issues to consider when you review EHR options associated with your PMS.

Your current PMS system may pose a number of operational and implementation challenges. The key problems are based on overlapping functions and the practical implications of using an interfaced EHR.

> **EXAMPLE**: Some PMS systems allow you to scan information on insurance cards into the PMS. However, the insurance card may be needed by the clinical staff to get prior authorization or check the payer's rules. As a practical matter, a variety of information is shared between clinical and practice management processes. These issues can impact your efforts to design a workable workflow and implementation plan. In some cases, you will have to work around both the EHR and PMS vendor to determine what is best for your situation.

All things being equal, you would want to buy the EHR associated with your PMS. However, EHRs are not equal. Common barriers to buying the EHR partner to your PMS include:

PMS Upgrades—Some PMS products require upgrades to various components. For example, you may have to move to a newer version of the PMS to support the EHR inter-

TABLE 3.3

EHR Partner	Description	Issues	Recommendation
PMS integrated with EHR	The PMS shares a common database with an integrated EHR.	Integrated products frequently do not support interfaces with other EHR products.	Closely review the integrated EHR in light of your needs. If the EHR product is not appropriate for your practice, insure that you have a reliable and cost effective interface strategy. The analysis should include the cost of the interface from the PMS vendor as well as hardware needed to allow you PMS and EHR systems to exchange information.
Companion and joint marketed PMS	The PMS vendor has a standard interface with an EHR product. The EHR product is jointly sold to the practice.	The existing interface with the companion or joint marketed product may be easily used by the PMS vendor to interface with the selected EHR. The EHR vendor may support interfaces with other PMS products.	Clearly establish responsibility for the interface with the EHR and PMS vendors. Insure that the PMS vendor will not change the interface (and disrupt your interface with the other EHR product) without adequate notification. Include protections for the strategy in your contracts.
Old technology	The PMS is based on a character interface	EHRs are primarily based on a graphical user interface like Windows. If you are currently using "dumb terminals" with your PMS, these users will have to be upgraded to PCs to access the EHR.	Set up a contingency in the budget for hardware upgrades to "dumb" terminals and a technology base. Carefully review the cost benefits of the current PMS system in light of these changes. Review the design and capacity of the current technology base to identify all upgrade costs.
Unsupported or not sold	The PMS is no longer actively supported or sold. The PMS product may have been superseded by another PMS offering from the vendor or you may be using a product that was discontinued.	PMS products that are discontinued expose the practice to a sudden loss of the PMS.	Seriously consider replacing the PMS system as part of your EHR effort. Critically analyze whether to further invest in an interface that may be used for a limited time.

— *Continued*

Continued from previous page

EHR Partner	Description	Issues	Recommendation
Not interfaced with an EHR	The PMS is not interfaced with any EHR products. The PMS vendor says that the interface will be built for whatever EHR you choose.	The practice could easily get caught in the middle of an effort by the PMS and EHR vendors to create an interface. Your practice could end up with a one of a kind interface with the selected EHR product.	Make certain that the EHR and your current PMS provides enough added value to be worth the trouble and cost. Check into the PMS product(s) that are sold with the selected EHR. In the long term, you may want to transition to one of the selected PMS products. Indeed, you should include such an option in your contract.
Old PMS version	Your practice has skipped one or more versions and/or upgrades of the current PMS system. The upgrade(s) may have been skipped due to cost of the upgrade, costs of hardware improvements needed for the EHR and/or lack of interest by your practice.	The "upgrade" to the newest PMS version may require changes to hardware and software as well as data conversion and retraining. The costs and efforts to upgrade may not significantly differ from those of a completely new system.	Include the PMS upgrade in your technology budget for the practice. Compare the cost of PMS upgrade with implementing a new PMS.

face and product. In some cases, your actually have to change to a different PMS system from your existing PMS vendor. For example, many PMS products may be sold by your PMS vendor, but only selected products (unfortunately, not your PMS) are interfaced with their EHR offering. **Hidden costs**: Upgrading your current PMS may require upgrades to your server, existing software (and new training), and, in some cases, your peripherals. You may need additional PMS modules merely to accommodate the EHR product.

PMS Interfaces—**Hidden costs**: Many PMS vendors charge for the interface module that allows you to exchange data with the EHR product. In some cases, separate charges may be required for each interface (e.g., patient demographics and appointments are considered two interfaces and charges a third interface). The interface modules may require a base charge and include a monthly maintenance fee.

EHR Features—The EHR companion product to the PMS product may not have the features you need. For example, the EHR partner for your PMS may not have the specialty clinical content you need for your practice. In other cases, the EHR may lack important features that you need, such as clinical messaging or transcription.

> ***TIP***: Be especially careful to insure the EHR meets requirements that you need to effectively use the EHR. Security, audit trails and Evaluation and Management coding tools can be easily overlooked when you are trying to fit your practice into the EHR of your current PMS vendor. In the final analysis, you should hold the companion EHR product to the same functional standard and requirements that you expect from any viable EHR product.

EHR Clinical Focus—Not all EHRs have the breadth of clinical content to address every type of practice. For example, some EHRs handle gastroenterology or ophthalmology but lack the clinical content for primary care and other specialties. And your practice may focus on a subspecialty that is not included in the clinical content of a more general specialty clinical offering. For example, a primary care focused EHR may lack the clinical content to support the cardiology specialty of one of the doctors. If the EHR of your PMS does not address your practice's clinical area then make sure you fully understand the effort needed to add the clinical content you'll need. You should be careful to itemize the scope and breadth of the clinical content needed by your practice. For example, a general ophthalmology practice will have different clinical content needs than a retina specialist. Similarly, general orthopedic clinical content may not be sufficient for a spine practice. Compare the effort needed to interface your PMS product with an EHR that addresses your clinical services "out of the box."

EHR Technology—Since many EHRs were not developed with a PMS system in mind, the EHRs are based on a completely separate technology base. Some practices find that the investment needed to buy and implement the PMS's EHR product is not cheaper (or even easier, in some cases) than buying a variety of other EHR options. For example, you may have to buy database user licenses for two databases: one for the PMS and another for the EHR. Similarly, the PMS and EHR may require a dedicated server for each module.

In the final analysis, you should not assume that the EHR partner with your PMS system is the best or less expensive strategy for your practice. Make sure that you fully understand the implications of using the PMS vendor's EHR product versus your other options.

COSTS OF CONNECTING YOUR EHR AND PMS

Connecting an EHR and PMS requires some investments in hardware and software. If the vendors have a working relationship, you must typically buy an interface module for the PMS as well as an interface module for the EHR. Such interfaces may cost from $3,000 to $12,000 or more for each interface. If you want to interface demographics, appointments and charges, you may have to buy 3 interfaces for the EHR and 3 interfaces for the PMS. Additionally, the interface may require an interface server (see Diagram 3.1, page 39).

Vendors that do not have a working EHR relationship will charge customization fees in addition to the purchase costs of their standard interfaces. If the vendor does not have a standard interface, you may have to invest substantial sums in a custom interface. Make sure you check the vendor's ability to accommodate other EHR products. Examine the costs to produce these interfaces, and contact customers who have such a working interface. The vendor should agree to a specific cost for any custom interfaces.

Additional interface implementation costs include technical assistance in placing the data that is being exchanged between the two systems, as well as the costs of testing the interfaces. Note that the initial loading of the data from the PMS to the EHR for the master files as well as loading the current appointments and demographic data may incur additional charges. Many interfaces will also require an annual maintenance fee.

> **TIP**: Be especially careful to insure that both the PMS and EHR vendors will appropriately support the interface and cooperate on resolving problems. Note that many of these interfaces do not post master file updates from the PMS to the EHR. You may have to separately enter the same master file record (e.g., appointment type, procedure code, diagnosis code) to the PMS and EHR systems.

Itemize the implementation costs and continuing support costs for the system that you desire. You will need to assign staff to test the interface, as well as train someone to troubleshoot the interface when inevitable problems appear in the future.

PRACTICAL ISSUES FOR REPLACING YOUR PMS

Replacing the PMS could have a significant effect on your plans for implementing an EHR. In general, most practices will want to replace the PMS before the EHR implementation effort begins. **TIP:** You need to insure that current administrative and billing operations are properly set up before you implement an EHR.

The practice needs to make sure that the replacement of the PMS is adequately accommodated in the schedule and budget for the practice. Between the effort needed to replace the PMS and settling into the new product, you may have to delay the EHR effort for 6 months to a year or more. The effect of replacing the PMS before you implement the EHR can affect the cost of the project since you may need to replace a lot of hardware and install the EHR infrastructure to move forward with the PMS.

Regardless of your PMS replacement product choice, the PMS implementation effort is not independent of your EHR effort or vice versa. PMS information drives patient demographics and appointment information and can affect your EHR. As important, EHRs generate charges which are posted to your PMS. For example,

> **Presentation of Patient Information in the EHR**—Most EHRs reference or interface PMS based demographic information. In some cases, the information in the PMS can differ from the EHR. For example, the PMS and EHR may use different coded sets of insurance information. Similarly, you may have user defined fields in the PMS that are not available or visible from the EHR.

Workflow Management—In most cases, appointments are made in the PMS modules and sent over to the EHR portion. If the appointment codes are not properly structured, the EHR office workflow management features could be undermined. For example, if the various doctors used six different appointment codes to classify a 15 minute same day visit (Ex. Acute 15, Same Day 15, SD1, etc.) then the appointment status viewing tools may be compromised since the same day 15 minute appointments would be difficult or impossible to monitor as a group.

HIPAA Privacy Information—HIPAA Privacy status and consent information is needed in the PMS and EHR. For compliance purposes, PMS users need access to the HIPAA status and the clinical staff needs HIPAA consent information to support clinical disclosures. If the HIPAA Privacy information is not viewable from the PMS and the EHR, monitoring disclosure could be difficult.

Patient Classification—the classification of patients and the patient information could affect the presentation of patients and even processing. For example, a patient type may drive pricing in the PMS, but be used to classify services in the EHR. If only the PMS type is maintained, then the EHR may not properly manage patient workflow and information.

Whether you keep you PMS or replace it, you need to make sure that the PMS information is structured to support the administrative side of the practice as well as trigger the appropriate handling of patients in the EHR. Otherwise, your practice will have to enter information in both systems and run the risk of triggering an unintended process due to the different ways the PMS and EHR use information to drive workflow and, ultimately patient service.

Compiling a Practice Focused Evaluation List

The evaluation list establishes the value and significance of the EHR features needed by your practice. An evaluation list can be very extensive or very brief. Some practices use evaluation lists itemizing hundreds of criteria, while other organizations are looking to fulfill a single requirement: get a world class EHR. Although a single criterion may be too general, an overly detailed list can flood you with details and complicate your decision. Regardless of the list length, your evaluation criteria should set an appropriate standard for your EHR as well as collect information that will be used as you proceed into the implementation phase.

The evaluation list establishes the expectation of the practice for the EHR as well as the measurement standard for EHR products. Set the expectation too low, and you may end up with many products that meet the standard but risk buying a product that will not meet your needs. Set the expectation too high and your practice may end up evaluating minutia but fail to get a grasp of the product practicality. For example, some evaluation lists itemized specific data items that the EHR should accommodate without including the features needed to capitalize on the data such as a report on the pending services for a patient. In some cases, the practice may search forever for the perfect product.

Many practices spend a tremendous amount of time looking at issues that are not necessarily EHR features but are necessary. Some EHR issues that are not product specific include:

Hardware Reliability—System protection is available through the hardware server purchased, regardless of the application. Your practice can buy hardware that is vulnerable to shutdown due to the loss of a critical component or you can purchase hardware that offers redundant components. Redundant disk drives, power supplies and fans are some of the redundancies that you can purchase for your server on a cost- effective basis. For an additional investment, you can buy fully redundant server hardware regardless of the EHR software. Workstations, communications, network components, tablets, printers, and scanner selections and strategies can also control your risks without necessarily impacting your software selection.

Tablets—Tablet devices are not specific to a particular EHR product. Tablet devices can access an EHR like a workstation or work through a terminal server that improves performance for tablets in remote locations. Some EHR vendors offer a variety of tablet options that include models with and without self contained keyboards. Know that your workstation and tablet decisions are not dependent on your software selection.

Internet Access—With the right equipment and/or communications, physicians and others can access the EHR over the Internet. Some products are optimized to work over the Internet directly, while other products require a server that lets Internet users access the EHR. For EHRs that require an Internet access server, you need an internet gateway and communications services that support such a gateway (e.g., Windows Terminal Server with Citrix.) In either case, you need a practical way for the remote user to access the Internet. For example, you may install a broadband connection at the doctor's home or access the EHR from the hospital connection to the Internet. EHR access over the Internet is not dependent on your EHR software. However, the ability to access your EHR through the Internet or a remote location is not specific to an EHR product. **TIP:** There may be a cost difference between the two approaches, but the ability to access the EHR is not product dependent.

The important issue is to focus on the features and capabilities of the product and not the hardware and communications that you will purchase to support the EHR. Hardware and communication issues can be addressed after you have chosen the appropriate software.

EVALUATION LIST FACTORS

Creating the evaluation list is a daunting task. The first challenge is identifying the important issues and features that you need. The second challenge is articulating a concise requirement that can be used to evaluate potential solutions. To gain some familiarity with the products, you should consider looking at a few products before you compile the evaluation list.

Compiling a list of important items is complicated by your reference point, the manual patient record and current workflows. It will dramatically effect what your practice will need in an EHR. Some questions to consider in compiling your list include:

- What are the specific clinical and treatment areas that the practice is active in?
- What are the specific subspecialty areas covered by the doctors in the practice?
- For primary care practices, which clinical conditions does the practice work in that would be considered outside of standard primary care area?
- What are the special aspects of the practice that need to be managed through the EHR?
- What information will be exchanged with patients over the Internet through the practice web portal?
- What are the supplemental services that the practice offers?
- How will the EHR be used at the front desk, clinical area, check-out and billing areas?
- What information is currently put in the paper chart?
- What supplemental information is kept outside of the patient chart?
- Where are the sources of patient information to be collected by the EHR?
- What are the testing, service and treatment orders tracked by the practice?
- What features are needed to properly serve patients?
- What information would improve the effectiveness of the PMS and administrative staff?
- Who accesses information from the paper chart and what information are they accessing?
- What are the supplemental logs, lists and diaries kept by doctors and staff to support clinical services?
- Where are copies of information from the patient chart kept? What are the copies used for?
- What is the expected patient flow with the EHR?
- What types of information and processes are involved in handing off patients among clinical staff?
- How will the EHR affect interactions with patients?

The evaluation list should highlight the issues that are important to you but not be so lengthy that you cannot practically handle or manage the list. For example, a list of hundreds of items will be difficult to evaluate and manage. Table 4.1 (see pages 56 through 76) itemizes the features that may be significant to your practice as well as the specific capabilities to look for in your evaluation. Review the table to compile an actual list in the next section.

TABLE 4.1 EVALUATION LIST

Feature	Significance	Look For
ARRA Support		
Certified EHR	Under the America Recovery and Reinvestment Act (ARRA), incentive payments are contingent on using a certified electronic healthcare record (EHR.) The definition of certified EHR was released at the end of 2009 and a certification process will be used to evaluate EHR products. **TIP:** Products that lack certification will be less desirable since any practice that is seeking ARRA Healthcare IT based payments will not be interested in products that are not certified. Therefore, uncertified products will be less competitive and may risk marketability.	Certification Representation from the Vendor to Meet the Current ARRA Certified EHR requirements. Plan for vendor to maintain the EHR to continue to qualify for EHR certification under ARRA.

Support ARRA Meaningful Use	ARRA Incentive Payments require use of a certified EHR and attaining meaningful use. Meaningful Use requirements currently consist of 25 aspects. However, the definition of meaningful use can change and evolve. Therefore, the vendor should be committed to supporting the current meaningful use standards as well as future extensions of meaningful use.	Features to Support:
		  Using computerized orders
		  Maintaining a Problem List
		  Checking Drug Formulary
		  Evaluating Drug Utilization Review
		  Using Electronic Prescriptions
		  Maintaining Medications and Allergies
		  Recording Vital Signs
		  Documenting Relevant Patient Demographic Information
		  Accept Lab Results into EHR
		  Report of Patients by Condition
		  Produce Reminders for Follow-Up
		  Document Progress Note
		Vendor commitment to supporting meaningful use

Basic Services		
Support	Vendors offer a varying array of support options. Some vendors offer standard working hours support with premium charges for off-hours support. Within three to six months of Go Live, your staff will probably know more about how the EHR system operates for your practice than your vendor. **TIP:** To get the most out of your vendor, consider establishing a designated support person or team that will be able to maintain "continuity of care" for your EHR.	Support hours meet practice working hours. Emergency support on demand. One-stop handling of hardware and software issues. The practice should be able to call a single support contact to coordinate hardware and software issues. Designated support staff for your practice to maintain continuity.

— *Continued*

Continued from previous page

Feature	Significance	Look For
	EHR vendors offer hardware support in a variety of forms. In most cases the support is coordinated with a third party support organization that the EHR vendor will contact to provide onsite support.	Specialty based support staff to address issues specific to your specialty. Annual user meetings and periodic seminars that allow you to meet other users to get ideas "from the field."
Documentation	The EHR system should be formally documented in paper and/or electronic help. Be certain that the EHR documentation is detailed enough to meet your needs. Thereby, you have a qualitative measure for any support or error issues you encounter. Note that some EHRs lack specific documentation and instructions. In some cases, the documentation consists of general information that does not contain sufficient detail to use the system. For example, the documentation may outline the screen flow but fail to explain whether the medication information is added to the patient medication list or a note is included in the E&M code calculation. **TIP:** Poor or deficient documentation may cause problems if you uncover a programming error since there may be a dispute about what the EHR does.	Clear and comprehensive documentation in electronic or paper form. Includes general directions, flow descriptions, and field-by-field explanations of EHR information. Specialty or area of medicine specific documentation that explains how the EHR works in you type of practice. Annotation notes that allows you to add practice specific instructions to the EHR documentation.
Upgrades	EHRs enhancements address evolving industry issues as well as generate new sales. New sales are needed to finance development and improvements. If new sales stop, then the vendor may start selling another product and not offer new features for your EHR system. Some vendors have specific plans and enhancement schedules, while other vendors do not release information on when the next release is or what will be in the release. **TIP:** Be wary of products that have new releases on a frequent basis. Frequent releases may indicate a new product that is still under development or has more serious structural problems. You should also be wary of vendors that have not released a new version within the past year. Lack of new versions may indicate a lack of research, development and investment in the EHR. Software releases can be costly for your practice. You may incur installation fees, disruption to operations for installation and database rebuilding, and additional training costs. The more organized the releases, the easier for you.	Review the history of software upgrades on a periodic basis (e.g., annual or semi-annually). Examine copies of release notes from recent releases. Look for enhancements and fixes. The lack of enhancements could indicate a product that is reaching the end of its marketing or support cycle. The lack of release notes may indicate a lack of planning or poor communications with EHR users. Review the release plans for the next version of the product. Note new features and look for indications that the product is making improvements and enhancements that will keep the product competitive and effective. Discuss the focus of new development by the vendor in areas of significance to your practice. Make sure that you focus on functional improvements as well as expansion of clinical content. For example, the next release may fulfill one of your evaluation list items.

— Continued

Continued from previous page

Feature	Significance	Look For
Backup Options	In addition to hardware and system backup, some EHRs are based on technologies that maintain a journal of all system activities. The backup journal may be used to update your previous backup to the point of system failure. Alternatively, the EHR technology base may support a backup hardware site. For example, the EHR vendor may send a file of the most recent updates to a remote Internet site every 30 minutes.	Maintains a backup journal of information posted to the EHR. The backup journal can be posted to update the last database backup and allow recovery to the point of the system failure. Allow for instantaneous transmission of all database activities to a backup system site. Access to a remote backup site in the event of a catastrophic loss of your system.
Security	EHR access should limit access, mobility or approval rights. Security issues are particularly important to an EHR since only an appropriate doctor or clinician can sign off on a chart note. As important, some chart notes require a physician signoff as well as a signoff from another party. **CAUTION:** Some EHR products do not differentiate between mid-level providers and doctors. If you have mid-level providers, you may need to have a separate signoff for the supervising doctor. EHR security controls will vary among practices based on size and workflow. Practices with large staffs and focused responsibilities require more specific security controls. For example, the clinical staff in the lab may be limited to lab order information and lab results entry. Smaller practices may not have a dedicated lab staff. EHR security should support compliance with HIPAA and allow you to establish access rights for groups of users. The EHR security should limit and control access to information as well as maintain the audit trails needed to monitor access issues (See Audit Trail).	A roles structure security model assigns access and entry rights by function (e.g., transcription, prescriptions, chart signing) by role or user class (doctor, nurse, technician). User roles can be defined to appropriately segment responsibility in the practice. For example, a large practice may allow a user to review a record, but not change the record. A smaller practice may not require specific controls. User roles can be supplemented at the user level. Additional capabilities can be added to a user profile and role-based permissions can be removed for a user. For example, new front desk staff may be limited to accessing only certain EHR features. Security controls access to clinical records by clinical-record area, entity, patient class and/or modality. Separate signoff authorities for mid-level providers and doctors. Supports automatic user signoff after a set-time period (e.g., 5 minutes-30 minutes). Requires user password changes within a set period of time (typically this occurs every 30-90 days). Allows users to quickly secure the screen from access, and facilitates returning to the previous EHR activity.
Practice Structure		
Entity	If your practice includes more than one legal entity, then you may be required by state and federal law to maintain separate medical records for each entity. For example, your practice and ASC may be separate legal entities that require separate medical records. Note that some states require separate medical records even for services that are provided by a single legal entity. For example, you may have to maintain a separate psychiatric file for a patient seen in a primary care practice.	Separate databases or database segmentation to keep information separate for each entity. For example, the EHR may be able to segment information by department (which could be the separate entity). An easy way for a user to switch among the entities.

— Continued

Continued from previous page

Feature	Significance	Look For
	Most EHR products are designed for a single entity. These EHR products require completely separate databases for multiple entities. Completely separate databases may prohibit sharing master file information and EHR setups as well as EHR information that is passed from one entity to another. For example, separate databases may complicate sending Evaluation and Treatment orders as well as progress reports between an orthopedic practice and the physical therapy center. **CAUTION:** Some EHR products suggest using an internal coding of the medical record to maintain separate charts. For example, ASC records start with "ASC", and clinical records start with "CLI." However, this strategy may prevent properly maintaining the medical record for each entity. For example, you may not be able to identify which items in the "clinical" record were also part of the ASC record and vice versa.	Tools to transfer medical record information from one entity to another. **CAUTION:** Some EHR interfaces pass "notes" that become notes in the receiving EHR database. However, these notes do not necessarily update prescriptions or procedure lists. Mechanisms to exchange setup information, master files and customization factors among entities.
Locations, Departments and Modalities	If the practice operates multiple operating units or locations, the practice may need EHR handling by locations and departments. Many EHR products focus on the doctor and not the location or department. For example, you can see the patient appointment status by doctor but not all appointments for several doctors in a pod or department (e.g., pediatrics, internal medicine) within a location. To verify the situation in a pod or department, the manager would have to separately access each doctor's appointment list. For larger practices this strategy would not provide management tools for the office or the practice. Some EHRs track patient office location in the appointment list and may allow the user to view all patients in a pod or department. Managers can track workflow by pod or department operating units. Tracking of locations and departments may be subject to the capabilities of the PMS appointment scheduler and/or the interface between the EHR and PMS. For example, a PMS schedule with the location in a comment would not be an effective reference point for an EHR that tracks locations.	Appointment list by specific location, as well as resource. Appointment list by a selected group of doctors defined by the user. For example, all doctors using a common pool of technicians and nurses. Appointment status includes a department and/or room indicator. Room and department indicators can be easily changed. Patient status and location are easily determined. Patient status codes can be customized for the practice and location. For example, a primary care practice may want a lab status while an orthopedic practice may want to flag a patient for x-ray. **CAUTION:** Some EHRs maintain a list of rooms and status for the entire practice and not for each location. For example, if you have 6 exam rooms in your largest location, you may define a list of 6 rooms, but the smaller location with 2 exam rooms will still see the selection of 6 rooms. Management tools coordinate patient workflow and clinical issues by location, department, doctor and user. Management tools can display combined lists of activities for a user defined group of doctors. EHR maintains user specific routing information for patients who may be passed among several doctors and staff in the course of a visit.

— Continued

Continued from previous page

Feature	Significance	Look For
Staff Collaboration	If your practice uses a collaborative patient service model, then the EHR needs to support and track the working relationship between the doctors, nurses and other staff. For example, patient intake may be performed by a nurse who passes the patient to a doctor and the doctor turns the patient over to another nurse for treatment. The EHR should allow doctors and staff to view the patient status and situation as well as interact on the patient's situation. Some EHRs limit those interactions and will hamper your ability to capitalize on the EHR. For example, some EHRs only support a single provider that is considered the source of all EHR information. Such products will not allow you to manage additional staff or allow retrospective review of clinical information entry. All clinical information is attributed to the doctor, regardless of the source.	Routing tools to transfer patients among doctors and staff. Forwards patient records and a note from the sending party to the next responsible provider. Indicates pending patient services to the selected staff and doctors. Supports and/or requires primary and secondary signoffs of a medical record. Audit trails indicate the source of information as well as the doctor who signed the note.
Ancillary Services	Physical Therapy Centers, Optical Shops, Coumadin Clinics, Urgent Care Clinics and Ambulatory Surgical Centers are examples of ancillary services. Ideally, practices should be able to offer patients more effective services through internal services and doctors should be able to more easily access patient service information. The EHR should allow the practice to simplify patient services and referrals to the ancillary service. The internal ancillary services should be more easily accessible and better coordinated than any outside service options. For example, the ancillary services staff should be able to access the relevant patient information and the doctor should be able to review patient status.	Accepts an order for ancillary services that will be performed by internal resources. Accepts service orders. Accepts and tracks status of services for current and future visits. Tracks service order items and associated patient information. Facilitates access to clinical information needed in the ancillary area. Facilitates access to the ancillary service information by doctors and others in the clinical area. Supports messaging and patient tracking between the clinical and ancillary service areas.
Diagnostic Services	Diagnostic services include radiology, lab, and imaging departments. Some specialties, such as ophthalmology, cardiology, plastic surgery and orthopedics may have extensive diagnostic imaging capabilities. Practices with diagnostic departments will need to manage the flow of patients and orders. The EHR should support order-entry assigned to the internal department as well as the routing of patients to the department. In some cases, the diagnostic equipment can receive the patient and order information directly from the EHR. Some diagnostic equipment will send information back to the EHR or provide the EHR with an reference identifier. The reference identifier may allow the EHR user to directly access the results on the diagnostic equipment.	Accepts and tracks diagnostic service orders. Diagnostic orders can be queued and tracked by department. Results can be posted to the EHR and tracked through the review by the provider. EHR can include diagnostic images in the patient's medical record. EHR can interface with the practice's diagnostic equipment. ***TIP:*** You should think ahead and buy diagnostic equipment that can interface with an EHR as soon as practical. You may want to include an interface option in the purchase.

— Continued

Continued from previous page

Feature	Significance	Look For
System Setup and Support		
Personal Digital Assistant (PDA)	PDA applications are used to provide a certain level of support to physicians outside of the office. The PDA offers a limited group of functions to capture information on patient services that can be uploaded to the EHR. PDAs may support charge entry, dictation, and prescription writing. PDAs may allow for brief notes and some order information. Typically, the PDA information is downloaded into a hold area for acceptance into the EHR. Some practices implement PDA applications and never move onto a full EHR implementation. *TIP:* PDA applications may be superseded by the ability to access the practice EHR through a wireless connection over the Internet. If so, physicians could access the complete medical record on demand. This option is becoming more practical as hospital wireless networks and other wireless options become available to doctors.	Records basic clinical information, including orders, prescriptions and a clinical note. Accommodates new patient information. Accepts dictation into the PDA for posting to the EHR transcription function.
Audit Information	The HIPAA Privacy and Security standards as well as your own tracking needs require appropriate EHR audit trails. Ideally, the EHR should maintain an audit trail of entry, edit, printing, and access activities. The adequacy of the EHR audit trails may also be determined by your practice organization and patient-service style. For example, practices that use physician extenders and have many staff members contributing information into the EHR. You may want to access the particular user who entered information even after the doctor has signed the note. Make sure you fully understand the audit trail that is part of the product. *CAUTION:* Some vendors have audit logs that are only accessible through system tools that are not part of the EHR application. Other EHRs only print an audit report. A number of EHR products track only the doctor who signs the chart note. Depending on your situation, you may need more accessible audit trails.	Record changes and additions are tagged with the user, date and time. Logs medical records access by patient and area/segment by user, date and time. Creates audit trails for the production and distribution of printed documents. Logs invalid security access attempts. Offers a print option to include the audit information in the patient note. Online access to audit logs with sorting and selection options for users, date, patients and information type. Includes audit log reports with user selection and sort options.
Practice Customization	EHRs offer varying levels of practice customization. Practice customization may include operational issues (e.g., Sequence of Templates), clinical content (Severity Levels), and selection options (Standard Medications). A number of EHR vendors support customization through specific programming for the practice and few "out-of-the-box" options. If your practice needs changes, the vendor will program the changes into your version of the system. Such accommodations are not the same as allowing you to select various options that are already built into the software.	Support customization of pick lists by the user. Allows for operational options selected by the practice including the order of information entry and clinical treatment standards. Allows the practice to flag clinical information that is required. Includes practice selected patient summary displays. Supports practice developed reports and documents that pull selected information from the patient EHR record.

— Continued

Continued from previous page

Feature	Significance	Look For
	CAUTION: Custom programming changes may have to be reprogrammed into future releases of the EHR. Make certain that you know how much it will cost you to keep your changes in the future. Practice-level customizations may allow you to establish EHR standards that can be further customized by users.	
Office/Location Customization	Practices with multiple offices may need to customize the EHR for the office or location. Location specific options may include patient status, rooms, task types, and procedures. **CAUTION:** Customization at the office level should be used with caution. Some office level customization could disable other EHR features. For example, office specific document types could complicate finding all radiology studies for a patient across the practice.	Supports office specific codes for patient status. Allows for office specific lists of rooms and services.
User Customization	Each user may have a different focus that should be reflected in his EHR views. For example, an intake nurse will want to see different information than a triage nurse. The surgery scheduler will need to see the list of procedures, while the billing clerk is primarily interested in dated chart notes. User customization includes information views as well as user specific pick lists for key information. For example, different providers may have specific lists of preferred medications. The user specific EHR view may be selected by the user, but many users will still need to access all EHR sections.	Maintains doctor specific codes for frequently used medications, procedures, orders by problem or diagnosis. Displays most frequently used information and templates for the user. Accepts user specific defaults for charting patient information. Facilitates quick identification of and access to templates and clinical information entry that the user most commonly uses. Allows user specific display of key patient information. Displays user specific workflow preferences (e.g., Display orders).
	Interfaces	
PMS Demographic Interface	The demographic interface between the PMS and EHR eliminates the duplicate entry of patient information between the two systems. **CAUTION:** The interface may be limited to PMS and EHR structural issues. For example, a single entity EHR may not be able to offer the flexibility needed for a multi-entity PMS. **CAUTION:** An EHR may not be able to deal with a practice that uses multiple billing systems. For example, a practice may have a separate billing system for the clinic and the ASC. Multiple billing systems could result in multiple patient records and a complicated interface. Significant differences may exist between the EHR and PMS demographic information. Key information including payer codes, patient class and billing type may use different coding structures and even have different effects on the two products. For example, the patient class may drive reports in the PMS but determine drug formularies in the EHR.	Insure that combined EHR and PMS products share the same demographic information. PMS demographic information should be posted to the EHR demographic file within a minute of posting to the PMS. Verify the ability of the EHR to translate key PMS demographic codes and data into comparable EHR structures. Key demographic information includes payers, patient types, and HIPAA Status.

— Continued

Continued from previous page

Feature	Significance	Look For
PMS Appointment Interface	EHRs use appointment information from the PMS to initiate and manage patient flow in the office. Once a patient is checked in, the practice will manage patient services through the EHR. Some PMS products include a basic tracking capability for appointments. These PMSs may allow the user to check the patient in, flag that the service starts, and check the patient out. **CAUTION:** The EHR may have a competing set of functionality. For example, the PMS may present the patient co-payment requirements at check-in, but the EHR presents outstanding health maintenance items. If the PMS is used to check-in the patient, the health maintenance screening may not be dealt with until the patient is seen. The doctor may not be able to service the patient since the basic health maintenance issue (e.g., blood test, diagnostic study) was not identified at patient check-in.	PMS appointment information should be posted to the EHR within a minute of the appointment entry in the PMS. PMS check-in information is posted from the PMS to the EHR. If check-in information is not posted from the PMS to the EHR, check-in desk staff may need direct access to the EHR. EHR appointment structures and codes can be mapped to the PMS appointment features. For example, the PMS appointment type and doctor codes may have to be translated into the relevant EHR codes to properly display the appointment in the EHR. **TIP:** Use of many appointment codes to accommodate individual doctors may affect the EHR. Ideally, you should standardize the appointment types in the PMS to simplify the patient flow tools in the EHR.
PMS Charge Interface	EHRs generate charges during the clinical process. EHRs may capture charge information as procedures are performed, as well as calculate the E&M code at the completion of the patient service. The transfer of charge information should be triggered by the approval of charges in the EHR. Once the charges are approved, the charges are sent through the interface from the EHR to the PMS. **TIP:** The formulation of charge information in the EHR does not leave a paper audit trail of the charges for the practice. The lack of a charge slip for EHR services has significant operational and audit implications for the practice. The specific audit procedures will depend on the EHR-to-PMS interface. For example, some PMS systems accept the EHR charges into a hold area that can be edited by the front desk before posting. Such strategies may require additional audit procedures.	Provides an E&M code calculator to accept information from the physician and calculate the level of service. Automatically calculates the E&M code based on the EHR charting process. Maintains an audit trail of the E&M code calculation. Accumulates procedure and testing information as the patient is served in the practice. Uses standard CPT and ICD9 codes to send the charges to the PMS. Includes modifier codes with the charge transactions. The charges are passed and posted to the PMS system in time to check the patient out of the office. Includes a daily charge report that can be used to verify PMS posting.
Lab Interface	To improve efficiency, and avoid problems, the EHR should have an electronic interface with your key reference labs, hospital labs, and/or lab information system. Some EHRs will interface directly with the lab equipment. Lab orders are entered in the EHR during the patient visit. Orders can be electronically transmitted to the appropriate lab system. Thereby, the doctor can view outstanding lab orders and status through the EHR.	Verify that the EHR can submit orders electronically to key reference labs (e.g., Labcorp, Quest Diagnostics) or in-house lab system (e.g., LabDaq or Orchard LIS.) Verify that the EHR can receive results electronically from your key reference labs and/or lab systems (e.g., LabDaq). Electronic results should be maintained in a hold status until the results have been reviewed.

— Continued

Continued from previous page

Feature	Significance	Look For
	Results are accepted from the reference or internal lab into the EHR. Results are saved to the patient chart for review. The EHR should track the review status of incoming lab results (e.g., pending, performed, received, reviewed, signed).	
Diagnostic Equipment Interfaces	As the repository for all chart information, the EHR should accommodate information and/or images from diagnostic equipment. Diagnostic equipment interfaces accept information directly from the equipment into the EHR. If the diagnostic equipment can generate an electronic record, then the information could be loaded into the EHR though an interface or saved as a standard image (e.g., pdf, bmp). Standard images can be saved as an EHR image. If the diagnostic equipment does not produce an electronic record, then the printout can be scanned into the EHR. The practice should insure new diagnostic equipment can be interfaced with the EHR. **TIP:** Any diagnostic equipment purchased by the practice should include an interface with the EHR. Additional interfaces with the EHR may require additional interface purchases from your EHR vendor. Some EHR vendors charge a set fee for each interface even for interfaces with equipment that has not been previously interfaced with their EHR. Other vendors charge a substantial amount of money for any new interfaces. Such interfaces could represent a substantial investment for the practice. **NOTE:** A number of EHR systems will store pointers to diagnostic images on your diagnostic equipment. The pointer is used to open the file using the diagnostic equipment's own software.	Compile a list of the current diagnostic equipment at the practice. Offers a variety of interface options including direct interfaces, and including a standard image file in the EHR record. Determine the availability of an interface between the practice's diagnostic equipment and the EHR. Develop an interface strategy for each type of diagnostic equipment.
Partner Interfaces	Some practices have electronic interfaces with a variety of business partners. Electronic interfaces could include downloads of information from a hospital, or other provider. For example, you may be able to download radiology reports from an imaging center. You may need to download results for a hospital lab.	Interface toolkit that simplifies and manages electronic exchanges of information including images. Offers a practical service to interface with other parties. Accepts downloaded clinical information for review and posting to the patient's EHR chart. Supports interoperability exchanges of data using standard transactions such as the continuity of care record.
Supports Interoperability of Patient Information	In addition to practice based EHRs, the healthcare system is developing mechanisms to exchange electronic information between practices and other healthcare providers. The facilities to support these exchanges are currently called Health Information Exchanges (HIE). HIEs can maintain a repository of information that can be accessed by all providers associated with an patient, and/or facilitate the exchange of information among healthcare organizations. Some exchanges act as a regional repository of shared information while other HIEs serve as the communications conduit between various systems. Practice based EHRs are the source of outgoing information and the destination of incoming information from HIEs. The key issue is buying a product that will be able to support the HIE initiative in your area.	Ability to create appropriate transactions and send the electronic information to an HIE. Support for incoming information from an HIE that includes holding the incoming information for review and the integration of the information into the practice's EHR. Produces and receives a Continuity of Care Record (CCR) and other healthcare transactions. Existing working relationships with Health Information Exchange (HIE) products in your area. If you have multiple entities in your practice, look for features that would allow your clinic to send information to the patient records in the other entities.

— Continued

Continued from previous page

Feature	Significance	Look For
HIPAA		
HIPAA Privacy Standards	HIPAA Privacy Standards address the handling and management of protected health information (PHI.) Practices are required to maintain information on the authority to use and disclose PHI. The EHR is the practice's repository for PHI. To guide practice staff, the EHR should control and track access to EHR information (See Security and Audit Trails). In addition to the consent form, the EHR should allow for highlighting and tracking any limitations as well as information on authorizations and disclosures. Disclosure tracking may include a log that the user fills out or an EHR audit trail. ***CAUTION:*** Some PMS products include basic information on consent forms. However, few of those products manage other aspects of HIPAA Privacy.	Maintains information on patient consent forms and status. Allows for limitations to be documented. Accepts a signed patient HIPAA consent or disclosure form that can be viewed through the EHR. Supports information on authorizations for disclosure of PHI. Accepts information on disclosures of patient medical information. The information may be manually entered by the user or electronically generated by the EHR. Maintains an audit log of printed and faxed information from the EHR. See Security and Audit Trails.

HIPAA Transactions	HIPAA Transactions include several standards that apply to an EHR:
	
	    Continuity of Care record includes key patient identification and problem information for patients that are being referred to another practice.
	
	    Additional Claim Information Transaction supports the exchange of clinical information, such as supporting documentation for claims or encounter reports to collaborating practices.
	
	    Service Review Transaction includes information on referral authorizations, pre-certifications and pre-authorizations.
	
	    Retail Drug Prescriptions could support exchanges with pharmacies.
	
	Although few clinical HIPAA transactions are being exchanged today, support for HIPAA Transactions and other EDI will become an increasing important EHR issue. At a minimum, the practice should understand the vendor's plan to support the EHR-related transactions.
		Produces and accepts Continuity of Care records containing key patient information.
		
		Generates Electronic Prescriptions from the EHR to a clearinghouse and participating retail pharmacies. ***TIP:*** Make sure that the electronic prescription service is connected to the key pharmacies in your area.
		
		Generates outgoing HIPAA Transaction Service Review referrals to payers.
		
		Posts incoming HIPAA Service Review referrals, pre-certifications and pre-authorizations to the EHR.
		
		Produces outgoing HIPAA Transaction Additional Claim Information for selected EHR information.

HIPAA Security Standards	HIPAA Security Standards allow for administrative, physical and technical safeguards for protected health information. Several HIPAA Security issues are addressed in the Security and Audit Trail Features.	Locks medical record to prevent any changes. Simplifies access and research of audit logs for access and updates to the EHR. Vendor offers a disaster recovery service.
Patient Information		
Patient Information Entry	Patient information entry accepts patient information directly into the EHR. The patient may enter the information through a Web Site, directly into a workstation (that has been secured from other EHR functions) or scanned in on a "bubble form." For Internet Entry, the patient is provided with a special code to enter information for posting to the EHR.	Includes patient specific signon facilities and passwords. Accepts initial HPI information through the Internet. Accepts Social and Family History through the Internet. Accepts Refill Requests through the Internet.

— Continued

Continued from previous page

Feature	Significance	Look For
	TIP: Patient interactions through a Web Site is gaining wider acceptance among patients. As important, interacting with patients through a patient portal is included in the ARRA Meaningful Use Goals. **CAUTION:** Some EHRs have a Web Portal for Messages, but the information is not accepted into the patient's electronic chart. For example, the Web Portal will create a message that a patient requests a refill for Celebrex, but the EHR user must find the prescription in the patient medical record to enter the refill. Additionally, the user must separately respond to the patient request. Other portals directly connect the refill request to the original prescription when the refill request is entered through the Web portal. **CAUTION:** Split vendor systems may pose problems for taking full advantage of patient interactions. For example, the patient would have to go to one portal to pay their bill and a second to submit a question for the doctor. Typically the doctor or nurse can review the information before the patient data is posted into the EHR. The doctor or nurse can correct and enhance the information as needed.	Supports Message Exchanges between Doctors and Patients. Identifies the information entered by the patient. Accepts information from the patient or another party (e.g., parent, guardian). Includes an indicator for the source. Information can be vetted and reviewed before posting to the EHR. After posting to the EHR, the actual source of the information can be viewed from the EHR.
Access Patients	The EHR will manage all patient interactions and services as well as act as a repository for your clinical information. A variety of options should be available to facilitate access to the patient by demographic information as well as access to the patients with a scheduled appointment or outstanding issues. Direct access to patient information from the list of appointments and/or tasks ensures the user is accessing the right patient information. EHRs that rely on an external email facility to manage patient issues and flow may not offer a direct connection to the electronic chart.	Accesses patients by name, medical record number, SSN, office and primary physician. Provides a list of patients based on appointment dates. Appointment lists can be viewed for date, location, provider and/or status. Presents list of patients with outstanding issues and to-do's. The EHR should facilitate access directly to the patient chart and/or document those who do. Tracks the status of current to-do's and maintains a repository of previous practice efforts and to-do's.
Patient-side Notes	The practice may need to highlight an issue that is not otherwise noted in the medical chart. The issue may be a continuing problem or a temporary issue associated with the patient visit (e.g., patient service issue). The EHR should allow for a patient alert to be maintained between patient visits, as well as a temporary issue that is only relevant for the current visit. For example, a patient who is discharged from the practice may get a special patient alert to indicate the discharge.	Establishes patient alerts that are displayed when a patient is accessed in the EHR. The alert can be customized for each patient. Supports a miscellaneous note on a non-clinical patient issue that is not saved in the patient chart.
Recalls	PMS systems support a basic recall capability. PMS systems may allow you to define a recall note and/or recall type that is entered with a recall date. Some PMS products also present the recall when an appointment is made. However, PMSs do not track whether the recall was actually fulfilled through a specific clinical action. EHRs may accept the patient return purpose and timeframe when entering the patient plan. However, this information is not commonly available in the PMS. In addition to the recall information, some EHR products maintain clinical treatment standards that are de facto recalls. The clinical standards in many respects are more powerful and useful than a recall.	Displays patients with recall instructions in the clinical plan according to user-selected parameters. Tracks completion of clinical recalls with appropriate clinical events. Generates general recalls for patients meeting a select clinical criteria based on diagnosis and specific findings. For example, a recall could be generated for all cataract patients without a visual field test in the past 12 months. Supports clinical standards that will be automatically assigned to a patient based on age, sex and conditions defined by the practice. For example, a cardiologist could establish an automatic EKG warning for all at-risk patients as well as patients older than a certain age.

— Continued

Continued from previous page

Feature	Significance	Look For
	For example, a clinical standard for a blood test in an EHR will only be fulfilled by the completion of a blood test. Non-EHR based recall systems do not typically track the completion of the recommended test or treatment.	
Clinical Chart Setup		
Clinical Content	Clinical content includes the specialty or primary care specific clinical information that is accommodated by the EHR. The clinical content that comes with the EHR may include a set knowledgebase of clinical findings, specific disease state templates and other clinical setups. Some products have a very specific clinical focus, while others offer a wide range of clinical content. For example, some EHR products focus on cardiology practices while several products are only sold to orthopedic practices. Note that the types of existing users will be a good indicator of the EHR clinical content. In the event that the EHR does not have clinical content for your treatment area, the vendor may offer to develop the clinical content or present the advantages of setting up your own clinical content. **Beware:** The setup effort may represent a substantial level of commitment. If you can find the clinical content you need, then you significantly mitigate the risk of failure.	Collect existing clinical forms. The practice should verify that the most common conditions are accounted for in the EHR clinical content. Itemize the various clinical areas and modalities that the practice will need covered in the EHR. **TIP:** Make sure that you include the specialties and sub-specialties that the practice works with to clearly define the clinical content. Review the EHR clinical content relevant to the practice. Ensure that the supporting clinical content includes documenting the clinical issues, access to additional clinical details and generating a relevant clinical report. **CAUTION:** You should not assume that your sub-specialty is covered if the vendor claims to cover the specialty area. For example, a product that has otolaryngology clinical content may not necessarily have audiology content.
Documentation Standards	EHRs can support the use of disease-based documentation standards. Documentation standards may be enforced through requiring entry of selected data and/or retrospective analysis of completed patient records. Documentation standards may also be managed with EHRs that calculate the E&M code from the data entered. If adequate information is not entered, then the code level will be affected. For example, the lack of a chief complaint could clearly be highlighted when the EHR calculates the E&M code.	Requires entry of selected information at the practice's option for selected conditions and templates. Reports on signed patient charts that do not meet the documentation standards.
Clinical Toolkit	Many EHR products include software tools to develop customized screens, lists, documents, or templates. The EHR toolkit allows the user to select the specific data items and entry options on the template. For example, the items to record a breathing problem could be selected by the user. EHR products that do not include a clinical toolkit may offer customized programming services.	Using a screen or template builder, the EHR clinical content can be customized by trained practice staff. Adding clinical findings to the knowledgebase by end users on demand. Document generator supports patient specific information into a letter produced by the EHR.

— *Continued*

Continued from previous page

Feature	Significance	Look For
	CAUTION: The vendor may reserve the right to make changes to improve the product and/or marketability of the EHR. Thereby, a serious practice issue may not be resolved if the resolution would not be applicable to a wider array of practices. Some EHR products are sold as is without customization tools. Even if you are pleased with the product now, it may be difficult to change the clinical content as you gain experience with the EHR and your practice changes.	Vendor demonstration on building a basic template or screen of information that you use in the practice. **CAUTION:** Insure that the template builder requires a level of technological competency that the practice can support. For example, some tools require little programming skill, while other toolkits are designed for use by a dedicated programmer.
Addendum and Amendments	Many practices are concerned with the permanence of a signed and un-editable EHR record. As a practical matter, the practice may need to revisit or amend the EHR record to account for test results or new information provided by the patient after the EHR note has been signed. The EHR should allow authorized users to amend the signed EHR note. The amendment may take the form of an additional note at the end or beginning of the note or changes that are actually entered within the clinical note. The previous information and changes should be clearly identified.	Addenda can be added to chart notes or existing notes can be annotated. Images can be annotated with a drawing tool. Changes to previous notes can be clearly identified. Maintains the content of the original note. Maintains information on original and subsequent contributors to the clinical note. Audit trail that differentiates the original document from the amended document.
Patient Summary Screen	The patient summary screen presents the key information needed for a patient. Summary information options include procedure lists, user preferences, outstanding tasks, image lists, encounter lists and chart note lists. Some EHR products have a static patient summary screen, and others allow the practice and/or user to select the summary contents. Patient summary options are useful since different practices may focus on different information. For example, a pediatrician may want to see immunizations while a surgeon immediately want to see the list of previous procedures. User specific summary options accommodate the clinical focus of various staff members and doctors. For example, the intake nurse may be interested in vitals and medications, while the surgical scheduling staff may focus on outstanding orders and the last visit note.	Verify summary screen includes key information on the current patient situation. Review the options for patient summary screen displays. Test the ability to navigate from the summary screen item to the relevant clinical item. For example, some EHR products force the user to access the prescription summary screen and then the individual prescription information instead of directly accessing the prescription record from the patient summary screen. Determine the sort and filter options for the patient summary information. Sort options may include date, item description and modality. Filter options may include selected dates and doctors. Verify the patient summary screen can be customized for users. The customization options should facilitate access to relevant information based on your practice staff. For example, a technician may need to see only the orders, vitals and current medications.
Clinical Charting		
Charting Patients	To minimize transcription and improve E&M coding, the EHR should be used to chart clinical records at the time of service. The look and feel of the EHR should be reviewed to ensure that the doctor and staff can easily navigate through the clinical content to chart the appropriate note. Ideally, a sample note from the practice should be used to test the charting process.	Practical screens to enter clinical data at the time of service. Support for WNL (within normal limits). Starting chart notes based on previous visits. Entry of structured chart notes using templates. Accepts as ad hoc notes and documentation.

— Continued

Continued from previous page

Feature	Significance	Look For
		Variety of documentation tools including templates, notes, drawing tools and reference materials. Allows for dictation into selected chart note sections.
Treatment Plans	Treatment plans are sequences of clinical services that are designed to address a specific condition. For example, a series of office visits and diagnostic tests over a 3-month period may be used for a patient with pneumonia. **NOTE**: Treatment plans and orders are included in the ARRA Meaningful Use Matrix. Treatment plans are patient specific. Most doctors will want to start off with a template for frequently encountered issues for the practice and modify the treatment plan for the patient's specific situation.	Accepts patient treatment data including procedure, performing provider and required date/delay period. Accepts a standard treatment plan that can be assigned to and customized for a patient. Treatment plans can be tracked by patient. Treatment plan items are separately managed for completion. Includes initial treatment plan setup for practice's area of medicine.
Clinical Protocols	Some EHRs manage treatment standards based on clinical protocols. The protocol can trigger treatment messages based on a variety of factors, including sex, diagnosis, risk factor, procedure and age. For example, a female patient older than 40 should have periodic pap smears and mammograms. The clinical protocols should be defined by the practice according to specialty and treatment standards. The clinical protocols should be verified with all patients who meet the protocol criteria, to catch issues that may not be triggered by treatment plans and recalls. Some EHR's will test the protocols on a periodic basis (Ex. Weekly) while other EHR products test the patient against the protocols on demand or when you access the patient's electronic chart.	Maintains practice specific treatment requirements based in diagnosis, age, sex, previous procedures and patient history. Tracks performance of treatment requirements by patient. Highlights clinical protocol issues for patients automatically. Reports on overdue clinical treatment protocols for all patients.
Transcription	A transcription facility with the EHR is important to most practices. In some cases, the scope of the EHR project is to make transcription available through the EHR. Other practices continue to offer a transcription option to doctors after other physicians are charting with the EHR. As a practical matter, you may continue to offer transcription for items that cannot be built in to the clinical content, such as extensive chief complaints and detailed analyses. The transcription facility should support tracking of the transcription process from dictation through distribution to outside parties. Some EHRs allow the user to insert voice dictation fragments into the EHR. The voice fragments are routed to transcription and inserted into the EHR chart note.	Accommodates a completely transcribed note or a brief insert into the clinical note. Accepts and tracks a voice (.wav or wave) file with the dictated note. Tracks status of transcription from entry to edit, approval and distribution. Identifies transcription without review by the doctor. Supports distribution of the transcribed document. Maintains a list of distributed documents. Accommodates working with a remote transcription service.
Image Storage	Every practice needs to store and track images, otherwise, a shadow paper file will be needed for non-electronic information (e.g., diagnostic images, ER reports, diagnostic reports).	Image classifications facilitate saving and locating images based on an image type and encounter date. Image description can be entered by the user.

— Continued

Continued from previous page

Feature	Significance	Look For
	EHR images may be stored with limited or extensive information. Some products merely assign an image type to the image. Other products allow for a free text description. A few products accept user specific indices that can vary by image type. For example, you could enter the hospital for a radiology image and the payer for a letter.	Practice specific indices (e.g., hospital, payer, study date) can be associated with the image description. Stamps each image with user, date and time. Images are listed in the several sort orders including by image type, date of service with other documents and user/doctor. Image status identifies images that are pending review by a doctor or other party.
Image Management Tools	EHRs will store images as they are received by the practice. Practices that scan the patient paper chart will store the original paper chart as an image group. The paper chart storage is a difficult challenge since paper charts were never designed to be scanned. The image management and annotation tools of the EHR will allow you to get the most out of your paper record images. Other images stored in the EHR include images from diagnostic equipment and incoming paper documents that are included in the patient's chart.	Image batch sorting tools allow reorganization of images. Image thumbnail viewer. Supports multiple image types including BMP, PDF, DICOM and digital camera images. Rotates images. Supports annotation of images with drawing tools. Pulls images out of one image file to save with updated annotations. Supports drawing on an image and saving the image with the annotations. Images can be printed within the associated clinical note
Clinical Drawing Tools	Many paper intake and clinical note forms include drawings of body parts and other illustrations to assist in documenting a patient's condition. For example. ophthalmology clinical forms include the right and left eyes. The user should be able to pick from artwork templates appropriate to the area of medicine. Specific and focused artwork should be available. For example, artwork for the bones and muscles could be separately offered. After selecting the artwork template, the user can use various drawing tools to document the patient's condition. In some cases, vendors offer specific drawing options for the area of medicine. For example, special drawing tools may be presented for various types of skin conditions for a dermatologist.	Clinical artwork for the area of medicine. Drawing tools to document information on the clinical artwork including shape and color options. Annotated clinical artwork is attached to the clinical note. Annotated clinical artwork can be printed on the patient encounter document.
Insurance Benefits Management	An EHR allows for entry and assignment of diagnostic and lab orders by the physician. However, some payers limit the studies that can be performed in a physician office. **CAUTION:** EHRs that include insurance coverage management are subject to the interface with the PMS.	Tracks insurance coverage limitations by payer. Notifies doctor on order entry of insurance coverage limitations. Supports ABN signature.

— Continued

Continued from previous page

Feature	Significance	Look For
Medication Entry	On patient intake, current patient medications are recorded. Current medication information may be incomplete or lack specifics. For example, the patient may not know the strength of the drug. EHRs should accept the information for other prescriptions at whatever level of detail is possible. **TIP:** The EHR should also accept the doctor and clearly differentiate between practice prescriptions and prescriptions from other practices. **CAUTION:** Some EHRs mix the patient medications list with the practice prescriptions. The mixing may impact the production of summary reports on prescriptions written.	Records information on medications from other providers with and without details. Accepts information on the prescribing physician. Medications are considered for drug interaction when new prescriptions are entered. Clearly differentiates between reported medications and prescriptions issued by the practice. Downloads prescriptions from a reporting service into the EHR prescriptions for a patient. The product should clearly differentiate between reported and prescribed medications.
Prescription	EHRs enable the production and documentation of prescriptions through a single process. Information entered as a prescription automatically is included in the clinical documentation. The same information is used to print, electronically transmit or fax a prescription. Typically, a preferred list of drugs can be maintained with the SIG, dosage and strength. The doctor can prescribe a drug from the doctor's preferred drug list, a list of drugs based on the patient's problem, or access the complete list of drugs from a third party drug database, such as MediSpan. In some cases, EHR vendors maintain their own drug database. Prescription information is stored in a separate table for each patient. Previous prescriptions can be accessed to record and manage refill requests from patients. Some systems support updating the original prescriptions. Other EHRs will generate a new prescription with a reference to the original script. In some cases, EHRs create an entirely new prescription without a reference to the original prescription. Reports can be produced to track prescribing patterns. Prescriptions written in the EHR may be subject to formularies by payer.	Accepts prescription information that is maintained in a list of patient prescriptions. Presents drugs based on disease state, provider favorites and/or frequently used drugs. Offers standard prescription orders for a doctor. Supports recording distribution of drug samples. Works with a drug database (e.g., MediSpan, First Data) that includes drug information. Highlights payer specific drug formularies. Considers allergy and disease interactions. Drug utilization review considers drug interactions. Submits prescriptions by fax. Supports electronic scripts (Ex. Surescripts.) Accepts and monitors refill requests. Discontinues prescriptions with a reason.
Lab	Lab orders entered in the EHR are used to document the patient plan as well as create a trackable order. Lab order information typically includes the lab test, current or future date and performing lab. Lab orders are tracked by the EHR through order, specimen capture, results receipt and results review. Incomplete, and/or overdue lab tests can be identified for follow-up. Operationally, the practice may need to check incoming lab results to ensure that all of the information is available for a patient visit.	Accepts lab orders including the date expected. Lab orders can be entered for a future date and periodic studies. Prints labels for specimens. Allows for tracking of labs performed by the practice as well as external reference labs. Tracks status of various lab steps: order, entry, draw, results and results reviewed. Highlights abnormal results. Supports electronic interfaces with reference labs or an in-house lab information system. Displays time series results in table and graph form.

— Continued

Continued from previous page

Feature	Significance	Look For
Procedure Orders	Procedure orders include the in-office procedures or procedures performed by others. The entry of the procedure is used to document the treatment plan as well as trigger service performance. The in-offices procedures may be performed by the doctor or other staff members. The procedure results will be documented in the EHR and included in the patient record. For future procedures, the EHR should facilitate tracking if the procedure is completed. The EHR should support locating incomplete procedures. ***TIP:*** Many EHR products assume that the procedures will be performed during the current visit. Make sure that the product can handle future activities without distorting the current visit note.	Accepts procedure orders for a current or future visit. Manages status for in-house and outside procedure orders including order entered, pending, scheduled, performed, and denied. Supports patient consent forms and signature directly into the EHR associated with the procedure order. Delegates the procedure to other staff and tracks procedure status and progress. Supports authorizations and consents for procedure orders. Includes documentation tools for procedures. Identifies outstanding procedures.
Diagnostic Studies	Diagnostic studies are currently recorded in the paper chart and supported with a written prescription. EHRs accept diagnostic studies as part of the plan for the visit. The entered study can be used to route the patient to the appropriate practice department or print a prescription. ***TIP***: Many EHRs assume that the study will be performed in your practice. If you refer patients to outside parties for studies, the EHR should differentiate between studies performed internally and externally. The EHR should track the status of the diagnostic study and support completion of the study upon review of the diagnostic results. The diagnostic results may consist of a message, incoming note or scanned image of a report. The EHR should track outstanding reports and practice staff should be able to easily identify diagnostic results needed for the next patient visit.	Accepts current or future diagnostic study orders. Tracks recurring diagnostic study orders. Prints prescriptions for diagnostic studies performed by other healthcare organizations. Manages status for in-house and outside diagnostic studies, including order entry, scheduled, performed, report received, report reviewed and report approved. Orders are tracked until fulfilled by the receipt, review and acceptance of the results. Supports authorizations for procedure orders.
Patient Education	Currently, preprinted patient education items are distributed to patients as needed. In some cases, the patient education items are bulk-printed documents from various organizations and, in other cases, the patient education is printed by the practice. EHR-based patient education materials can use a wide array and range of materials. In addition to computer-based content from a subscription service, you may be able to add practice developed materials and items from other sources. The EHR may support producing the education materials directly from the EHR and recording the distribution activity as part of the clinical record.	Includes a database of clinical patient education covering the practice's area of medicine. ***TIP:*** Make sure that you check the breadth and depth of the clinical content in light of practice services. Allows for practice developed patient education. Supports customization of patient education content for a specific patient situation or clinical condition. Documents distribution of patient education materials to a patient. Supports online patient education products and demonstrations.

— Continued

Continued from previous page

Feature	Significance	Look For
Surgery Scheduling	The surgery order and scheduling process involves co-ordinating clinical and administrative tasks for a patient. Surgery scheduling tasks include pre-surgery testing, medical release, consent forms, payer authorization, physician scheduling and facility coordination. Currently, practices use a form to track the surgery schedule status. Unfortunately, numerous clinical and administrative staff must compete for possession of the patient surgery scheduling information or keep their own copies of the surgery form. The surgery scheduling information is an important component of the EHR record. The list of surgery items and status should be maintained in the EHR. Then all of the staff involved with patient scheduling can track the status of each patient surgery through the EHR.	Accepts a procedure order with diagnosis for a future surgery. Includes a note area for doctor preferences and surgery details (Ex. Anesthesia, type of implants, etc.) Tracks user defined action items and issues to complete the surgery scheduling process. The action items can be customized for each patient, and include insurance, facility and clinical issues to support surgery scheduling. Surgery action items can vary by surgical procedure. Scheduling features support surgery scheduling, including appointment location, appointment note, appointment status (to flag completed surgery scheduling versus pending surgery scheduling efforts) and wait-list appointments. Supports patient consent forms and signature directly into the EHR associated with the surgical procedure.
Product Sales and Distribution	A number of practices may sell products to patients to support treatment and clinical services. For example, dermatologists may sell skin treatments, pediatric practices may sell lactation supplies and orthopedic practices may sell DME. The EHR should record the product as part of the treatment plan and manage the associated charge posting to the PMS.	Maintains a list of products sold by the practice. Records product sales in the EHR as part of the treatment plan. Passes relevant transactions for posting to the PMS. Includes reports to support inventory tracking and usage. Tracks inventory usage and levels.
Quality Reporting	PQRI and other quality reporting requirements are generated from clinical data. PQRI standards from Medicare include deterministic items as well as items that may require research. By capturing the quality reporting factors through the EHR, practices will be able to easily review the backup for the reporting items.	Supports entry of PQRI quality measures in the EHR. *TIP:* Some EHRs even select the appropriate PQRI measures based on the service and patient condition. Sends the quality reporting codes to the billing system with the charges. Offers reports that can be reviewed by the practice to monitor performance.
EHR Workflow		
Patient Flow Management	Patient flow management includes tracking the patient status and location. Typically, the user can maintain several pieces of data in the patient appointment list such as location, status and/or a comment. In some EHRs, the user sends the patient chart to the next user with a note or instruction.	Includes a list of scheduled appointments and patient status (e.g., arrived, roomed, in service, checked-out.) Doctors and staff can pass a patient to another party with a forwarding note.

— Continued

Continued from previous page

Feature	Significance	Look For
	Some EHR products do not adequately support the flow of patients in the office. In some cases, vendors suggest the use of a dummy paper chart for each patient in the office or a flag/light system for the office. Unfortunately, this strategy does not allow the practice to optimize operations or develop the management strategies available with computerized patient flow. For example, a paper "token" to manage patient flow will not keep management informed of any bottlenecks or delayed patients. An EHR workflow tool allows managers to view patient flow from another location or for all offices in the practice. Patient flow tools should include a location, department and practice-level views to allow managers to monitor patient flow and proactively address problems	Doctors can monitor status of their patients in the office. Records current status and location of a patient to facilitate patient services by doctors and staff. Maintains an audit trail of patient flow activities for management review. Presents management level views to monitor current practice patient flow.
Workflow Tools	An EHR informs the doctors and other clinicians on the wide range of patient issues and visit activities. The EHR must manage and support tasks and messages including patient messages, patient office movements and staff services. In a collaborative patient service environment, physicians and staff need to be able to check on the status of a particular patient as well as the status of a doctor's schedule. For example, patients queued for radiology services are important to the radiology department, the doctor who sent them and the PA awaiting the results and returning patient. Office managers may review real-time office status to manage patient flow and allocate resources.	Task management accepts information on patient specific and general items for users. Maintains information on patient status that can be viewed at the patient, department (e.g., lab, radiology, diagnostic testing) and doctor levels. Includes a manager function to monitor task status and performance. Displays overdue tasks. Supports performance tracking including tasks completion statistics, tasks by status category and time to complete tasks.
Task Management	A paperless office must manage the same avalanche of incoming issues and paperwork found in the paper-based physician office. Telephone messages, incoming results and documents and miscellaneous patient related queries must be recorded and tracked. An EHR is superior to paper-based messaging since the task is attached to the patient EHR chart upon entry. Some EHRs also maintain a direct connection to the appropriate document. For example, an incoming radiology study will be directly accessible. The message or task instantaneously appears on the user's workstation. When the user has a few moments between patients, the clinician or doctor can select the task; instantaneously access the patient EHR chart or incoming item. Tasks can dramatically cut the response time to patient inquiries and issues.	Supports task information including message, task type and priority. Assign tasks to a particular user or a group of users. Forwards tasks to other users or replies to the originator of the task. Allows for tasks to be completed at a future date. Monitors task priority and due date to inform appropriate parties and management.
Sign-Off	In many situations, other staff may enter information or serve patients that require physician signoff. For example, a PA may perform a post-op exam that is signed off by the physician.	Assign staff authority to enter notes but not sign the notes. Supports signing authority for different levels including doctors, and mid-level providers.

— Continued

Continued from previous page

Feature	Significance	Look For
	The sign-off capability enables the use of triage strategies and mid-level clinicians. The appropriate staff treats the patient and the medical record is automatically forwarded to the doctor. The EHR enhances patient service and supports the use of physician extenders. *CAUTION:* Some EHR products do not differentiate between the signing of a chart by a doctor or a mid-level provider. *TIP:* Some EHRs combine the signing authority with the audit trail. In these cases, the signer is assumed to be the source for the entire note.	Presents unsigned notes for sign-off by designated doctor or supervisor. Displays unsigned note list for doctors and practice management.
EHR Analysis Tools		
EHR Reporting	Discrete EHR data is a specific finding or data item that is accessible to a reporting program. For example, a temperature data item with a value of 100 can be reported if you select all temperatures higher than 99 degrees. However, a note that says "patient temperature is 100" may not necessarily be found with certainty. *TIP:* Searching for discrete information within text is not as accurate as seeking specific data items. A reporting feature should allow for generating detail or summary reports for patients meeting a user-defined selection and sort criteria.	Supports graphing of flow sheet information. Custom reporting of patients based on selected clinical data including patient summary data and chart details. Presents active patient list screens to access relevant patient records. Offers flow sheet option for selected clinical data. Generates lists of selected patients in user defined sort and grouping orders. Produces statistical reports based on user selection criteria and reporting formats. For example, total prescriptions by drug for a selected date range.
Quality of Care Factors	The EHR should provide tools to track, manage, and analyze the clinical information. Forms and knowledgebase EHRs may maintain specific information on patient conditions and services. To capitalize on the information, the EHR should provide tools to analyze and check the clinical records.	Requires documentation standards for clinical conditions. For example, the EHR allows the users to require entry of vitals for primary care visits. Supports clinical documentation surveys to determine clinical records that may not meet compliance and/or treatment standards. For example, a list of patients on Coumadin without a blood test during the office visit could be produced. Supports statistical surveys of patients who meet a specific clinical condition and services panel.
Collections Support	The practice must supply clinical records in support of claims on a frequent basis. Payers may require documentation for certain E&M codes as well as procedures and other selected services. In the absence of a paper chart, the insurance collections staff will need access to the clinical record. The EHR should support quicker access to the clinical information needed to support claims.	Supports read-only access to selected EHR information. Easily creates clinical note with patient identifying information for claim justification. Allows information to be directly faxed from the EHR to the payer with a cover note. Maintains a log of faxed information and destinations.

— Continued

Feature	Significance	Look For
Clinical Reporting	In the absence of a paper chart, all outgoing reports are produced from the EHR. The EHR collects a large amount of discrete information on a patient visit, but outgoing documents may include only a limited or selected amount of clinical information.	Clinical reports can be generated with selected information or all information according to a user option. Clinical reports include information from the clinical note as well as prescription, order and other EHR information. Allows information to be directly faxed from the EHR to the selected party with a cover note. Maintains a log of faxed information and destinations.
Letter Writer	Using discrete data, the EHR can generate letters with selected information. For example, the practice could design a letter with information plug-ins that report on a particular aspect of patient care or that it's time to make another visit. *TIP:* Some EHRs pull the entire clinical note into a word processor for editing. The user would edit the letter, and then save the letter in the EHR as a separate document. However, letter editing can lead to inconsistent presentation and incorrect information (e.g., deleting a critical word.)	Includes a self contained letter generator based on clinical information. Maintains an audit trail of distributed letters and the letter contents.

PRACTICE AREA SPECIFIC EVALUATION CRITERIA

In addition to general requirements for an EHR and the specific clinical content needed by your practice, you should also consider features that are specific to your specialty or practice area. Table 4.2 (see page 77) presents some of these features.

CREATING THE EVALUATION LIST

The evaluation list should consider the factors and issues described in the preceding sections. You should create a specific list that includes the nuances of your practice as well as general EHR requirements. For example, you need to insure that the EHR includes clinical content for your specific clinical services and area. A primary care practice with cardiology and OB/GYN specialists will not be satisfied with general internal medicine clinical content.

The Evaluation List is used to record the feature analysis of the EHR product. The analysis may consist of the following columns:

Feature—Features itemize the specific requirements for the practice.

> *TIP*: Strive to be as specific and concise as possible. The features should be structured to evaluate all of the selected products. Be careful about

TABLE 4.2 PRACTICE AREA SPECIFIC EVALUATION CRITERIA

Practice Area	Features to Look For
Allergy	Accommodates allergy testing. Supports serum formulation and tracking. Quickly documents allergy shots. Tracks shot treatment programs.
Cardiology	Tracks device use by patient. Supports stress tests. Manages Nuclear Camera Studies. Accommodates Cath Lab. Includes Coumadin Clinic Management.
Dermatology	Manages and Tracks Biopsy Results. Supports Product Sales. Documents in-office procedures. Accommodates Anesticians.
Gastroenterology	Stores colonoscopy results. Manages long term recall for screening colonoscopies.
Endocrinology	Supports specialized growth charts.
Internal Medicine	Includes sufficient clinical content for doctors in selected specialty areas. Supports sick patient visits. Tracks compliance with well patient services. Manages outgoing referrals.
Neurology	Interfaces with EEG testing equipment.
OB/GYN	Tracks prenatal care trends. Tracks pregnancy progress. Supports mammography results. Manages tracking patients with abnormal pap smears.
Oncology	Manages Chemotherapy Regimens. Tracks Inventory and Treatment Preparation. Supports Administration of Treatment.
Ophthalmology	Interacts with Optical Product Sales. Coordinates with Optical Lab Work. Supports Contact Lens Sales and Fulfillment. Accommodates ASC Services. Interfaces with Diagnostic Equipment.
Orthopaedics	Interfaces with a PACS system. Tracks Evaluation and Treat Orders. Accommodates ASC Services. Supports Physical Therapy Services. Supports Occupational Therapy. Tracks DME.
Otolaryngology	Manages working with Audiologists. Supports Audiograms. Supports Hearing Aide Sales. Manages Hearing Aide Service.
Pediatrics	Handles Sick and Well Child Conditions. Easy handles ad hoc "family" add ons for a patient visit. Maintains Immunization Information. Supports Lactation Counseling. Tracks Immunization Standards. Includes Growth Charts.
Radiology	Interfaces with a PACS system.

using terminology or features that will tilt the evaluation toward a specific product. Consider the following feature composition suggestions:

Simplify the Requirement—You should balance the need to keep the number of evaluation features manageable with your need to practically score the item. A focused feature will have a limited number of measurable aspects. For example, a feature that states "supports medications from other providers, sample drug distribution and refills" will be difficult to review and score. The feature could be split into 3 different items and include more details about each of the three aspects.

Avoid the Trivial—Many requirement lists include items that every product needs to have, and are basic requirements. Trivial items create a lot of work, may obscure the product differences and inflate scores. For example, a patient name, and address may not be as significant as the ability to annotate a clinical image.

Eliminate Common Standards—Although few products do everything, you should minimize the commonly available features that are included in virtually every product. For example, the existence of diagnosis, procedure, provider and patient files are common standards for EHRs. These items are needed to support other features.

Articulate the Practice Need—The features should clearly identify the practice needs and not include items that are not relevant. For example, one practice has the doctors performing all patient services without physician extenders. A simpler workflow feature should be used. If a practice has a very specific workflow requirement, it should include the specific workflow item in its feature's list.

Include Required Components—The feature may include the specific manner in which you want to handle an item. For example, a practice with some new diagnostic equipment may include specific interfaces with the specific vendor equipment in the feature list.

Minimize Specific Design—The features should avoid specific design issues and strategies, unless the design is a feature requirement. For example, you may require customized templates without dictating the tools to support the templates.

Evaluation—The evaluation assigns a feature score for the reviewed product. The scoring scale can be based on any system you are comfortable with. You could use words (e.g., None, Poor, Fair, Good, Excellent), characters (A, B, C, D, E), or numbers (1–10). However, you should be careful to use a scale that can be easily used and summarized. Steer away from a finely graduated scale. For example, a score with 15 different gradients may have such fine differences, that the scoring and interpretation will be difficult to determine. Summarization is best done with a numeric scale. Indeed, practices that use non-numeric scales frequently convert the scales to numeric values to arrive at a total score. An easy scale to measure the capability of a product follows:

0—Does Not Support the Feature—The EHR does not have the feature you desire. If the vendor currently lacks the feature but is releasing the feature in the next release, you should still award a '0,' but note the coming enhancement in a comment.

1—Does Not Fully Support the Feature—The EHR partially provides the feature but is missing a significant component. In many cases, the partial fulfillment is based on a workaround in the EHR. However, you should be certain that the workaround is practical and actually useful.

2—Fully Supports the Feature—The EHR fulfils the feature in a straightforward manner. If there are any questions on the feature, review the handling and capabilities again.

3—Exceeds the Feature in a Meaningful Way—The EHR product contains an additional capability that enhances the EHR in light of the practice's needs. The evaluation should not include an enhancement that is not significant to the practice. The additional capability should be documented in a comment.

Importance—Importance prioritizes the features in your evaluation. Although each feature may be significant, some features will be more important than others. For example, the interface with a specific PMS product may not be important to the practice, if you are not happy with the current PMS. Importance can be assigned any scale you wish subject to the scoring issues for the evaluation. A scale to consider follows:

4—Critical Requirement—The lack of the feature would prevent the practice from meeting its EHR goals. For example, the lack of a workflow feature would undermine the usefulness of an EHR in a collaborative practice. Practices that have a unique workflow style may require features that support the current workflow.

3—Important Requirement—The feature is needed to achieve operational efficiency. For example, the inability to track incoming patient appointments may require PMS system appointment management by clinical employees.

2—Nice to Have—The feature would help the practice but is not a key requirement. For example, some specialty practices may not need clinical recall features.

1—Optional Requirement—The feature is not necessary for the practice to use the system. For example, the interface with the PMS for charge entry may not be as significant for practices that have complex coding and modifier posting issues.

Comments—After spending a significant effort evaluating products, most people find it difficult to recall the specific capabilities of the product. To preserve key information from you review, consider recording a brief note for each feature. The note should indicate the key reason for the evaluation score. For example, you may include a note with a "0" evaluation that the vendor promised the feature would be in a future released. A comment for a "1" evaluation may state that outside providers are not entered in the medications' list. A "2" evaluation comment may state the workaround used to meet the requirement. A "3" score may be accompanied with a note that the EHR product is the companion product to the current PMS.

The following table presents a template for your own Evaluation List. Below it is an example of an evaluation list. *Caution*: This example should serve only as a starting point for you to develop your own evaluation list, not as your complete list. There will be specifics about your practice that should be taken into consideration in modifying this list.

TABLE 4.3

Feature	Evaluation	Importance	Comment

TABLE 4.4

EHR REQUIREMENTS	Evaluation	Importance	COMMENT
General Technology and Business Issues			
1. Support - Vendor should offer a full range of support services including hardware, software, and training.			
2. Certified EHR - Product has been certified under the ARRA Healthcare IT program.			
3. Meaningful Use - Features support the meaningful use of standards to qualify for Stimulus Payments.			
4. Ease of Use - Product should be easy to use and easily accommodate the needs of individual users.			
5. Audit Controls - Maintains adequate audit trails and allows access to the audit trails.			
6. Security - Access is controlled at the system and user level.			
a. Security can be based on user-defined groups of users.			
b. Access can be restricted at the functional level (i.e., prescriptions).			
7. Privacy Standards - Existing Features Support HIPAA Privacy Requirements.			
8. Security Standards - Existing Features Support HIPAA Security Requirements.			
EHR Patient Access			
7. Interfaces with Practice Management System (PMS) - The EHR accepts demographic and patient scheduling information from the PMS.			
8. Access Options - Patients can be accessed by Account Number, Patient Name, and Chart Number.			
9. Schedule Access - Patients can be accessed through a list of patients who have checked into the office. The access list tracks the patient from check-in to check-out.			
Clinical Records			
10. Images - Stores images and scanned correspondence for reference.			
11. Practice Specific Records – Practice specific screens with clinical information can be established and maintained.			
12. Content - Clinical forms, images, and content supports clinical practice areas.			
13. Patient Summary Screen - Key patient information is displayed in a user definable screen to highlight clinical issues and needs.			
14. Patient Questionnaires - Accepts information from patient questionnaires into the medical record.			

— Continued

Continued from previous page

EHR REQUIREMENTS	Evaluation	Importance	COMMENT
15. Transcription Tracking - Tracks transcription from entry to approval and distribution.			
16. Prescriptions - Accepts patient prescriptions and monitors refill activities.			
a. Accommodates prescriptions from the practice and other doctors used by the patient.			
b. Records drug samples.			
c. Tracks refills.			
d. Includes online information for drugs and dosages.			
e. Supports online formularies by insurance company.			
f. Maintains preferred drugs based on physician and/or diagnosis.			
g. Tracks interactions.			
h. Supports electronic, faxed, and printed prescriptions.			
17. Lab			
a. Exchanges Orders and Results with Reference Labs.			
b. Manages the status of lab orders.			
c. Accepts and tracks results from the lab. Supports alarms and/or flags for critical values.			
d. Supports flow sheet views of lab tests.			
18. Procedure Orders			
a. Tracks Procedure Orders.			
b. Prints Procedure Order for Outside Provider.			
c. Prints patient information on preparing for the procedure.			
d. Manages the status of a procedure order.			
19. Diagnostic Study Requisitions			
a. Tracks requisitions for diagnostic studies by practice departments and other providers.			
b. Prints Order for Outside Provider.			
c. Manages the status of diagnostic requisitions.			

— Continued

Continued from previous page

EHR REQUIREMENTS	Evaluation	Importance	COMMENT
d. Stores diagnostic images.			
e. Electronically interfaces with diagnostic equipment.			
20. Patient Education			
a. Prints patient information from a handout library or customized items.			
b. Maintains a log of distributed information in the patient's medical record.			
Workflow Support			
21. Office Flow - Records the progress of a patient or issue (i.e., refill request, lab results).			
a. Supports dated "to do" lists with future ticklers.			
b. Patients can be transferred between doctors, clinical staff and clinical units.			
c. Supports Physician Sign-off of Medical Records from services provided by mid-level staff.			
d. Addenda and notes can be added to patient records.			
22. Facilitate User Activities - Includes features that help users identify pending tasks and patient service items.			
a. User desktop helps manage patient service items (Ex. Messages, Reports)			
b. User desktop manages patients in the office.			
23. Charge Transfer - Charges can be transferred from the EHR to PMS.			
Management Reports			
24. Graphs - Graphing tool allows trend and comparison graphing of clinical information.			
25. Clinical Based Patient Searches - Supports searching for patients matching treatment and/or diagnosis.			
26. Report Writer - Users can define custom reports by selected content, records, and sort criteria. Information queries can be based on demographic and clinical information.			
Letter Writer			
27. User Letters - Clinical information can be merged into a user-defined letter.			
28. Log and Image – Sending logs and images of letters sent are maintained by the system.			

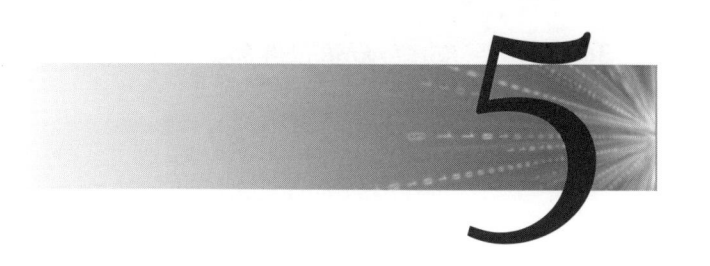

EHR and Malpractice Risk

According to the publicity, EHR adoption triggered by the Stimulus Package will improve patient care, cut healthcare costs and mitigate malpractice risk. Unfortunately, cutting malpractice risk is not just a matter of using an EHR. You also must protect your practice from risks that are inherent in the move to and use of EHRs.

In fact, EHRs present a variety of new malpractice risks that we do not have today as well as exposes our organizations to malpractice issues that are a direct result of how we adopt and deploy EHRs. Indeed, each step in the use of an EHR must be taken with an eye towards the strategies and processes that will yield better operations and control our malpractice risk. Keys areas that could increase your risks included:

Selection—Surprisingly, the product selected can affect malpractice risk. Not all EHR products are the same or have the same capabilities. For example, some EHR products lack the workflow tools that are needed to keep track of patient service issues and problems. If you select an inappropriate EHR, you may have to make compromises or workarounds that undermine your services. For example, an ineffective order entry feature may necessitate tracking future tests in a message that is not part of the patient's clinical record. In the event of a malpractice challenge, you may be hard pressed to prove your efforts to manage the standard of care or be challenged on the disconnect between service messages and the patient record contents (which does not include the message.) Indeed, you may not be able to determine the status of a particular care recommendation since the order is in the EHR patient medical record, while the follow-up details are in the messaging items which, in that particular EHR, are not part of the patient record.

EHR Customizations—Many EHR products are based on customized components or modules that are used according to your specific needs. The custom programming may create significant differences or problems with that same "product" used by other healthcare organizations. For example, your customized clinical standards may have a problem calculating the patient return date for a periodic check on a patient hip replacement or a chronic condition. In the event of a problem, your practice could be held accountable for not meeting the standard of care that you thought was programmed into the EHR.

Product Design—EHRs have a variety of product design aspects that can affect malpractice risk. The entry, reporting and storage of information that is the basis of every EHR product must be considered as you design your strategy to analyze and use EHRs. For example, EHRs dramatically differ in how amendments to a patient record are recorded. In a paper chart, you may record, sign and date a supplemental note that may result from additional patient information, a test result or a wide range of issues. Depending on the EHR product, an amendment may consist of a note at the bottom of the original encounter note, as a new note with a different date, as a supplemental note that is not connected or referenced in the original encounter note, or any number of other ways. In a malpractice case, you may have difficulty explaining how your staff and doctors knew where to look for the most current patient information or whether they were aware of important subsequent information.

Data Conversion—Regardless of what a practice plans to do with the current paper records, an EHR requires information that will enable the EHR to properly process and manage the patient. For example, immunization schedules will generate unnecessary EHR warnings if you have not entered a patient's immunization history. Similarly, if you have not recorded the fact that a patient had cataract surgery, the EHR will not be able to automatically warn your practice that a patient is due for an annual check. In the event of a malpractice claim, you need to be able to prove that the lack of access to the paper chart information did not impact patient care and that the EHR based patient chart correctly reflected the patient's condition. In the transition from the paper chart to the EHR, the practice needs to assure and maintain the continuity of care information.

Usage—Adopting and deploying an EHR requires redesigning virtually every process and interaction in the practice. In order to succeed, the practice must have the governance and management structure that will facilitate the various transitions that are the foundation for a successful EHR effort. Unfortunately, many organizations have implemented only part of an EHR or use the product differently within the practice. For example, a physician practice only uses the messaging module of the EHR while using the paper record for all other patient information. In the event of an error, a practice would be hard pressed to prove that providers and staff had access to the complete patient situation since the messages were not integrated within the paper record, and medical issues were being addressed outside of the paper record which contains specific information on the patient condition and history. When EHRs are used in an inconsistent basis, standard EHR tools may be misleading or confusing. For example, some EHR products only allow for one set of vitals per visit. If additional vitals were recorded elsewhere in the record, the other vital information would not appear on the EHR patient summary sheet. During malpractice discovery, key patient information that is not consistently and appropriately displayed in the EHR could open the door to challenges of the efficacy of information and whether the patient condition was properly presented.

The adoption of EHR systems in your practice will necessitate a dramatic change to the way you work in your practice and interact with patients. However, you need to methodically approach each step of the selection and implementation process to insure that your understand the appropriate way to use the EHR to serve your patients and improve your practice as well as mitigate the possibility of a clinical or service lapse.

Keys to EMR/EHR Success is full of strategies, processes and directions to guide your efforts to use EHRs and avoid increasing malpractice risk. However, there are a wide range of risks that you need to be aware of and mitigation strategies that will protect your organization from encountering a problem. The table at the end of this chapter itemizes these challenges in detail and presents strategies to help take advantage of EHRs to improve clinical services while lowering your risk profile.

EHRs can help address a number of the patient service and operational risk issues faced by medical practices. However, failure to methodically select, implement, and use EHRs can lead to additional malpractice risk. The following table identifies some of the risk factors associated with the use of EHRs by physician practices. A mitigation strategy is presented for each issue. Thereby, the practice can insure that the use of an EHR produces effective results, improves patient service, and cuts the risk of encountering problems.

TABLE 5.1

Factor	Description	Issue	Mitigation Strategy
Selection Issues			
Incorrect Practice Selection	Practices may select an EHR that does not offer all of the features and capabilities needed by the practice. Practices need to insure that they purchase an EHR with appropriate workflow, patient service, and clinical content features. The specific needs of the practice are affected by practice size, number of locations, patient service style, area of medicine, services provided, and a wide range of other factors.	If a practice does not select an appropriate EHR product, it may resort to inappropriate workarounds that could affect the accuracy of the patient record and patient safety. For example, a system without appropriate health maintenance items for the specialty could miss key treatment requirements such as diabetic A1C tests.	Verify that the selected product addresses the clinical, workflow and management needs of the practice. (See Chapter 6 on Selecting an EHR)
EHR Selected by Another Party	Some practices are implementing EHR systems that are selected by other organizations for reasons that are not focused on the practice and patient safety. For example, a hospital or PHO may choose an EHR that is offered or, in some cases, forced on the practices. In some cases, practices are deferring EHR selection and implementation to their billing services which may have to consider other clients and issues in the EHR strategy.	Not all EHRs have the same capabilities and features. An EHR product may be chosen by a hospital in order to facilitate exchanges of information with doctors, but the underlying information and structure may not be appropriate for the practice setting. For example, some EHRs lack workflow tools that may be needed by the physician practice, but are not an issue for the hospital sponsor. Similarly, continuity of care tools such as health maintenance items and long term treatment plans may not be important to a hospital focused on episode of care issues.	EHR options from hospitals or other parties may be considered with other product options. However, the practice is responsible for picking and using a tool that meets the practice's needs. If there are problems with the offered product, consider documenting the issue and seek resolution through the EHR sponsor. If a solution cannot be found, then the offered product may not be the best EHR for the practice.
Product Design Issue Examples Note: A wide range of product design issues can affect the risk factors associated with EHRs. The following examples are some of the potential EHR issues.			
Maintaining Entity Specific Patient Records	Each separate entity is required to maintain its own medical record. Some practices consist of separate legal entities for the clinic, and ancillary services. For example, some orthopedic practices maintain a separate entity for physical therapy or an MRI machine. Ophthalmology practices may have an optical shop in	EHR products have two general strategies for dealing with multiple entities: Separate Databases for Each Entity—Many EHRs require a separate database with separate clinical information for each entity. In cases where information is shared among the entities, the information must be separately transmitted or entered. For example, you may have to print the report from the ASC to be scanned into the clinic's EHR.	If the organization has multiple entities, make sure that the EHR will maintain a separate patient record by entity. The vendor should document the strategy and you should verify your ability to access the appropriate patient record for each entity. Note that

Continued

Continued from previous page

Factor	Description	Issue	Mitigation Strategy
	a separate entity. In some states, an ASC within a practice must maintain a separate medical record.	However, such a process could lead to incomplete processes since the report may be classified as not reviewed in the clinic when the doctor reviewed the report in the ASC. Source Entity within a Database—A number of EHR products accommodate multiple entities within a database by tagging each item with a source entity. However, tagging each item with the source is not the same as identifying the patient's medical record for an entity. For example, the procedure report for the patient may be sourced from the ASC, but the report is also part of the patient's clinic record. Similarly, the original justification for surgery may be sourced from the clinic, but is also part of the ASC's patient record. In these cases, the entity may have to select the items that will be included in their patient record, but lack the audit trail of care activities taken on behalf of the patient.	you should document the multiple entity issue and feature in your contract.
Document Creation	The final documentation generated by an EHR may be subject to a variety of translations and other changes. For example, some EHR products have a document creation module that can create different documents from the same clinical data. These documents are created based on a separate script that may formulate information, label information differently from the underlying EHR information, and/or compile a statement based on analysis of several pieces of information.	Since many EHRs produce documents of selected information through a programmable document feature, the scripts that generate the documents could transform the same information on different reports in different ways. For example, a clinical finding could be described according to a set text fragment that is included in the EHR, or, through programming, be transformed to a completely different text. Indeed, a prescription drug name could be translated into a generic drug class. The lack of consistency in presentation and the translations completed by the document creation could create a situation where the medical record in the EHR differs from the documents distributed to the patients and other parties.	You practice should verify the clinical content and the resulting documentation as part of your implementation process (See Chapter 10—Implementing an EHR.) Any future changes to the creation of documentation should be similarly tested and verified by the practice.
Document Creation Scripts	Many EHRs use documentation scripts that are can be modified over time. Changes could be needed to refine the text, adjust data, or allow for additional options. However, EHRs do not keep time sensitive information on the changes to the program. For example, it may not be possible to recreate the exact same document from the underlying clinical visit information at a future date.	Different clinical documents for the same clinical condition may confuse clinical staff and patients as well as undermine the ability of the practice to establish, maintain, and prove the standard of care provided to patients with a particular problem. The underlying clinical data that is used to produce the document may be amended or modified without forcing document recreation. For example, the physician may become aware of additional information that warrants an amendment to the clinical information, but the generated document is not updated. Thereby, anyone who accesses or distributes the document will be accessing the clinical information before the amendment.	A practice should strive to limit the presentation and documentation variables. In the absence of a clinical issue, a common documentation base should be used. If the EHR product does not trigger new document creation when information changes, a procedure should be established to identify dated documents and coordinate updates to the documents as well as redistribution to appropriate parties.

Continued

Continued from previous page

Factor	Description	Issue	Mitigation Strategy
Document Retention	EHR products widely vary in how clinical documents are generated, handled, and saved. Some EHR products merge data with a word processing product, while other products have a document generator. A number of EHRs directly produce the document.	Some EHR products require the user to save a copy of the document, or the document as it was sent will not be available in the EHR. This strategy is particularly serious since some document generation strategies allow for last minute editing of the document. Interestingly, many of these vendors suggest that the user can merely regenerate the document, while the regenerated document could be based on a different set of data or even a change to the document generation process.	Users should be trained to always save the document to the medical record. A verification procedure should be established to make sure that outgoing documents are also in the EHR, and/or that a document has been saved for each office visit.
Programmable Clinical Content	A number of EHR products are based on programmable clinical content that may be maintained by the practice and/or the vendor. The programmable clinical content can change the data contents, presentation and usage. For example, some EHR products allow change to programs that calculate clinical measures and recommended treatment plans. Some vendors sell clinical content that is customized for the practice.	Changes to clinical content must be carefully designed, effectively programmed, and thoroughly tested before patient care is charted in the EHR. Otherwise, the changes may not effectively operate, or even collaterally damage the existing data in the patient's EHR record. For example, relabeling a screen field could result in the mislabeling of historic information and invalidate document generation scripts. Additionally, changes to clinical content programs could create continuity of care issues in the patient record. For example, a single labeled field that is split into two fields could create unintended changes in the health maintenance standards that use the modified labeled fields. Note that changes to the clinical content can also cause diversion from the standard clinical content provided by the EHR vendor. In these cases, the practice may have to retrofit the new clinical content into their customized clinical content or reinstall their changes into the new release of clinical content.	Any and all changes should be verified and tested using a formal and structured clinical verification process (See Chapter 10 on Implementation.) Future changes to clinical content as well as new clinical content released by the vendor should be similarly tested and verified by the practice.
Image Management	Many EHR products do not store the actual images within the EHR database. The EHR product stores a pointer to a file that is managed outside of the EHR database. For example, the EHR may reference a file name in a directory that is used to store EHR images.	The image pointers are not verified with the file. As important, few EHR products maintain links to confirm that the file pointer references the correct contents. For example, files could be switched in the system and the information would be attached to the wrong patient. Similarly, files could be corrupted or deleted without detection until a user tries to access one of the missing files. Indeed, thousands of image files could disappear without anyone noticing the loss. The lack of integrity and error checking in the image files could expose the practice to loss of information that documents care and patient status.	Establish a backup retention strategy to mitigate the chance that images could be lost. The strategy includes keeping more periodic backups (Ex. Weekly backups for 4 weeks) and checking on the number of files in the image directories on a periodic basis. For example, you may verify that the number of files in closed image directories does not change before rotating a weekly backup out of the stored versions.

Continued

Continued from previous page

Factor	Description	Issue	Mitigation Strategy
Reported Medication Entry	Many EHR products do not directly indicate reported prescriptions. For example, some vendors suggest using a note in the patient's record or a dummy doctor name. Ideally, the EHR should accept the name of the prescribing doctor and a clear indication that the prescription is reported.	If the practice does not record reported prescriptions in the EHR, then the drug utilization analysis will not be based on all drug information. If the practice records reported prescriptions in a manner that obscures the source of the prescription, it may be difficult to determine that the practice has not prescribed the drug and a refill could be issued for the reported drug.	The practice should establish a clear and consistent procedure to insure that reported medications are properly indicated if the EHR does not explicitly indicate reported medications. Additionally, all staff and doctors should be completely trained to verify that a prescription was prescribed by the practice before issuing refills.
Third Party Applications	Many EHRs have relationships with other products to fill in application gaps or extend the product. For example, some products do not have a complete prescription program and rely on a third party drug prescription product such as NewCrop.	Third party programs can create treatment risks since the split information may undermine basic functionality. For example, a chemotherapy program sends regimen treatment reports to an EHR, but the EHR does not have the detailed orders contained in the chemotherapy program.	The practice should work with the vendors to create a proper interface that correctly and completely records information in the patient EHR record. If a proper interface cannot be designed, then the practice should consider more appropriate EHR options.
Order Management	Orders are the plan items recommended by the doctor to maintain or improve patient health. Lab tests, radiology studies, physical therapy and surgeries are examples of orders. Orders represent the key instructions for the patient to follow and are a significant factor in the ARRA Meaningful Use standard. Many EHR products accept order items for the current visit, but not order items for a future time. Other EHR products only accept orders for practice services, but not orders for third party providers. In some cases, the EHR product will help the doctor create a note containing the order, but require a second step to create a task to track the order.	Orders are typically recorded in the patient chart to document, but not to manage care. The PQRI requirements and ARRA Meaningful Use standards require physicians to manage and monitor patient orders. Thereby, the physician will be in a position to reinforce patient wellness and care. The key issue is the extent to which physicians will be held accountable for communicating and managing patient wellness. For example, an order for a radiology study may be a significant care issue for a patient that must be monitored by the practice.	The ability to record future orders and orders performed by other parties is a key requirement for most practices. The practice should discuss the problem with the vendor and arrive at a practical solution before the implementation of the EHR. Otherwise, the practice should consider other product options.
Amendments	Many EHRs do not allow for amending the patient records to record relevant patient information. Other EHRs accommodate amendments in a manner that undermines the patient record. For example, some EHR products require creation of a completely new note that starts off with the contents of the signed note to be amended. A user	The nature of the amended note should be clearly visible to the clinician. Otherwise, the amended information will not be properly used and could lead to a clinical error. For example, some amended notes only allow for a text note at the bottom of the patient record. If the user operates off of the initial information, they may miss an	Doctors and staff should be carefully trained on the procedure to amend a record as well as the way to identify such a record. Amended records may require each user to enter additional information to highlight the changes to an amended document in an EHR that does not adequately track such changes.

Continued

Continued from previous page

Factor	Description	Issue	Mitigation Strategy
	could easily reference the original note instead of the amended information.	important amendment. In other cases, the user cannot determine that the note has been amended at all. Indeed, the original contents of the note cannot be differentiated from the new note in a number of EHRs.	
Record Keeping Limitations	Some EHR products limit the number of values or readings. For example, some EHR products only allow one set of vitals per visit. Similarly, readings for blood sugar levels (BSL) may be limited to two or three readings per day.	Depending on the area of medicine and services, a practice may need to record numerous readings in the course of patient treatment and service. If the user runs out of locations for information, then the additional information may be recorded in another area of the patient record that is not contextually connected to related readings. For example, the third BSL reading may be entered in a message since the EHR only accommodates two BSL readings. A review of standard EHR patient record may not clearly indicate that other readings exist and computerized searches of patients meeting specific criteria will not consider the third BSL reading.	Any recording of information outside of the standard information structure poses a wide range of patient care and reporting problems. In addition to working with the vendor to address the issue, any workaround should include a clear way to indicate that additional information was recorded outside of the standard data structure. For example, the user may enter a free text note at the beginning of the section that additional information is located in a note.
Record and Document Status	Some EHRs do not maintain discrete information on the status of a clinical document or image. For example, some EHRs assume scanned images have been reviewed and accepted into the patient record. A more effective approach is to allow the practice to set a status that can indicate whether the image has been reviewed and accepted by the practice.	The lack of status for each document does not adequately support the workflow and medical records management needs of a practice. For example, management cannot identify those records that have been actually reviewed by a doctor and those records that remain outstanding. As important, tracking the flow and nature of a document without a status is not reliably managed by the EHR.	The practice should document the status of every document in the patient record. Options may include using tasks to document image status, or notes in the document summary screen. The practice should be careful to insure that the method results in a reliable and auditable trail.
Contract Issues			
EHR Termination	Many EHR contracts identify a variety of termination triggers that expose the practice to the possibility of immediate loss of access to the EHR records. In many cases, vendors can notify the practice of termination of the EHR license without providing adequate notification to allow the practice to move to another EHR product.	According to the HIPAA Security standards, a practice has to maintain a contingency plan for events that could result in loss of access to the EHR records. Any loss of access to the EHR records could compromise patient safety and significantly disrupt practice operations. Any problem that could be traced to the occurrence of such a loss and the lack of a contingency plan could compromise the position of the practice.	Contract terms that limit access or could result in termination should be eliminated. The contract should include an exit strategy that allows for adequate time to convert to another EHR and requires the vendor to support the conversion effort. The termination trigger and exit strategy should allow sufficient time to make the transition as well as allow access to the old EHR for as long as necessary.

Continued

Continued from previous page

Factor	Description	Issue	Mitigation Strategy
Tail Issues	When a practice is closing, the practice may be responsible for continuing maintenance of the patient medical records under state and federal laws.	The computer hardware and software may require continuing investments to maintain access to the patient data. For example, the practice may have to maintain the EHR records according to the retention requirements through upgrades by the vendor to the software as well as transitions to new technologies and hardware. Throughout the retention period, the practice would have to pay for these upgrades even though no new information is being entered. Otherwise, vendors will not take responsibility for supporting the product and addressing access problems the practice may encounter.	The EHR contract should allow for an access only option to accommodate tail issues at a minimal cost to the practice.
Implementation Issues			
EHR Setup Options Driven by Other Parties	In some cases, other parties are setting and establishing health maintenance items and treatment strategies. For example, some software vendors establish treatment options based on their interpretation of the best practices strategy. In other cases, a hospital or PHO sponsor is establishing treatment protocols that will be required for use by all practices using the EHR.	Treatment and documentation protocols established by other parties do not allow the practice to customize strategies for the appropriate standard of care considering the practice's patient base. For example, the practice may choose to use a more stringent recall cycle due to the nature of the patient population.	The practice is responsible for managing patient care and its own standards based on clinical conditions. The practice is ultimately responsible for protocols, treatment plans, documentation and the use of the EHR. The contract for the EHR as well as the implementation strategy should not cede this right to any other party.
Use of Clinical Content	Clinical content is developed by EHR vendors to support areas of medicine. However, many practices use clinical content without an analysis and acceptance process. In essence, the practice is accepting the documentation standard established by the EHR vendor. For example, the clinical content of some EHR vendors include recommended drug, and treatment steps for the patient. The practice that uses these recommendations without a formal acceptance process, could be considered to not exercise due care in the use of protocols that the EHR vendor has provided.	The physician practice is responsible for the accuracy and representation of conditions and treatments recorded in the EHR. If the practice is using an EHR, the practice needs to verify that the documentation tools and standards are clinically appropriate and within the practice guidelines. For example, some EHRs purport to create an appropriate level of service note for the patient's condition. However, if the doctors do not verify the appropriateness of the documents and the setup tools, the use of the EHR will increase the risk that a treatment plan not supported by the doctors could be assigned. Similarly, a patient condition could be incorrectly documented and classified.	The practice should verify and accept the EHR clinical content. This process should fully engage physicians and insure that the practice fully understands how patient services are recorded as well as the documents that are produced from that process. See Chapter 10—Implementing an EHR.

Continued

Continued from previous page

Factor	Description	Issue	Mitigation Strategy
Incomplete Implementation	The EHR has been partially implemented and patient medical record information is split between the paper record and the EHR. For example, a practice may use the EHR for messages, a web service for prescriptions, and a paper record to store documents and transcription.	Split records can lead to confusion and continuity problems. In many cases, the lack of a single place for patient information can undermine continuity of care issues and context of patient problems. For example, a doctor may prescribe a drug that conflicts with other drugs that the patient may be taking since the doctor is working off of the paper record and does not have access to the web based prescriptions.	The rollout and use of the EHR for all doctors and staff is a key strategy to avoid risks associated with incomplete implementation. The practice must commit to the EHR strategy and insure that the implementation plan is comprehensive and complete. See Chapter 10—EHR Implementation.
Data Conversion Issues			
Incomplete Data Conversion—Loading Data	EHR systems need patient specific information to operate properly. In many cases, practices are not analyzing the information needed to initially describe a patient to the EHR. For example, key conditions, treatment and historical information is needed to flag the patient for health maintenance items or trend analysis in an EHR.	When a practice does not load essential historical information into the EHR, the EHR may provide incorrect warnings or advisories to physicians. For example, missing immunization information may result in warnings that patients require immunizations according to treatment protocols and could result in misleading compliance reports. A missing diagnosis could prevent the system from warning the doctor that a patient is due for treatment.	The loading of patient information is a clinical decision that should be analyzed and decided by and for the practice. The practice needs to define the information that is needed to properly set up the patient in the EHR and then develop a procedure to accurately and effectively enter the information. See Chapter 10—EHR Implementation
Incomplete Data Conversion—Paper Records	The disposition of paper records after an EHR is implemented could expose the practice to record retention compliance issues. Unfortunately, many practices do not fully understand the record retention compliance requirements. For example, many malpractice attorneys recommend retention of patient medical records for 10 years after the last time the patient is seen. For pediatric patients, some attorneys recommend that the record be kept for 10 years after the last visit, or 1 year after the patient is 18 years old whichever is later. A key detail is that the clock resets for the entire patient record each time the patient is seen.	Many practices believe that the paper record will not be needed after a certain number of years on the EHR. However, the retention requirement is specific to the patient and not easily tracked in the paper record once the EHR is in use. The disposition of the paper record and insuring continued access to the patient record on an as needed basis could result in a compliance violation or a treatment problem. For example, the doctor may treat a patient with a birth defect or serious condition that predates the EHR. Lacking access to the original documentation in the EHR, treatment decisions may be delayed or inhibited by lack of access to the patient's complete record. The inability to get access to the historic paper record could lead to unnecessary risk and compromise patient safety. On the compliance front, the practice may be violating the HIPAA and state requirements if they cannot produce the complete patient record which includes EHR and paper components.	The disposition of the patient paper records should be carefully and completely analyzed in light of the clinical and compliance issues. The final decision should result in consistent and reliable handling of the patient paper record while maintaining the patient medical record to meet care and retention requirements. Failure to seriously review all options (including scanning some or all paper chart information) may limit access to key patient information or present a view of information out of context to the patient's situation. See Chapter 10—EHR Implementation

Continued

Continued from previous page

Factor	Description	Issue	Mitigation Strategy
Conversion of Patient Information from one EHR to another EHR.	Each EHR product is based on a data structure and design that, in many cases, significantly differs from the structure of other EHR products. These differences could result in translations and transformations to record the old EHR information in the new EHR. Such translations could change or distort the meaning of the original EHR record. Additionally, the new EHR may have different features and structures.	When practices are moving from one EHR to another, the data conversion design may undermine or distort the information being converted from the current EHR and may not appear in the new EHR the same as if the patient information had been entered in the EHR. For example, an old EHR attached notes to scanned images while the new EHR did not connect the notes to the scanned images. The converted notes were not associated with the underlying images in the conversion strategy proposed by the vendor. Additional collateral damage to the integrity of the EHR included tagging contents as if the items had been reviewed by the physicians when they were not reviewed.	Conversion of electronic information from one EHR to another product is a difficult task. The portability of such information should be part of the analysis of EHR options and the conversion strategy decided before agreeing to purchase a product. The strategy and costs should be documented in the contract. As important, the practice needs to verify the conversion of each class of information (Ex. Prescriptions, notes, images) in a test conversion as well as before accepting the converted data for use in the new EHR. See Chapter 10—EHR Implementation.
Usage Issues			
Documenting Expected but not Performed.	Some EHR products offer documentation that is based on a standard strategy (i.e., Bright Futures.) The template note is then modified by the doctor and clinical staff to focus on the patient situation. Unfortunately, the documentation may not accurately describe the specific services that were provided to the patient. For example, the analysis of the patient problem may not require reviewing a system that already has results recorded in the standard note.	Presenting a note that documents services that were not provided could have serious risks and implications. For example, a patient could develop a problem in an area that is extensively covered in the standard note, but was not reviewed by the doctor since the patient's situation did not warrant further examination. In some cases, generated notes could misrepresent the patient's situation and condition. These misrepresentations could be sent to other providers and be included in a patient record in community health information systems and other clinical repositories.	The key to avoiding problems is to fully understand how to document patient services and the documentation produced by the EHR. The practice should have a formal process to review, validate and accept the clinical content initially as well as conduct similar reviews for future releases and changes. See Chapter 10—Implementing an EHR.
Documentation of Patient Visits	EHR products may have a number of different options to document various aspects of a patient visit. For example, some systems consider messages part of the patient record, while other systems do not consider messages part of the patient record. If a doctor records significant clinical information in an	All staff and doctors must understand and use the documentation strategy that has been designed by the practice. Otherwise, significant patient information could be missing from patient and practice analysis. For example, a prescription refill that is entered in a patient message will not update the prescription records or be included in survey reports.	The practice should decide how and when information should be recorded in the EHR. User and doctor training should focus on the standard way of documenting information and establish the expectations for documentation quality and timeliness. Procedures and review strategies

Continued

Continued from previous page

Factor	Description	Issue	Mitigation Strategy
	EHR message that is not part of the patient record, the information will not be presented when a user accesses the patient medical record. For example, a doctor may note an important clinical issue on a message, but not include the information in the clinical notes of the EHR. A search of the medical record contents will not include the message for many EHRs.		should be established to verify compliance and maintain consistent use of the EHR.
Inconsistent Use	Frequently, EHR systems are not consistently used in a practice. Inconsistent usage may be a result of allowing various doctors and staff to use the system according to their own desires, or failing to completely roll out the EHR. Indeed, many practices lack a practice focused standard governing the use of the EHR.	If doctors and staff are not using the system on a consistent basis, then information may recorded incorrectly or not at all. More importantly, other users may assume that the patient information is correct and complete, when in fact information is not accurately represented. For example, most EHR products allow information to be recorded once and used many times. A physician order for an MRI to be done in six months will be displayed in the original exam note, on the patient face sheet as an outstanding order and on a list of incomplete orders for all patients. However, if a doctor or staff person were to record the MRI order as a note within the exam note, the order will not be displayed on the patient face sheet or on the list of incomplete orders. Other users may justifiably assume that the patient has no outstanding orders since none appear on the EHR face sheet. Such an assumption could delay or bypass important patient care issues.	Reporting tools should be used to verify appropriate use. Deviations should be analyzed to help users meet expectations and maintain a reliable patient chart. Otherwise, the practice will not be able to rely on the accuracy or appropriateness of information for reporting or analysis. More importantly, EHR features that rely on specific information to flag situations and present information will not be reliable.
Documentation Options	EHR products may not directly document all of the relevant patient service information. In many cases, the physicians and staff resort to work around strategies which can have unintended effects on the patient record. For example, some EHRs cannot document patient orders that are not performed by the practice	In the absence of features that deal with all aspects of medical services, practices will resort to using shadow paper charts or try to document the information in another area of the EHR. For example, some EHR systems include medications and prescription lists without proper handling of issued and reported prescriptions (from another doctor.) Thereby, the practice could accidentally refill a prescription which was never prescribed by the practice. Additionally, practice analysis of prescription drugs would not be able to focus on those prescriptions from the practice.	Any documentation deficiencies should be discussed with the vendor before the EHR purchase. Ideally, the problem should be fixed before the product is implemented. In the case where a problem cannot be addressed, a formal and consistent strategy to address the problem should be designed and implemented for the practice. Such workarounds may require audit procedure to verify compliance and proper use.

Continued

Continued from previous page

Factor	Description	Issue	Mitigation Strategy
Loss of Service	EHRs are based on components that may fail as well as be affected by problems with electricity, communications, the environment and software problems. In the event of a loss of the EHR, the practice may continue to see and serve patients. Indeed, every practice should have a fall back plan to continue operations during the EHR outage. Of course, the practice can invest in backup and fail safe technologies that mitigate the chance of such an outage.	Many practices do not have an organized plan to deal with the loss of an EHR. As important, when the EHR is restored, the practice needs a formal procedure to update the patient records for activities that occurred during the outage. Updating the EHR insures that the various patient tracking and service features will be accurate and current. For example, prescriptions issued during the outage should be entered into the EHR as well as treatment plans provided to patients. Otherwise, patient care issues may not be properly managed by the EHR. For example, an incomplete medications list could lead to a prescription problem. In most cases, the recovery effort should document the entire patient visit in the EHR to properly maintain the patient record. Unfortunately, many practices will scan the paper documents used to record patient visits during the outage which does not properly maintain the EHR information, standards, or treatment plans. In these cases, the patient record would not properly display the result and changes that would typically be recorded for the patient visit. For example, an outstanding order would still be outstanding even though the patient visit during the outage fulfilled the plan item. Similarly, new plan items identified during the patient visit would not appear on the patient order list.	The practice should have a procedure to continue operations without the EHR at any time. This procedure should be verified on a periodic basis. However, the practice should also periodically review the EHR to identify evolving problems and vulnerabilities on a continuing basis. The practice should review strategies to address vulnerabilities and implement cost effective solutions to potential problems. The practice should maintain a written recovery plan to guide recovery efforts in the event or a loss of service.
Support Issues			
Loss of EHR Support	Most EHR contracts allow the vendor to stop supporting the EHR with a notification period of thirty to ninety days. Interestingly, many EHR contracts allow the practice to similarly terminate support. However, the right to support termination by a practice has limited use, since the practice has the obligation to maintain the patient's medical record	Due to market forces or other issues beyond the control of the practice, the vendor may stop supporting the product. Alternatively, the practice is at risk of the business failure of the software vendor. In the event of a suspension or termination of support, the practice is at risk of not being able to access any of their records. As important, the practice may not have a practical way to transfer patient records on the EHR to another EHR or even paper.	The contract should include adequate notification of support changes as well as an appropriate exit strategy. See Chapter 9—Negotiating a Contract.

Continued

Continued from previous page

Factor	Description	Issue	Mitigation Strategy
Inadequate Backup of Information	As the primary repository of patient clinical information, the practice has an obligation to maintain current backups of the EHR data to support recovery of the clinical information in the event of a catastrophic failure of the computer system, or access problems to the location of the EHR computer.	Many practices do not maintain appropriate backups of their EHR data that could support recovery of the EHR system. In some cases, practices do not maintain offsite backups of EHR data. Other practices do not have a full backup of their information to support recovery. In the event of a system failure, the practice could lose substantial amounts of information. Many practices think that they are properly backed up but in fact are not. For example, some practices have accumulated more information than can be accommodated by their backup facilities. In other cases, the EHR backup is failing, but no one is checking on the successful completion of the backup strategy.	Backup procedures should be reviewed and verified on a periodic basis. Additionally, test recovery of backed up information should be undertaken every year.

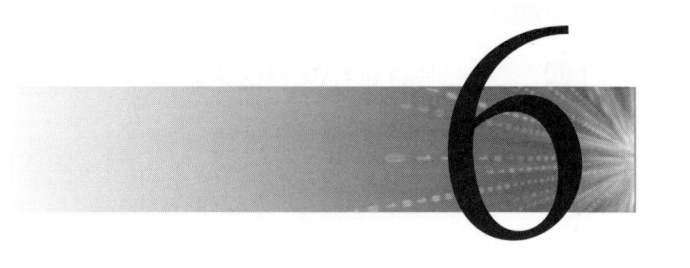

Selecting Products to Review

With more than 400 EHR products and a steady stream of new EHR offerings, the options present a daunting task for the average practice. In some cities, you may have dozens of EHR vendors competing for your business. Some practices spend years looking at systems and options without making a decision. Many practices look at a wide range of products and cannot differentiate between the products reviewed. In many cases, you find an exhausted staff with little to show for their effort.

Before selecting products to review, you need to consider several initial filtering strategies to cut the number of EHRs and focus your effort. Much like any other product, a particular EHR product will not satisfy every practice. Some EHR products are focused on a specific specialty or on primary care. Other EHR products are designed for practices where the doctor independently serves the patient. A number of EHR products are appropriate for a practice based on size alone.

IDENTIFYING CANDIDATES

Once you have decided to explore an EHR, you will be quickly inundated with materials and sales people for a variety of EHR products. In larger cities, you will encounter dozens of options. Indeed, you will be contacted by a host of new vendors as you proceed through the selection process. Your current PMS vendor as well as perspective PMS vendors will be soliciting your business. The current PMS vendor will seek to capitalize on their existing relationship with your practice, and prospective PMS vendors will be seeking to get on the short list to serve all of your technology needs.

Identifying potential candidates should be a fairly open process to insure you will consider products that are of interest to your staff and doctors. In essence, you are trying to identify viable products as well as preemptively address questions that will surely arise as you proceed in your decision making process. When you come across a vendor, you should catalog the vendor name and briefly evaluate the appropriateness of the product for the practice. In many cases, you will be able to quickly eliminate the product. However, you should document the rational for the decision to not seriously consider the product.

You will not necessarily take a detailed view of all the products, but include the products in your list of EHRs that your could look at. In general, you will come up with 8 to 15 different products that people in your practice, local, or specialty area are talking about. You can gather potential solutions from the following sources:

Systems of Interest to the Doctors and Key Staff—Practice staff and doctors are an excellent source of information on potential EHRs. EHRs are a hot topic among practices and healthcare industry professionals. Doctors and staff members may have seen one or two products that piqued their interest. You should account for the products that are being discussed by your physicians and employees. If you account for these systems, and fairly consider potential options, you may be able to avoid "buyer's remorse" after you make your decision. Presenting thoughtful reasons for not reviewing a product will instill confidence in the process and gain credibility for your final decision.

Colleagues in Your Area—Local practices are good sources of information on EHR vendors. Local practices can help you identify EHR products sold in your area, as well as the support capabilities of the vendors. You will probably encounter a local EHR vendor with a limited install base that is used by a local contact. **TIP:** Make sure the local vendor has a viable product before you consider the EHR for your practice. For example, the product should be used in a practice that is of similar size and/or services. Many such initiatives are still in the development stage and may require your advice to develop and your expertise to test the capabilities of the EHR.

Colleagues in Your Specialty—Other practices in you specialty area can help identify products that were sold to organizations in your specialty. Be especially careful to verify the specific subspecialties and services that the other practice provides as well as their ancillary offerings.

Colleagues in Practices of Similar Size—Similar size practices can help you identify the types of products that are used in practices of your complexity and volume. For example, a practice with more than one legal entity will need a more sophisticated EHR selection and setup. Similarly, a multi-office practice has a number of coordination and management issues that are not issues for practices with a single location.

Systems Supported by Hospitals—A number of hospitals are offering EHR products to their medical practices who work at the hospital.

CAUTION: These initiatives vary widely from buyer discounts to an entire EHR system controlled and managed by the hospital. In some cases, you control your EHR and in others, the hospital makes decisions for your practice. In any case, you want to check into these options. In the event that you buy into an EHR solution that is controlled and managed by the hospital, make sure that you have a clearly defined exit strategy in the event that the hospital leaves the EHR business at a future date, or your practice changes. Looking back on the problems some practices encountered when some hospitals shut down their MSO organizations, an EHR exit strategy is prudent and necessary to protect your practice and your patients.

TIP: Practices that have relationships with more than one hospital should carefully evaluate the implications of following one particular strategy. Indeed, some practices are being torn between the conflicting and differing product offerings. **CAUTION**: Do not try to use more than one EHR product for your practice. Such an approach may make your hospitals happy, but undermine your practice operations and services.

TIP: In any event, you should make sure that you end up with an effective solution for your situation regardless of the preferences of the hospital(s.)

Systems Supported by Key Partners—Some local associations or regional healthcare networks may use or endorse an EHR vendor. Be careful to fully consider the product situation in your analysis. For example, some groups may back a particular EHR to encourage adoption among their members to improve their physician networks. In other situations, you may find out that a referral fee is being paid for your business.

CAUTION: Some physician networks are requiring use of a particular product as a condition of participation. Note the conflicting problems discussed about hospitals apply to other practice relationships.

But before you go too far with whatever a key partner may be using, quiz the partner on these two elements:

Selection Process—You may discuss the EHR selection process and how they chose the product. The other products considered and their final decision will help you refine your process and focus. For example, they may have eliminated a product for an issue that does not apply to you such as the influence of a closely related healthcare organization. In other cases, they may have bought a system for a reason that is irrelevant to your practice.

EHR Status—In some cases, practices may be in the middle of installing a system or have yet to fully deploy a product. For example, one closely related practice of an internal medicine practice was "completely installed and operational" when in fact only a single doctor was using the EHR to chart his patient visits. The EHR report was printed out and placed in the patient chart. The current status of the implementation can tell you what may be a good candidate as well as which strategies will not work in your implementation.

At the end of collecting potential products, you may have eight or more EHR products that you could consider. Next, focus on the products that have a good chance to meet your needs.

SITUATIONS TO AVOID

With the large number of existing vendors, the number of new and evolving entries is surprising. New products are coming out from a variety of companies. Although you may be tempted to buy into a new product or extension of an existing product for a number of reasons, make sure that you are fully informed of the level of effort involved and what, if anything, you will get out of the investment. *Here are 5 warning signs to be wary of.*

1. Small Installed Base–

Dozens of products have small numbers of installed systems. The vendor may have few installations due to the nature of its target market, continuing development, and/or early product lifecycle issues. In some cases, the EHR business is ancillary to the main business of the vendor. For example, some PMS vendors have sold a limited number of companion EHR products. The PMS product is the main business, and the EHR merely rounds out the product line.

These vendors have been successful implementing and supporting a limited number of EHR installations. In some cases, the small installed base allows the vendor to focus attention and resources that have been significant attractions to the EHR customers.

In these situations, you need to concern yourself with the longevity of the vendor and how long the business can operate with limited revenues and resources.

> **TIP**: In the event that you resolve to purchase a system with a limited number of users, make sure that the contract protects your practice in the event that the product is not viable in the long run.

2. Develop an EHR product–

A number of physicians and practices feel that there are no adequate EHR products. The PMS and EHR market clearly proves this point. The initial development of many of the more than 1,000 PMS, and 400 EHR products was initiated by a doctor who was frustrated with the products available in the marketplace.

If your practice cannot find the right product, you may be tempted to get involved with the development of a new offering. Typically, the practice teams up with a software developer to design a new product. In many cases, the software developer is new to healthcare.

However, the development of an EHR product can consume a significant amount of resources and time. EHR product development cycles of 2 or more years are not uncommon. During that time, you will be expected to provide subject matter expertise, testing resources and even real life testing support for the new product.

Unfortunately, at the end of the process, you may not end up with a marketable product. Even if you successfully complete an EHR for the practice, you are not assured that other practices will buy the product. The final product may specifically reflect the needs and operations of your practice, but may not be sufficiently flexible to work for other practices. In the end, you risk having a customized system that is only supported and maintained by and for your practice.

> **TIP**: Before undertaking such an effort, verify that the new EHR product will represent a dramatic competitive advantage for the practice. Thereby, the risks associated with creating and maintaining a custom product will be offset by overwhelming benefits to the practice and patients.

3. Enhance the EHR Product–

Some practices get involved with an existing EHR product that requires substantial enhancements and changes. The changes may include adding features practices want, or repairing mistakes from the initial implementation. For example, an EHR product may lack a lab module for practices with internal labs. **Beware**: Some EHR products lack drawing tools and imaging modules. A number of EHR products do not include workflow or patient health management tools.

Enhancing an EHR product can be even more complex than creating a new product. Initially, you need to catalog the necessary enhancements to meet the needs of your practice. The software publisher needs to analyze the changes and determine a workable way to add the capability to the EHR. The practice and EHR vendor have to agree on the specific implementation of the enhancements, timeframe, and, in some cases, cost. Unfortunately, changes may add complexity and appear awkward. For example, you may have to access another screen to enter additional information that is not part of the current EHR.

Regardless of the out-of-pocket costs, the EHR vendor will frequently look to your practice to define the changes and collaborate on the design, development, and testing effort. Depending on the level of enhancements, the effort could consume a lot of your and your staff's time. Do not underestimate the time that you may need to support the design of the enhancement and the extensive amount of time needed to test the changes. For example, adding additional information to the patient intake screen would require testing of the data within the screen as well as the effect of the date on the exam documents, E&M coding and even the follow-up list of patient services.

4. Develop Clinical Content–

Some EHR products may have a reasonable functional offering, but have not been implemented in your specialty. Typically, the EHR is in use in a primary care practice, but has not been installed for your specialty. The clinical content for your specialty may be present at a very high level, but the depth of details needed by a specialist is not available. In other cases, a product targeted to a specialist may lack the breadth of clinical content needed to work in a primary care environment.

The practice will be expected to work with the EHR vendor to improve the clinical content to support the specialty, sub-specialty and/or primary care clinical areas. You will be expected to develop clinical content that comprehensively addresses the specialty/primary care area in a manner that could be applied to a wide range of similar practices. If you are a sub-specialist, you may need to develop content that you may not typically use. For example, a hand surgeon may have to develop general orthopedic content before adding the hand surgeon subspecialty.

The EHR vendor will rely on the practice to provide subject matter expertise, develop the content and support the testing of the clinical content. In some cases, the practices may be expected to support marketing to other practices for compensation based on sales. These issues may be part of the contractual obligation of the practice and often complicate the negotiations of a contract. For example, your practice may be obligated to support marketing activities and allow your name to be used in advertising.

Before you agree to support the enhancement of clinical content, make certain that the basic functionality and capability of the EHR meets your needs and that the resulting clinical content will be worth your investment.

5. Market Segmentation–

The practice marketplace is highly segmented, and, in some cases, highly specialized. Practice structure, size, patient service styles and other factors determine the capabilities of the EHR. As such, you should be very wary of EHR products that do not have a presence in your type or size practice. The product may lack features, clinical content for your clinical area, and even operate in a way that will not work in your practice. For example, interfaces with diagnostic equipment may be an important factor for your practice, but the EHR's target market may not have such equipment.

The lack of comparable practice installations may lead to offers to enhance the product or enticements for your expertise to customize the EHR. However, these offers should be critically evaluated in light of the level of effort that you will have to invest in the development effort and the scope of the development effort.

> **CAUTION**: Before committing to any product that will require your expertise and time, you need to clearly understand and define the level of effort that the practice and the vendor will invest, as well as what the end product will look like. In the final analysis, the decision to use a product with these issues may be a great benefit to your practice. However, there are many practices that have pursued similar initiatives without achieving the goals and results they expected.

In the final analysis, the less you have to do to make the product work for you, the better off you are. For example, you may be better off going with a product that meets your needs than buying into the development of a product that requires additional work. However, in the absence of an appropriate product, you should not avoid situations and products that will provide you with a substantial benefit and competitive advantage.

PARING DOWN YOUR EHR PRODUCT LIST

Completing a detailed analysis and review of every product that you identify will be an expensive and time-consuming task. Even if you were to review all of the products, your selection team would have difficulty remembering the specific capabilities of each product reviewed. To pare down the list to viable candidates, perform an initial analysis of the potential products.

As you analyze the product options to pare down the list, you should keep notes on why each product was not further considered and the rational for not performing a detailed review. Then you can account for options and be prepared to itemize why a particular product was not granted a detailed look. The documentation will come in handy when your doctors and/or staff review the selection process, and/or query on the viability of a particular product. Consider the following 5 issues to reduce the list to potential vendors:

1. **Certified EHR**—ARRA has started a process that will create a class of acceptable EHR products for those practices seeking to meet the meaningful use standard. Regardless of your position on ARRA and the stimulus incentives, many practices will be limiting their search to certified products. If the product is certified, include the product on your list. If the product is seeking certification, then you may make your final selection contingent on certification. If the product is not seeking certification, then you should seriously consider the viability of a product that will be excluded from consideration by any practice that is seeking ARRA Incentives, and meeting meaningful use standards.

2. **Practice size**—A number of selection criteria depend on the size of the practice. Location management, workflow tracking, and patient service issues can be significantly impacted by the size of the practice. When you initially consider a product, determine if the vendor has installed his product in ex-

isting practices that match your size and structure. The key criteria would include the number of physicians, staff and locations. Taking an EHR in use in a solo practitioner's office and trying to use that same product in a 7-doctor practice with a couple of physician extenders runs a number of significant risks. Key questions:

- Is the EHR used by practices with a similar number of providers and staff?
- Does the EHR have current installations with as many or more locations?
- Do the EHR practices use similar ancillary and diagnostic service offerings?
- Do other EHR users have the same type of staff and doctor composition?
- Do other practices use the same type of clinical support strategies for the doctors?
- Does the product support the entity structure of the practice (Ex. separate clinic and ASC entities)?

3. **Clinical Areas**—Some EHR products focus on selected specialties and/or types of primary care. Clinical focus may determine the types of features as well as the specific clinical areas covered by the EHR. For example, a primary care focused EHR may lack surgery scheduling support. You may even uncover a number of odd nuances depending on the original practice that started the clinical content. For example, an ENT focused product may lack audiology documentation tools and not accommodate hearing aid orders. Key questions:

- Which specialties does the EHR currently serve?
- What are the specific subspecialty areas covered by the EHR?
- What are the specific services or disease states that current EHR practices focus on? For example, a sports medicine practice would have different needs than a general orthopedic practice.
- What ancillary services are supported by the EHR?
- What diagnostic services are supported by the EHR?
- What products are distributed by the other practices?

4. **Patient Service Style**—EHR systems are built around one of several different patient service strategies. Some EHRs are structured as the personal documentation tool of the doctor. The EHR assumes that the doctor records and approves all information. Some EHRs assume that the patient is initially seen by a nurse, and then treated by the doctor. Not all EHRs support patients being handed off between ancillary services, diagnostic services and other staff during a patient visit. If the practice uses physician extenders and has a wide range of patient services offered in various practice departments, you need to verify that the EHR will support your patient follow strategy before you invest a lot of time in a detailed analysis. For example, one practice

purchased an EHR that did an adequate job of documenting a visit, but assumed that the doctor would call the nurse in to transfer responsibility for a patient. The practice was using an EHR top document with the old flag system to manage patient flow. Key questions:

- What is the model patient flow strategy supported by the EHR?
- Do the EHR audit trails include tracking of a collaborative patient service process?
- Does the EHR support the various types of clinical staff and doctors involved in patient service?
- Does the EHR facilitate supervision of mid-level providers working under a designated doctor?
- What is the assumed EHR process for incoming patient issues, such as messages, follow-up, and test results?

5. **PMS Interface**—Depending on your PMS situation, you may want to insure that the EHR product includes an established interface strategy for your PMS. You can choose to require an existing interface with you PMS product or a mutually workable strategy. For example, some PMS and EHR systems have interface toolkits that support standardized interfaces with other products. **CAUTION**: Some EHRs and PMSs only interface with selected partner products while other EHR vendors have established a toolkit to interface with any PMS product. **TIP**: If an EHR product does not offer an interface strategy, you should seek out other EHR options. Key questions:

- Does the EHR have a standard interface with your PMS?
- Does the EHR receive demographic information and appointment data from PMS products?
- Does the EHR send charges to PMS products for posting charges?
- Does the EHR support additional data exchanges with the PMS?

Notice that price is not listed as a major qualifier in the selection of EHR candidates. Price driven decisions do not insure that you will get value for your investment. In too many cases, practices primarily qualify EHR solutions based on the "cost of the system." However, without completing an analysis of the product and its pricing structure, you will not be able to determine the real cost. For example, a cheaper or basic EHR without the tools to manage your workflow, or allow for images of documents, may be substantially more expensive with the necessary modules. **TIP**: The mix of purchase and support costs can also distort a cost-based criteria. For example, a product with a low acquisition cost but higher annual support cost may be more expensive than a product with a higher acquisition cost, but a low annual support cost.

At this early stage of your search, vendor estimates are based on general assumptions and unspecific estimates. Many vendors will present a general quote based on some undetermined estimate. Such quotes lack any realistic basis for you practice and make untenable assumptions. For example, a practice with various mid-level staff could be facing substantial additional charges for vendors that classify mid-level staff as fully licensed providers. The analysis of initial cost estimates are hampered by a number of factors including . . .

- A less expensive EHR that does not allow you to support a paperless operation may require continuing paper medical record costs.
- Significant issues are not included in a preliminary estimate. Without a detailed proposal, you will not be able to determine a realistic delivered cost for any product. Important components that could be easily missing from any preliminary quote include conversion services, appropriate licensing, diagnostic equipment interfaces and additional software.
- Vendors significantly vary in their pricing strategies and options. A focus on license costs could be ancillary to significant differences in support, training, and service costs. For example, an inexpensive license fee could be offset by more expensive support fees from the vendor. Such fees could offset any license cost benefits in the first few years of EHR use.
- Half of the costs for a typical EHR in the first 5 years are attributed to hardware and support fees. In many cases, buyers focus on the license fees and installation fees and exclude significant cost components. For example, some vendors include the first year of support in the license fee while other vendors start charging support fees when the system is delivered.
- Time based services are frequently used for support and implementation services. Usage based costs reflect the standard implementation services that the vendor provides without considering your specific situation. **TIP:** A vendor that includes fewer hours is not necessarily a cheaper system. For example, the vendor is not in a position to include integrating their system into your current computer network until the current equipment has been analyzed in light of the EHR hardware requirements.
- Service and hardware exclusions distort the true cost of many vendors. Vendors may have varying degrees of costs for key services and hardware issues you may need for your EHR. **Beware:** For example, off-hours implementation and training may be charged at premium rates for practices that want to work on EHR implementation outside standard working hours. Similarly, an EHR Vendor with extended service hours may prove cheaper than a vendor with additional charges outside of a shorter standard service hour window.

In general, pricing concessions in the negotiation for purchasing an EHR can frequently cut the cost differences between competing products. For example, vendors may offer discounts for larger number of users, significant hours, or products bought at the same time. Indeed, comparable products are frequently priced within a fairly narrow margin. **TIP:** Product cost differences will only become clear when you take the time to specify your needs to insure the vendor includes all of the hardware, software and services needed for your EHR effort.

After you have focused your attention on a couple of viable EHR products, you can proceed to get workable proposals and evaluate them to produce a comparable cost comparison.

4 EHR PRODUCT TYPES

Not all EHRs are created equal. EHRs are based on a couple of underlying strategies that can have a substantial impact on your implementation and use. EHR products come in several different models:

Document Management

Document Management EHRs are designed to work with other products that develop the clinical information. The finished information is tracked and managed by the Document Management EHR. For example, you may use Word to document a patient visit, or a drawing tool to document a patient condition.

As you are saving the document or image, you invoke the Document Management EHR which allows you to associate the document/image with a patient record, description, and/or date. In some cases, you can assign specific information to a document. For example, you may be able to assign the hospital to a procedure report. Examples of document management EHRs include SRS, NG Cabinet and TouchChart. **TIP:** Some EHR vendors will sell the document management module as a standalone product.

Document management systems may actually store the file with the clinical information within the document management database, or save a pointer to the file that you have created. The original file may be accessed through the document management system, and, in some cases, the original software used to create the file (e.g., Word).

In some cases, document management based EHR strategies are used with paper-based forms to collect new patient information. The patient form is scanned into the document management systems to add information to the medical record. Of course, document management EHRs could also accept documents from other applications and documentation tools. For example, you could use a drawing tool with an image of your existing intake document to fill out an electronic version of your intake form. The intake form could be saved in the document management product.

EHRs that support paperless medical records include a document management feature. A sample screen from the document management module of Sage Intergy EHR follows (see Figure 6.1).

Forms

Forms-based EHRs use a screen-design tool to create a checklist like a typical flowsheet or intake form used by many practices. Instead of checking boxes on a paper form, the Forms based EHR allows you to define the screen based on your existing forms or some other standard. Some forms-based EHRs allow conditional handling and data entry. For example, data entry may differ for male and female patients or the form could automatically trigger the printing of a prescription when you check a drug in the treatment area. Similarly, a Forms Based EHR could automatically date and time stamp the template and print a consent form for a patient procedure.

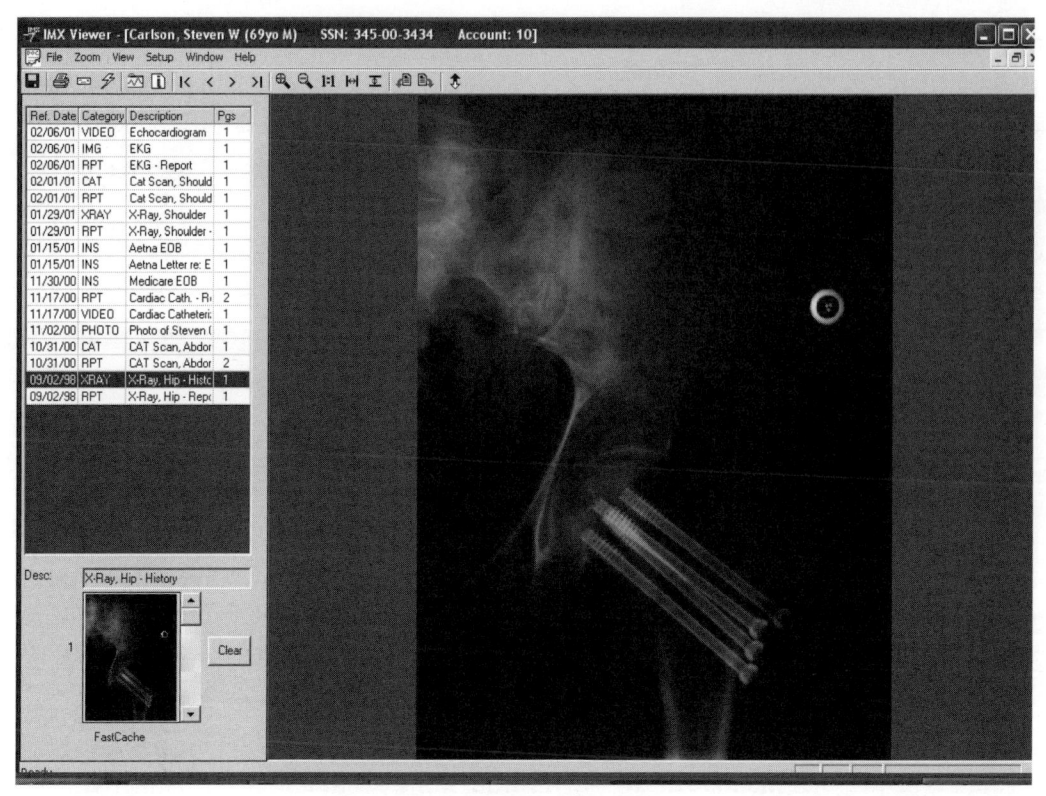

FIGURE 6.1

Forms-based EHRs may be particularly attractive to practices with an extensive base of flowsheets and precise clinical workflow requirements. Depending on the capability of the form design tools, you can program specific activities, and workflows directly into the template. For example, an intake record could automatically generate the lab task for a patient that meets certain clinical data entries. The template could be programmed to conditionally trigger the lab test, and route the patient.

Some forms-based EHRs are programmed by the vendor only, and other products include tools that can be used by practice staff. Some knowledgebase EHRs include a form-building tool to support a specific checklist for the practice.

Most forms-based EHR vendors offer specific clinical content for selected specialties and clinical areas. Additional clinical content may be available from third party and other practices. NextGen EHR and Centricity EHR are examples of forms-based EHRs. A sample screen from NextGen, a forms-based EHR is shown in Figure 6.2.

Knowledgebase

Knowledgebase systems use extensive lists of findings or conditions to document patient visits. The most widely used knowledgebase is Medcin. Medcin contains over 300,000 items that the user can choose from. Several other knowledgebases exist, and some vendors design and maintain their own knowledgebase. Of course, selecting findings from such a list is a massive undertaking.

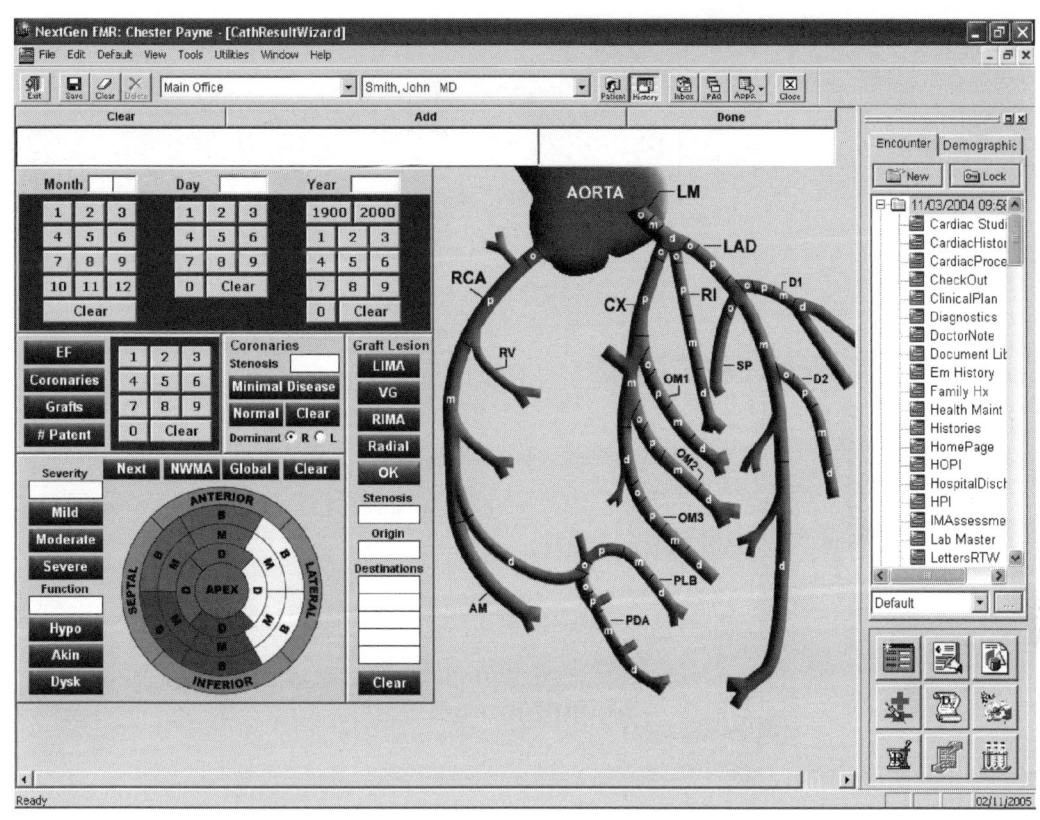

FIGURE 6.2

To simplify the use of the knowledgebase, knowledgebase EHRs include a variety of tools and classifications to focus your selection. For example, most knowledgebase EHRs include search tools that help you locate findings based on keywords as well as organizational structures to categorize findings into clinical areas. Knowledgebase EHRs include user-defined lists, and, in some cases, templates of findings that allow you to organize the findings you most commonly use.

Knowledgebase EHRs generate documents from the findings into SOAP structures, and/or user-defined letters.

Allscripts Professional EHR, Electronic Healthcare Systems, and Purkinje are examples of knowledgebase EHRs. A sample screen from Allscripts Professional EHR is shown in Figure 6.3.

Notes

Free form note tools are another form of EHR. Information, such as transcription and notes, entered by the doctor may not offer the same access and search capabilities as a knowledgebase or a form. Knowledgebases and forms consist of discrete data items that have a specific definition. In a free form note, the significance of information is driven by the context. For example, you can electronically search knowledgebase or forms EHR data item search to compile a list of your patients with diabetes. If you search a large number of notes for the word "diabetes," then you will end up with a list of patients that have the word di-

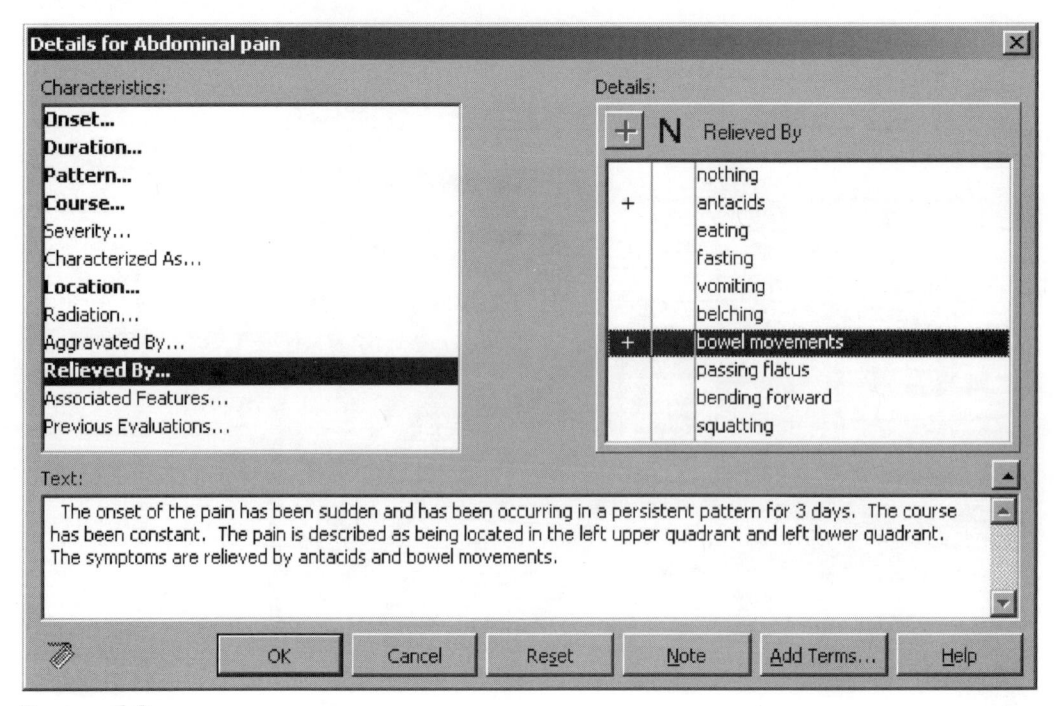

FIGURE 6.3

abetes in their note, but do not necessarily have disease (Ex. A relative has diabetes.) Natural language processing presents an interesting development in notes based EHRs. Natural language processing paired with notes based EHRs may provide a way to derive specific information from a patient note and present discrete data to the user or be used to populate specific information. For example, the order details or E&M evaluation may be derived from note text through natural language processing and offer a hybrid note and selected data presentation option to the user.

Several hybrid systems include a mix of these different EHR models.

You should consider the types of EHR in your short list to insure that you have a variety of structures or that you exclude product types that will not meet your needs. For example, if your doctors do not want to chart at time of service than you may want to focus on note and document management based EHRs. If you are interested in performing computer assisted analyses of your clinical data, then you need to insure that the EHR will store and manage the specific information entered.

MANAGEABLE LIST OF CANDIDATES

Ideally, you want a manageable number of products to start the detailed review process. Too many potential candidates will be difficult to keep track of, and too few product options may result in a limited view of your choices. *TIP*: Keep your short-list to 3–4 products. Many on the initial lists could be eliminated based on the paring strategy.

Using the cataloging and elimination strategies in this chapter, you should feel confident that the products on your short-list are viable candidates worthy of your detailed review.

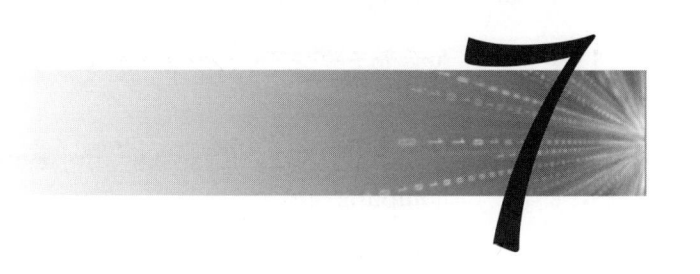

Reviewing Products for Your Practice

Ideally, your EHR product reviews can be completed within 2 months. Some practices stretch out the process for months. Unfortunately, the longer process can risk derailing your efforts and cause fatigue within your entire review team. Other risks of extended reviews include:

Additional product releases may require updates, and, in some cases, force a reexamination of the original review.

Over time, you may forget product specifics. Indeed, some vendors jockey for the last demonstration of the product to make the most lasting impression.

Physicians and staff may lose interest in a project that drags on.

EHR REVIEW PREPARATIONS

Initially, the practice should select who will review the EHR products. A comprehensive EHR review requires technical, clinical, operational, and user interface analysis. In addition to viewing the demonstration, the reviewer(s) needs to analyze what is being done and how the product works. In some cases, practices use outside consultants to review the EHR products. If the review will be performed by internal resources, you should appoint a small review team to look at the products and measure them against your evaluation list. The team should include a strong clinical person who understands charting needs as well as an operational person who understands current patient service and workflow issues. If possible, the team should also include a person knowledgeable in computer applications.

The review team should meet before any demonstrations to review the evaluation list and discuss what the practice needs. The team members should discuss what they are looking for in each item as well as the relative importance of each one. The team should examine some sample screen shots (see some examples later in this chapter) and other materials on each product to gain a general understanding of what they will be looking at. Some vendors even have demonstration disks or websites that your team can view. **TIP:** All of the reviewers should take advantage of CDs and Web sites to become familiar with the products to be reviewed in detail. The initial effort will help you make the best use of your detailed analysis.

To complete the evaluation, you should have a clear strategy for the vendor demonstration. Many vendors want to show you their highlights, but may avoid getting into the details of their product. You should notify the vendor upfront on the general areas that you want to discuss and see demonstrated. For example, you can tell them the key clinical areas that you want to review as well as the ordering system, workflow, prescriptions and other items. **TIP**: Give them actual clinical examples and see how the product performs under each scenario.

You can utilize several different methods to help the vendor set up for the demo:

Limited information—Many practices give no information or demonstration requirements to the vendor. Unfortunately, this gives the vendor an out for any items that the product cannot handle. If you give the vendor guidelines upfront, you can use the evaluation list to challenge the vendor on missing capabilities. For example, if you don't challenge the vendor, the vendor may avoid showing you how the system functions with a certain subspecialty. If you give vendors information to focus the demonstration, and they cannot address your scenario, then the product may not be appropriate, and/or their sales process is not designed to address your needs. **ALERT:** If the product cannot be made to look good in a demonstration, then you should be concerned with what will happen when you try to install the EHR.

Evaluation list—Giving the vendor your evaluation list is your choice. If you give the vendor the evaluation list, the salesperson may fill out the list for you and challenge your analysis. If you do not give the vendor the list, the vendor may claim that they are not prepared for your question or require more resources. Either way, you or your consultant should score the product independently for each evaluation criteria. **TIP**: You are welcome to use the vendor evaluation as a reference, but you should assign your own scores to each item. For example, the vendor may use a task to track a clinical requirement and tasks may not be visible from the patient record when you open the chart. Such a design would complicate identifying important clinical issues for a patient.

Scenario list—Consider sharing a scenario list with the vendor instead of your evaluation list. The scenario list itemizes various processes or activities that demonstrate the flow of patients in your practice. The scenario may cover the handling of patients at the front desk and the handoff to the clinical area. In the clinical area, the scenario may cover the collaboration of nurses and doctors as well as patients receiving various tests and ancillary services. The purpose of the scenario is to walk through a familiar process on the EHR. You'd get a feel for the use of the clinical content and EHR flow. A sample scenario list follows:

- Demonstrate How the Doctor Knows a Patient is Waiting
- Review Initial Patient Information
  — Patient Summary Screen
  — Outstanding Clinical Services (Ex. Tests and Immunizations)
  — Records for a Previous Visit
- Chart Visit
  — Document Chief Complaint
  — Record Previous Medications and Conditions
  — Note Information Available for a Primary Care Visit
    - Record Subjective Primary Care Findings
    - Record Objective Primary Care Findings
    - Document Primary Care Analysis
  — Demonstrate the Information Available for a Cardiology Visit
    - Record Subjective Cardiology Findings
    - Record Objective Cardiology Findings
    - Document Cardiology Analysis
- Complete Clinical Visit
  — Record Plan
    - Lab Orders
    - Diagnostic Study
    - Treatments
    - Prescriptions
    - Recalls
  — Record Charge Information
    - Discuss Support for E&M Codes
- Distribute Patient Education Information
- Sign Chart Note

Be sure to explain to the vendor the importance of the demonstration structure. You should consider telling the vendor how you chose them for a detailed analysis and emphasize the seriousness of your process. The vendor will know that it's on a short list and involved in a serious selection process. In some cases, vendors will be inspired to prepare for your practice and conduct a productive demonstration. Some vendors will not prepare for the demonstration regardless of the amount of information you provide. Failure to prepare under your guidelines should raise a red flag on the capabilities of the product and/or vendor.

EHR SCREEN SAMPLES

Conducting the review and gathering information on your evaluation items requires some familiarity with general screen contents as well as the product your are reviewing. This section presents selected sample screens and general comments on items you should look for. The screen samples are not an endorsement of any particular product; they are used for illustration purposes only.

Patient Summary Screen—The patient summary screen displays a list of the pertinent documents and key information that is stored in the EHR. The user should be able to access the detailed information from the patient summary screen. Verify that you can access the key care information that you need for a patient. For example, a pediatric practice needs to access pending immunization or checkup information while an orthopaedic practice may need to access outstanding orders and incoming MRI results. Some products allow the practice or each user to select the specific information that will be displayed on their patient summary screen. Thereby, nurses can see key information and vitals, while doctors may be more interested in presented results and continuity of care issues. The following sample patient summary is from the Greenway Medical PrimeSuite (Figure 7.1).

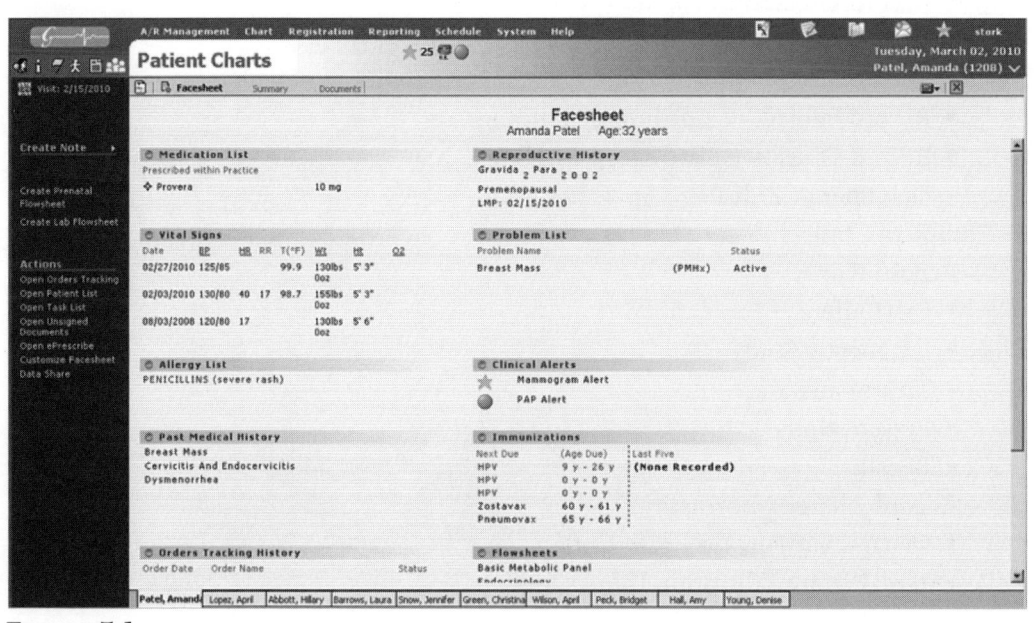

FIGURE 7.1

Workflow Screen—The workflow screen displays pending work items as well as the status of patients in the office. The list of current patient appointments should directly access the appropriate patient chart. The outstanding to-do's should support more extensive information on the patient issue. Depending on your practice size, you may want to view workflow screens for individual people, doctors, and/or practice units (Ex. Locations, pods, modality, department.) The workflow screen is a key component of the EHR since your staff and doctors will be constantly referencing the screen to identify the next patient or issue to work on. Note that some EHRs only focus on doctors in their workflow screens. The following sample workflow screen is from e-MDs EHR (Figure 7.2).

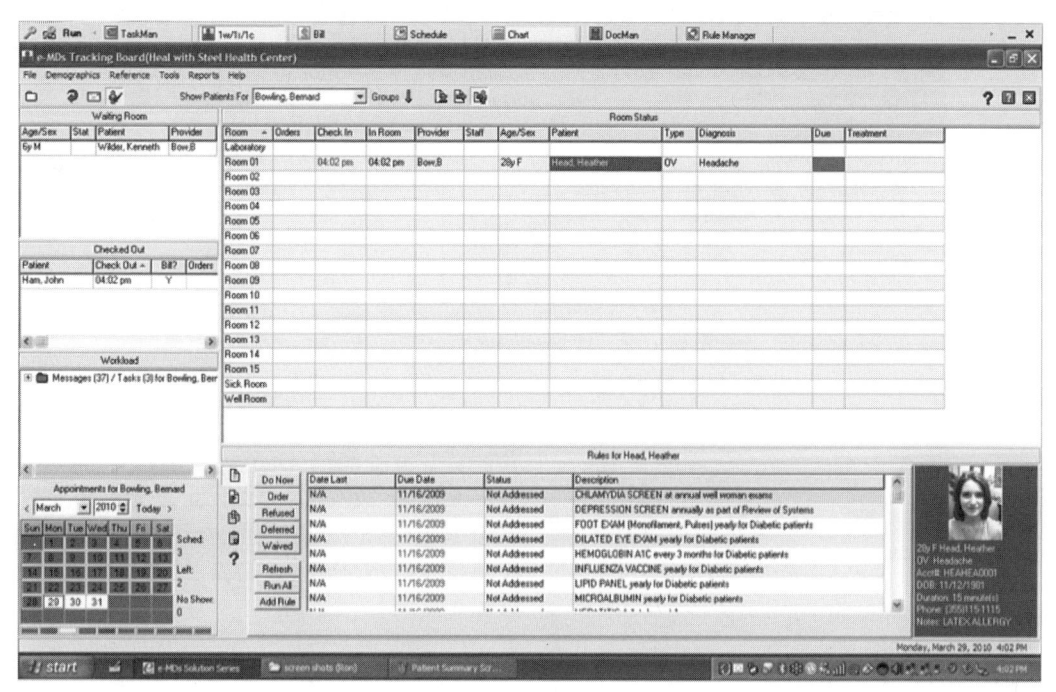

FIGURE 7.2

Patient Information Entry—Patient information entry screens allow patients to enter information that can be posted to the EHR. Practices should be able to customize the patient information entry screen to meet their specific needs. Some EHR products have self contained patient entry screen while other EHRs work with an Internet application to accept information into the EHR. Typically, the information entered by the patient is accepted into the EHR by an authorized user. Patient information entry is an important tool to improve efficiency since it allows the practice to accept information from the patient without having to reenter information from the patient information and intake sheet. This feature can also speed up the doctor since they do not have to dictate the patient information that has been accepted into the EHR record. The following sample patient information entry screen is from Allscripts Professional EHR (Figure 7.3):

Message/To-Do Screen—The message/to do screen is used to enter information on outstanding items for patients. The to-do's may be associated with a document (e.g., a radiology study) that triggered the to-do. To-do's may be assigned to specific resources or groups of resources (e.g., nurses). Some EHRs consider the messages as part of the patient's medical record, while other EHRs exclude messages from the patient medical record. A few EHRs allow you to optionally accept selected messages as part of the patient record. The role of messages and their relationship to the patient's record can have a big impact on workflow. For example, if the EHR optionally accepts the messages into

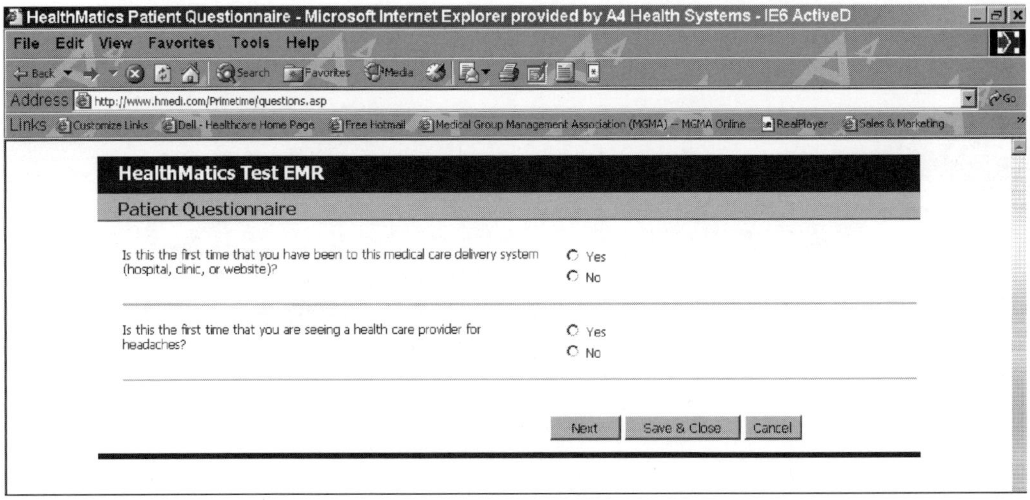

FIGURE 7.3

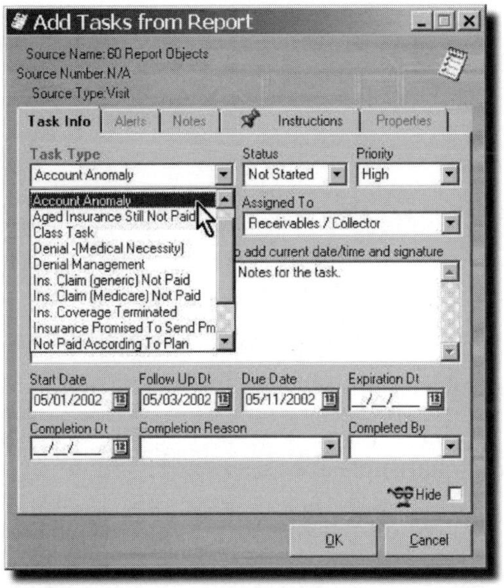

FIGURE 7.4

the patient record, then you need a specific standard and protocol as well as disciplined staff to properly maintain the patient EHR records. The following Message/to-do screen is from the NextGen EHR (Figure 7.4).

Clinical Charting—Charting of patient care at time of service is the key to more effective E&M coding, as well as the elimination of transcription. The charting screen should support most of the information that you need to record directly as well as offer the ability to enter a note for information that is not accommodated by the EHR. Make sure that you understand the inclusion and implementation issues of the clinical content for the EHR product. Some vendors sell a defined set of tools to address selected clinical areas, while other vendors provide access to a library where their users can share clinical content. A brief test of clinical charting should be conducted as part of your evaluation. Ideally, you should take a sample note and review the charting process for the note. Make sure that you review the actual note that is produced by the EHR and compare their note to your sample. You should also verify the document production and distribution (Ex. To PCPs, Case Managers) mechanism for clinical information to internal and external parties. The following sample clinical charting screen is from Allscripts Professional EHR (Figure 7.5).

Image Review Screen—Practices accumulate large numbers of images in the EHR. Images may come from scanning of the patient's paper record as well as incoming doc-

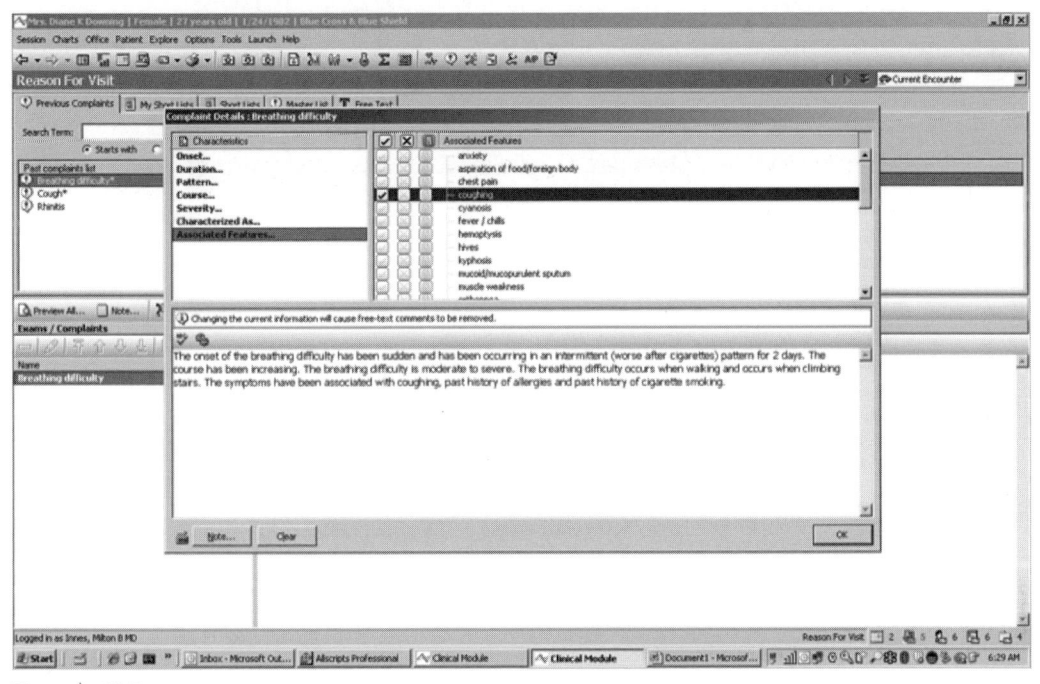

FIGURE 7.5

uments and faxes. The review screen allows the user to select images from a list of patient-related images. Images may be identified by a document type and a description. The EHR should provide viewing options as well as the ability to note issues and items on the image. The following sample image review screen is from SRS (Figure 7.6).

Prescription Screen—Prescription screens are used to record patient medications and produce the appropriate script for the pharmacy. The prescription is automatically entered in a medications' log, as well the patient chart note for that date of service. As a practical matter, the EHR should allow you to enter and track medications from other doctors as well as over the counter drugs being used by the patient. The prescription screen should facilitate the handling and approval of refill requests. The following prescription sample screen is from the Allscripts Professional EHR (Figure 7.7).

Lab Order Screen—This screen accepts information on lab orders and is used to manage the lab test and track the review of results. Lab orders should be managed for lab tests done by the practice as well as lab tests performed by outside parties. Lab modules should also offer a flow sheet view of lab results and a graphing option. The following sample lab order screen is from Allscripts Professional EHR (Figure 7.8).

Diagnostic Testing Order—Diagnostic tests are entered as part of a patient treatment plan. The EHR should track the diagnostic test through the receipt and review of results. Diagnostic tests may be ordered for recurring issues and patient monitoring. The EHR should monitor tests with a future date as part of a treatment plan. For example, the doctor may want the patient to return with a test in 3 months. Diagnostic tests may be

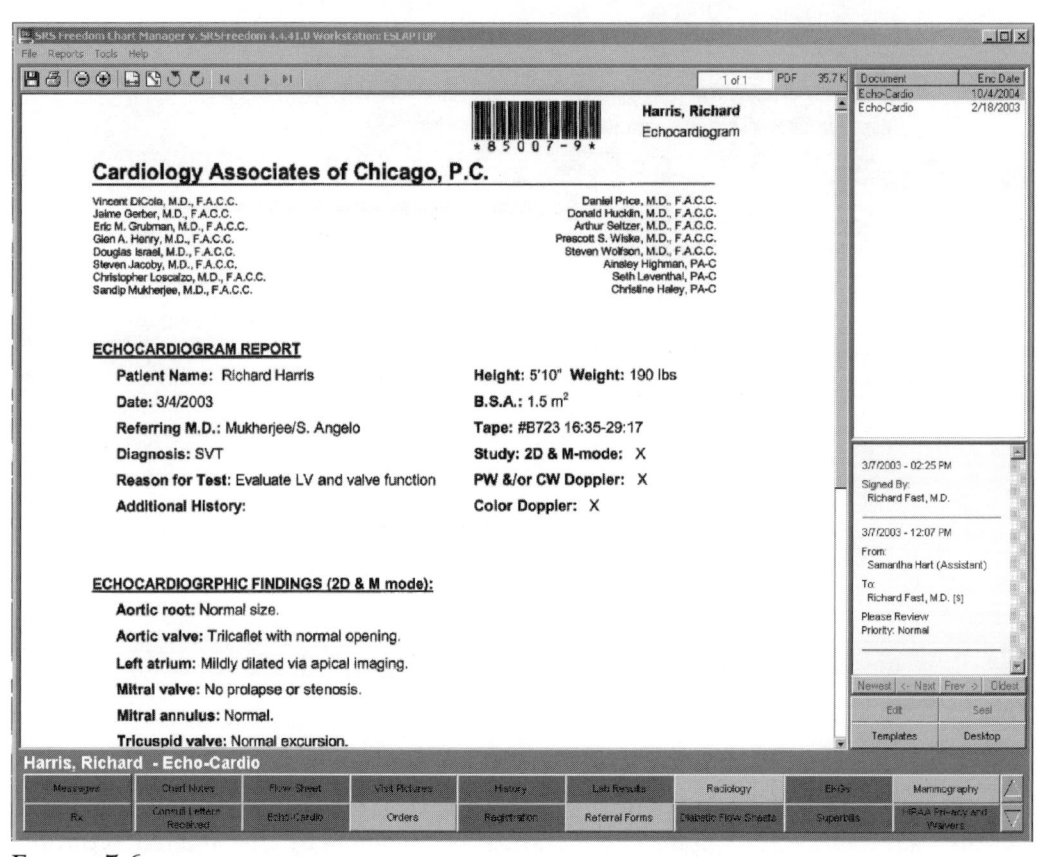

FIGURE 7.6

FIGURE 7.7

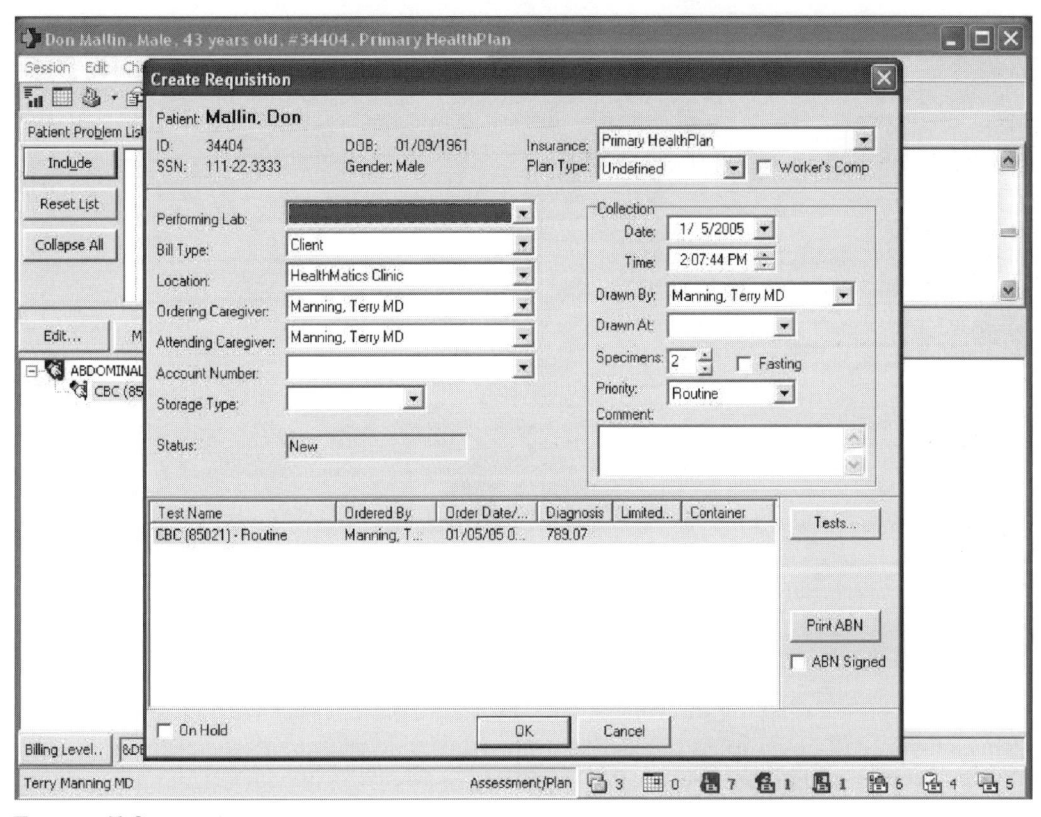

FIGURE 7.8

performed by the practice or an outside party. The following sample diagnostic test screen is from Greenway Medical PrimeSuite (Figure 7.9).

EHR DEMONSTRATION

The product demonstration has a number of conflicting objectives. You want to quickly review the product, but you also want to get detailed information. The participants will want to see how the product would work in a clinical setting, and everyone wants to pose various permutations. Ideally, you need at least 2–4 hours to go through the basic operation of the EHR as well as get your questions answered. Based on the number of specialties, complexity of the practice and number of participants, you may be lucky to get the demonstration done in a day.

At the start of the demonstration, some vendors like to talk about the superiority of their company. They may discuss the company's history, number of employees, revenue growth and client base. Although this is useful information, the introduction should only consume a few minutes. Some vendors have a canned demonstration and others will ask you what you want to see. In the event that the vendor takes too long talking about their company, feel free to ask them to move onto the demonstration.

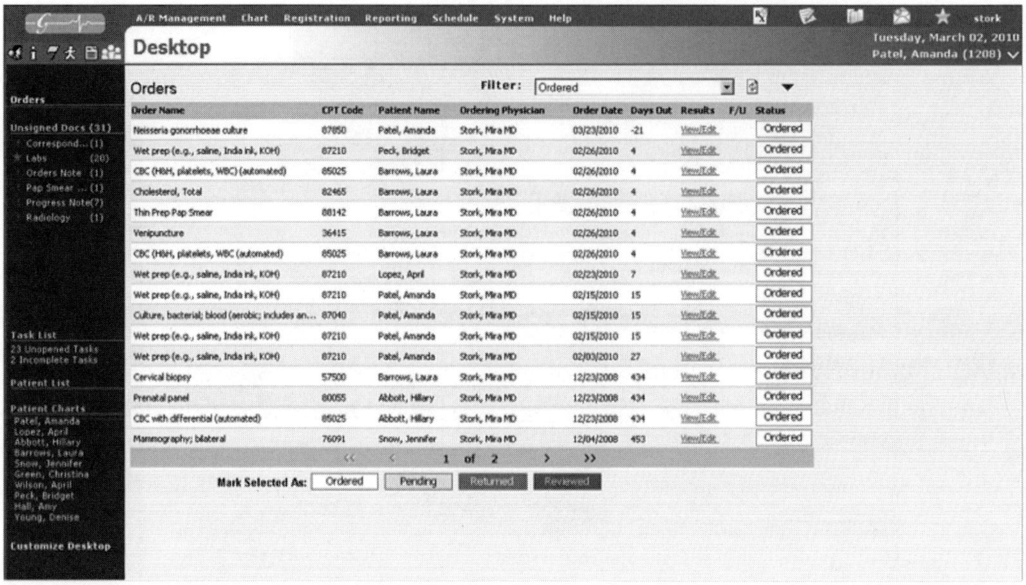

FIGURE 7.9

You should consider having the vendor run through a patient visit without interruption. Although you will be tempted to ask questions, the evaluation team should just sit back and get a look at the flow of the product. **TIP**: Remember to take advantage of their CDs or Web site to prepare for the demonstration. In some cases, practices may perceive that the system is slow and hard to use since they never saw the optimal flow and use of the system during the demonstration. **CAUTION**: If you let the vendor drive the product run-through, you could end up with an impractical "sunny day" scenario. In order to get the most out of you demonstration, the vendor should be provided with a scenario and note that represents a real visit to your practice. **TIP**: After the uninterrupted run-through, have the vendor repeat the demonstration more slowly and stop at each key point in which you need a clarification or additional information. The initial run-through prepares you for a more detailed discussion of the product in the second viewing of the process.

Using your evaluation list, you should methodically grade each item against the vendor demonstration (see Chapter 4—Compiling a Practice Focused Evaluation List). As you work through the evaluation, make a note for each item that satisfies your evaluation list. Comment on any problems you uncover as well as any particularly effective or impressive features you see.

The note will help participants remember the details of the demonstration. The note is also useful to refute challenges from vendors, doctors and staff, if and when, you discuss any problems. For example, you may award a "1" for a product that had a workaround that was difficult to use, or for an item that would require an excessive amount of work. Ideally, each staff member who is on the review team should take his own notes. The various areas of expertise will assure that your get a comprehensive view of how the product would work. For example, a vendor may suggest using a clinical note to track surgery scheduling, but the surgery scheduler may notice that the note would be manually copied when the surgery is assigned a schedule slot.

In the course of the review, make sure you work through each evaluation item. As you analyze the product, insure that you understand how the product meets the requirements for these issues:

Limited Data—Too often, a vendor conducts a demonstration that does not contain the information of setups to address your questions and issues. Demonstration databases that are not realistic, setups for a different kind of practice, missing clinical content for your area of medicine, and inappropriate examples do not provide an effective and adequate view of the product. This limitation indicates a failure on the part of the vendor to prepare for your practice. ***TIP***: If the vendor does not have the demonstration set up to address your issues, evaluate the product on what you see, and not what the vendor claims.

Product Customization—In the event that the vendor offers to customize the product to meet your requirements, you should seriously consider whether any credit should be given for the requirement. Some vendors admittedly are developing their product by adding new features requested by other users. But not all features require the same level of effort. For example, an allergy shot chart is easier to add to an EHR than a workflow management tool. Promises of customization may get a note, but deserve a score of "0." However, you should note any customization commitments for additional analysis if you choose the product. ***TIP***: Include the customization requirement in your contract with the vendor.

Upcoming Enhancement—In some cases, the evaluation criteria will be addressed in a forthcoming release by the vendor. You should make a note of the release containing the feature. However, the evaluation should be based on the current capability of the product. ***TIP***: Similar to customization, upcoming enhancements could be included in your contract.

Qualify Workarounds—In some cases, the EHR will not be able to do what you are asking and the vendor will suggest a workaround using another feature or more general capability. For example, the vendor may suggest "to-do's" or a note to track pending procedure orders. However, the EHR may lack a connection between the pending order and the supporting note. You would have to monitor the procedure order in the medical record as well as the "to do." Getting from the note to the procedure task could be complicated. In many cases, the workarounds may not be practical to deal with your issues. If the workaround is obscure or does not meet the requirement, you should not give full credit. If you understand and can live with the workaround, credit the vendor accordingly.

Complexity of Features—When the vendor is demonstrating a feature, note how easy the vendor can access the information or demonstrate the capability.

If the vendor makes it look difficult or explains the problems with the feature, then you should be concerned with how easy the product will be. For example, the vendor may have to go to 3 or more screens to document a basic issue on your evaluation list. In situations where the product looks difficult, you may want to verify your impression with another viewing of the process. If the product meets the requirement in a complex and difficult matter, you should not award full credit for the criteria.

Comparable Vendor Examples—Solicit comparable practice examples from each vendor. You may solicit these examples indirectly by asking how similar practices deal with one of your key issues. For example, you may ask "show us how primary care practices track immunization shots with the EHR" or "how does the doctor notify the surgery scheduler of a patient treatment need." The lack of examples may indicate that the product cannot handle your requirement or the vendor lacks comparable practice clients.

Verbal Explanations—Sometimes vendors verbally explain how the product works but cannot demonstrate the capability. **ALERT:** In some cases, you are viewing screen shots of the EHR and are not even seeing the actual product in use. Common excuses are that the vendor does not have the current version of the software or lacks the clinical content for your specialty. **ALERT:** Verbal explanations are a red flag. You should request another demo with the correct version or base the evaluation score on the capability you observed through the software.

Defer to the PMS—Some EHR vendors suggest that certain features should be handled by the PMS. For example, a vendor with an EHR that lacks a patient flow feature may suggest that the patient be tracked through the PMS. However, you are evaluating the issue as part of your EHR selection process and you should verify that you have a workable EHR solution. For example, the recall information may be recorded in the clinical note but not be accessible to the appointment scheduling module when a patient is scheduled for an appointment. Indeed, one vendor suggested giving the patient a post-it note to give to the check-out person for appointment scheduling. Even if your PMS has a certain feature, the PMS should not affect your EHR evaluation—or all of the reviewed EHRs get credit for your PMS' capabilities, which doesn't make sense.

Outstanding Issue—In some cases, the vendor may not have any answer for your evaluation item. The vendor will promise to get back to you. The evaluation items should be scored without the explanation and issue noted. **CAUTION:** In some cases, vendors just do not have an answer to your requirement but want to stay competitive. In other cases, you may receive promises but never get an answer.

When you have completed going through the evaluation list, review the items to insure that all of the evaluation items have been scored. Outstanding issues may result in a change to your evaluation but you should verify that all of the issues have been discussed.

Before completing the demonstration and evaluation session, be sure to cover the following additional issues:

Upcoming Releases and Enhancements—The vendor should supply information on upcoming releases and enhancements. For example, you may request a list of the enhancements in the last release as well as enhancements in the next release. You may need specific feedback on enhancements that meet some of the evaluation list items. Such explanations should be in writing and may be included in your contract. For example, a vendor may be adding a drawing tool to the EHR but you will need to know what the drawing tool will offer and how it would work with the image module.

Support Strategy—Have the vendor explain its support strategy. You need to understand how it will address hardware and software issues. Note the support hours and the expected level of expertise in the practice. For example, some EHR vendors limit support contact to a practice employee who has passed a vendor test. A number of EHR vendors have limited support hours or offer a questionable off-hours support strategy. The support strategy should be reviewed against your own support plan and approach. For example, if your practice has a dedicated EHR support person, you will want access to someone who is capable of supporting your EHR point-person. Practices have been frustrated with vendor support staff less knowledgeable about the EHR than the practice employee making the call. Ideally, the vendor should offer contact with a high-level person to insure you get the appropriate support.

Implementation Strategy—The practice should understand how the vendor intends to implement the EHR. In addition to its standard methodology, you should understand how the vendor will deal with your practice's issues. For example, you should be able to discuss how the EHR vendor works with your hardware vendor. Similarly, you need to verify that the vendor can support an implementation strategy that fits your needs. Many vendors require practice staff for management and implementation efforts that should be clearly understood by the practice. Some vendors only offer training services during regular business hours. Thereby, you can prepare your doctors and staff for the time and effort needed to support the implementation process. The vendor should have a clear plan for working with a practice of your size and complexity. For example, an implementation strategy that requires training at the vendor site for all staff may not work if the vendor training facility is far away. **CAUTION**: Some EHR vendors assume that the practice handles hardware, training and even software installation. By understanding your implementation obligations for each vendor, you will avoid surprises later. Knowing your implementation responsibilities could affect the cost of a system. For example, some vendors include implementation of hardware in their installation fees. Your practice would incur additional expenses with another product that would require more resources and costs.

Training Options and Program—You should discuss the various training options (e.g., Train-the-Trainer and direct-user training) offered by the vendor. You should understand the type of training offered and the ability of the vendor to train the people on your staff. Most vendors offer a single set of classes that may not allow you to focus your program on the training needs of your various staffers. You should also review the materials offered by the vendor that can be used to train and support your staff. A number of vendors have developed Web based training programs and CDs that are an integral part of their training services. These options provide flexibility for your practice, but require that each employee have the time and resources to access and participate in the training program. **TIP**: Be certain that you can use the training materials to develop your own.

Online Help and Documentation—You should review samples of online help and printed documentation. Be especially careful to determine the level and quality of the documentation. Some vendors lack sufficient documentation to explain their product. Specialty-specific clinical templates may lack any documentation. **ALERT**: Poor documentation may inhibit your ability to justify an error in the EHR.

At the end of the demonstration, the vendor will typically ask how the product measures up to what you are looking for. You can provide as much information as you wish but you should avoid getting involved in an informal exchange of information outside of the formal review process. Upon hearing of a problem, some vendors may verbally explain the EHR features that address the problem. You are welcome to reopen the demo, but you should not change your evaluation, unless you actually see the solution work.

After the demonstration, call the review team together to compare notes—without the vendor present. **TIP**: Schedule the meeting as soon as possible after the demo. A delay of a few days may undermine your final evaluation. The team should review each evaluation item and develop a consensus evaluation by line item. The consensus evaluation should be the basis for making your final decision and selection.

REQUEST FOR PROPOSAL

A request for proposal (RFP) solicits an EHR product that meets the specifications from your evaluation list. The RFP kicks off the formal EHR selection process. The RFP is typically sent to a selection of EHR vendors to qualify the vendor for further consideration. In some cases, you send the RFP to every vendor. In other cases, the vendor must be prequalified before it gets the RFP. A number of larger companies require the use of RFPs for major purchases. For example, practices that are units of a publicly held corporation may require the use of an RFP. **TIP**: Most private practices do not use the RFP process.

TIP: To save you time, and to focus on getting vendors to respond, determine viable vendors for your practice (see Chapter 6—Selecting Products to Review) and send the RFP to these vendors. Otherwise, you may spend time working with and reviewing vendor proposals that have no chance of winning your business.

Be aware that your RFP could scare off vendors. For example, a large practice that seeks an inexpensive product typically used in solo practices may seem illegitimate to vendors.

Regardless of the number of vendors you select, some will not respond to your RFP. To increase your change of getting a response, send RFPs to at least 5 vendors. Certainly limit your RFP distribution to 10–15 vendors.

Begin the RFP by introducing your organization. Describe the number of employees and locations as well as the services you offer. The RFP will continue with an explanation of the selection and evaluation process. The composition of the evaluation team and schedule for the evaluation and implementation process may be included. The RFP articulates the scoring and review process as well as the proposed contract terms and, in some cases, a project plan. The scoring plan will include the specific scoring scales as well as how the scores will be awarded. For example, the RFP may include the weight item for each evaluation list entry as well as the relative value of the evaluation list, implementation plan, support strategy and price in making the final decision.

RFPs can vary widely in length, from a few pages to 50 or more. To increase your chance of getting a response from a vendor, make your RFP concise and direct. Ten to 20 pages should be sufficient for most practices. Don't spend more than a page or two describing your organization, and devote the bulk of the rest of the RFP to your evaluation criteria. The scoring process and contract terms should only be included if your practice or parent organization requires this information in its RFPs.

The RFP may include the evaluation list and, in some cases, detailed information on specific capabilities and features. For example, the RFP may require an interface with a selected PMS system and specify interface data. The RFP also includes information to support the creation of a cost proposal for the EHR purchase. For example, the RFP may list the sites, number of employees by type and volume of business.

Vendors are expected to indicate their ability to meet the features and requirements as well as to submit a cost proposal for the requested products and services. Vendors are expected to comment on any contract terms and conditions that may be a problem for them. As a practical matter, know that vendors do not necessarily always provide the information you seek.

EHR vendors are not going to invest a significant amount of time responding to an RFP that will eliminate their product from further consideration. Some vendors will not respond to RFPs at all since they have other potential customers. Some vendors see the RFP as an opportunity to get their foot in the door of a practice and answer all of your questions in a skewed, positive light.

Although RFPs may have problems, they allow the practice to screen a large number of vendors at a relatively low cost. The vendors who respond to the RFP are considered interested and those vendors who did not respond can be easily eliminated.

After receiving the responses from the vendors, the practice will compile the results to compare vendor proposals. The RFP responses will be compiled and evaluated in much the same way information is compiled from the demo results.

Based on a review of the responses, a select number of vendors will be invited to demonstrate the product for the selection team. This demonstration should be managed using the same strategies described above.

For many practices, an RFP will not necessarily help you advance the EHR project. The results must be verified through your own demonstration. However, the RFP process may be useful, if not required, by larger organizations that may need to engage in an open-selection process.

CHECKING REFERENCES

Reference checking is complicated by the vendor's involvement. References from the vendor may be useful, but keep in mind their references are probably practices that are happy with the system. Ideally, you should seek out references through your own networks and resources. You may call practices you have working relationships with, as well as associations that you may be familiar with. **TIP**: Call the references provided by the vendor and ask the references for other practices they know that use the product. If they mention ones that don't appear on the vendor's list, be sure you contact these practices.

Talk with at least one and preferably two people in the practice. For example, the clinical manager and a doctor may speak with you. The actual reference check should be conducted at a scheduled time and cover:

> **Practice Description**—You should exchange information on your practices. You should get information on size, specialty and clinical focus. For example, practice workflow may not be as important to a smaller practice. You should discuss their operation, patient service style and services offered. You should also verify the use of the EHR in light of your expectations. For example, a reference site may be using the PMS portion, but may be working on installing the EHR. The interaction between the EHR and PMS should be discussed. You want to verify the viability of connecting your PMS with the reviewed EHR.
>
> **EHR Process**—Discuss their selection process and implementation experience. Get the names of key vendor players and comments on their performance. You should seek out the identity of knowledgeable support staff, project managers and other vendor staff. You'll identify key vendor staff that can help your EHR effort. You may also get a whiff of any employee turnover problems within the vendor, which can tell you something.
>
> **EHR Use**—You should discuss the use of the EHR in the practice. Ask about information on workflow changes, successes and failures as well as strategies used to succeed. Gather information on charting, workflow and paper medical records. Make sure you follow-up on any of your concerns and special issues.

Current users of the EHR may have more practical advice and solutions than the vendor trainers and support staff.

A sample form for reference checking and site visits is contained at the end of this chapter.

CONDUCTING SITE VISITS

Site visits are useful to review an actual implementation of the EHR, as well as familiarizing yourself with the potential of the EHR. Site visits are expensive due to the loss of office time, and in some cases, travel expenses. However, site visits allow you to see the product in action, and to interact with someone who has gone through the process.

Before committing to a site visit, you should conduct an interview similar to a reference check. Make sure that the practice is a comparable operation. Ideally, the practice should be of similar size and clinical focus to yours. You should also verify the use of the EHR in light of your expectations. For example, an office that is not paperless may not be a good site visit for a practice that wants a paperless medical record.

Make sure you talk about your practice's situation and objectives. You may also discuss their selection process, implementation experience and the objectives of your visit. You should explain the size of your site visit team and verify that the activities that your want to see will be taking place while you're there. For example, avoid a day when few patients are scheduled and the doctors are in surgery.

Your site visit team should consist of at least one clinician and one operations person. The site visit should allow the team to view the current operation and use of the EHR. The visit should include viewing the use of the EHR during a patient visit, as well as how information flows in the office. Ideally, your team should run through the entire operation and view all areas where the EHR is in use.

After each site visit, your entire EHR evaluation team should meet to discuss the findings and observations of the site visit team. The key successes and problems should be noted as well as strategies that the practice should use in its continuing EHR efforts, including possible additional site visits.

EHR REFERENCE CHECK/SITE VISIT QUESTIONNAIRE

Practice Name: _____ Phone: _____

Type: _____

Number of: Doctors: _____ Staff: _____ Locations: _____

Contact: _____ Position: _____

What were 3 key compelling reasons that the practice bought the product?

1.

2.

3.

What were 3 areas where the product has exceeded the practice's expectations?

1.

2.

3.

Cite 3 areas where the product has not met your practice's expectations.

1.

2.

3.

Evaluate the following vendor services:

Implementation: ❏ Poor ❏ Average ❏ Good ❏ Outstanding

Why? _____

_____

Training: ❏ Poor ❏ Average ❏ Good ❏ Outstanding

Why? _____

_____

Continuing Support: ❏ Poor ❏ Average ❏ Good ❏ Outstanding

Why? _____

_____

Date product was used as the primary source of your medical record information: _____

Was the date above: ❑ Before   ❑ On   ❑ After the expected activation date?

Why? _____
_____

Has the practice eliminated paper medical records? ❑ Yes   ❑ No

If yes, how long did it take to eliminate paper medical records and what were the key issues/problems you ran into:
_____
_____

If no, what are the reasons that you still use paper medical records:
_____
_____

In what ways is the EHR superior to paper medical charts?

1.

2.

3.

In what ways is the current EHR not as good as paper medical charts?

1.

2.

3.

What were the key strategies used to transition the doctors to the EHR?

1.

2.

3.

If you could go back through the implementation of the EHR, what would you change?

_____
_____
_____

What advice do you have for our practice in implementing the EHR product?

_____

_____

_____

Please rate the effect of the new EHR in the following areas:

Patient Service	❏ Less Effective	❏ Same	❏ Improved
Clinical Workflow	❏ Less Effective	❏ Same	❏ Improved
Staff Productivity	❏ Less Effective	❏ Same	❏ Improved
Doctor Productivity	❏ Less Effective	❏ Same	❏ Improved
Record Accuracy	❏ Less Effective	❏ Same	❏ Improved

How long did it take before things calmed down (non-chaotic) after EHR implementation? _____

Why? _____

_____

What specific items were done to help speed this process? _____

_____

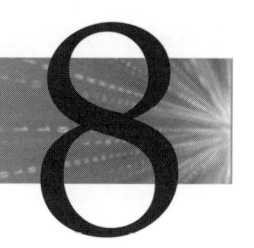

Making a Final Decision

The final selection of the EHR is rarely a slam dunk proposition. If that were the case, far fewer that 400 different options would be offered in the marketplace. Typically, the EHR decision is mostly a choice between closely matched product options.

To make a final decision, you need to focus on the key differences between the products based on the information you have compiled. If you try to rationalize 100 or more items, then you may have difficulty working through the analysis.

Your final decisions should be based on an analysis of your product evaluation as well as a clear understanding of the costs of each EHR.

SUMMARIZING THE EVALUATION

Compiling the information from your evaluation into a meaningful summary is a challenge. You could have hundreds of data points and many comments. You need to create an easy to understand metric from a complex set of information. Considering the detailed evaluation backs up the summary, you can simplify the comparison as follows:

> **Eliminate Criteria When all Products Met the Standard**—To highlight the differences between the products, you could ignore items where all of the products met the requirement. For example, if all of the EHR products have interfaces with your PMS, then the evaluation criteria could be ignored. Items where product scores differ would not be eliminated. Eliminating these criteria would highlight the quantitative difference between the products. For example, say, three prod-

ucts scored between 200 and 220 in total based on the evaluation effort. If 80 points for each product represented meeting the same exact features, then the difference in scores is actually 120 to 140. The 20-point difference is then more significant as a percentage of the total score.

Categorize Results—Categorizing results helps you focus on areas where the products differ. The total score could obscure issues that may be important for you. For example, serious deficiencies in workflow may be offset by a good training program. The results can be categorized using the categories from your evaluation list. You may compile summary scores for technology, HIPAA support, workflow, interfaces, clinical content, patient order management, patient service, training, reporting, cost and support.

Weighted Scores—A weighted score is calculated by multiplying the evaluation score by an importance factor. You may assign importance factors to each evaluation item or to the category. For example, you may use a weighting factor of 3 for critical requirements, 2 for general items and 1 for nice-to-have features. The weighted scores ensures that a less important requirement does not offset a more important item. For example, you may assign a low weight to PMS interface and a high weight to workflow capabilities.

Occurrence Summaries—Occurrence summaries are counts of the number of scores received by each product in each scoring category (e.g., 10–0s, 21–1s, 57–2s, and 26–3s). The occurrence summary quantitatively presents the number of deficiencies and does not shield problems with outstanding scores in other areas. For example, missing lab order features will not be offset by outstanding workflow features. Occurrence summaries will help you identify the product that met the most requirements.

These various scoring methods are not mutually exclusive. You may calculate and consider all of these measures in making your final decision.

HARDWARE PROVISIONING

In a typical EHR purchase, hardware represents 20%-40% of the EHR cost. EHR implementations frequently result in massive changes to the current practice technology base. You may have some existing hardware that you intend to use with the system but you will **probably not have the number of workstations needed** to support an EHR. Most practices will need to buy the main EHR computer server, additional workstations, tablet devices, scanners and a whole host of equipment and system licenses. Indeed, you may have to replace substantial portions of your technology infrastructure to handle the EHR.

How these changes are implemented and who is responsible for these changes will be part of your final decision process. Excluding all other issues (including cost), you would prefer to have a single vendor and point of responsibility. However, hardware provisioning varies widely among EHR vendors. Some EHR vendors sell all of the hardware you need directly, while other EHR vendors have a preferred hardware vendor. Several EHR vendors do not sell any hardware. Some EHR vendors are not competitive on price, and many vendors do not want to accept responsibility for your existing hardware.

Depending on your situation, the practice should decide from whom the hardware will be purchased. As a practical matter, you have three options: (1) Buy all hardware from the EHR vendor, (2) buy all hardware from another source (e.g., local systems integrator) or (3) purchase the server from the EHR vendor and other hardware from other sources.

If you have a current hardware supplier, you may be tempted to buy equipment from it. Since your existing vendor knows your system, the vendor will be able to more effectively analyze the changes that are needed. **ALERT:** However, your existing vendor may lack experience with the EHR product. Nonetheless, some practices have gone to the expense of keeping their local supplier involved in the EHR project. Continuing involvement may include paying the local vendor to get trained on the setup of the EHR and your new hardware as well as serving as a technical advisor to the practice. Under this arrangement, you maintain a local resource that may be able to more quickly respond to problems and more easily keep track of continuing advancements for your system. An added benefit of using the local vendor is that the local resource can serve as a sounding board for any technical issues raised or specified by your EHR vendor. For example, you EHR vendor may sell one brand of hardware since they get the best deal, but another hardware vendor may have better support in your local area. Similarly, the EHR vendor may have limited experience with high availability systems that you may choose to use. **CAUTION**: If you change hardware vendors or use the EHR vendor for your hardware, you will have to pay the new vendor to learn your system.

Some EHR vendors have working relationships with select hardware vendors. Depending on volume, the EHR vendor may or may not have much influence with the hardware vendor. In some cases, the hardware vendor may not have a good support system in your area and you may end up with hardware support from a local third party. The EHR hardware vendor may not understand your current hardware system or setup. **CAUTION:** Many hardware vendors may come into your practice and recommend a number of changes. In some cases, the recommendations will not improve your situation, but will bring your system in line with their "standard products." For example, the vendor may prefer a different backup device and software product even though your existing backup system may be adequate or even more widely used. Unfortunately, the "standard products" usually aren't better that the products you have currently installed.

If your practice buys hardware components from a variety of sources, you may encounter problems holding anyone accountable for problems. A variety of vendors can be particularly vexing when you are trying to solve a problem. For example, one practice couldn't get their tablets from one vendor to work with the practice's wireless network from another vendor. All of the tablets had to be replaced. Interestingly, the replacement was not technically necessary, but the two vendors could not agree on a workable solution and strategy. Due to these problems, the project was delayed several months.

Similarly, practices that try to mix and match equipment may have problems getting the entire system to work together.

You could end up paying several vendors to learn each other's products and solve your problems. **CAUTION**: On occasion, the only way to solve a problem is to have a representative from each of the vendors working on the problem together in your facility and billing your account. To avoid such problems, the practice should have an in-house or local advisor to maintain current information on the system and act as the practice's advocate in dealing with the various vendors. For more technical issues, you may even have a more experienced local technical resource to supplement your own staff for more complex problems.

The best strategy is to limit the variables and vendors. If you have a local hardware support group, you may be better off letting it handle your computer network, workstations, tablets, scanners, network infrastructure and installation. Of course, if you have an internal IT support staff, you are in a better position to mix and match hardware sources. **TIP**: Another way to limit issues is to assign support for the EHR server to the EHR vendor. The EHR vendor is responsible for managing the one point in the system where your alternative hardware vendor may lack expertise. The clear line of responsibility will help you keep the vendors accountable for their areas and limit the points of dispute.

The hardware purchase should be supported by the hardware standards from the EHR vendor. In comparing various vendors, you will find that most EHR products use the same basic hardware. However, products may differ in their hardware requirements. For example, some vendors require separate test and production servers, while others may require a separate server for the EHR and a dedicated server for images. A few products can even put the entire EHR setup on a single server. EHR vendors may also require different types of access to your system and control over the various aspects of your installation. For example, some vendors will not provide the passwords to administer their EHR servers. **TIP**: Make sure that the EHR vendor has published hardware specifications that you can rely on to configure the hardware for your specific situation.

Your hardware selection and strategy reflects your tolerance for a system loss. This strategy can affect the cost of a system. Your hardware strategy may include the following.

High-Availability Hardware—High availability hardware includes redundant components that allow the EHR to operate in the event of certain hardware failures. For example, a power supply failure will not affect a system with redundant power supplies. Cluster servers offer an even higher level of availability by providing you with "twin systems" to support the EHR. If a component fails in the main server, the clustered server immediately takes over. Due to continued drops in cost, cluster server setups are available for under $30,000. Additional protection is available by allowing for multiple servers in your network to manage system resources and performance. For example, a network uses an active directory server (ADS) to keep track of what all the users are doing. A problem with the ADS could cause a complete system failure. However, for a relatively modest additional investment, you could add a second ADS to your system. A variety of other components (Ex. Routers, Tablets, Workstations, Scanners) can be protected and backed up according to your tolerance for failure balanced with the cost of the additional protection.

Server Hosting—Your EHR and other servers could be placed with a computer-hosting or co-location organization. The computer-hosting facility typically provides power generators and batteries to avoid problems due to power failures as well as redundant communication lines. The hosting facility will also be secured and include environmental controls for your system. In some cases, the hosting company will provide backup hardware in the event of EHR server failure. Hosting fees would be included in your cost comparison. For example, one vendor may have an arrangement with a hosting facility that is less expensive that the other vendors. **ALERT:** Hosting facilities typically charge a monthly fee and may have usage-based fees. You may also incur additional expenses for communications expenses from the main office (that would have severed as the EHR-server location) to the host site. **TIP**: A number of communication companies that you buy your data lines from may offer co-location services at a discount when you buy a package of services.

ASP (Application Services Provider)—Many EHR products are available through ASPs. Software as a Service (known as SaaS) is similar to an ASP offering. ASPs provide the servers to support selected EHR products as well as the hosting facility. The ASP charges are typically based on users and provider-based fees on top of the hosting fees. The ASP strategy will minimize your upfront license cost since the ASP owns the licenses that they rent to your practice. **CAUTION**: ASP offerings vary widely in what is included in the fee and what your practice gets for the fee. For example, some ASP costs do not include training and initial implementation costs. **TIP**: If you choose the ASP option, make sure that you fully understand the "exit" strategy in the event that you switch to another product in the future, or decide to bring the EHR inhouse.

Backup Sites—Some EHR vendors now offer backup sites that could be used in the event of a catastrophic loss of your system. On a periodic basis, your new data is sent to the backup site and posted to an operational version of your database. In the even of a system loss, your users would be switched to the backup site and have access to your data as of the last update. Note that updates could occur with every transaction, every hour, or within any other period you choose.

Backup Servers—Blade servers allow you to quickly replace a defective server with an operational server. Blade servers are less expensive than cluster servers and can be swapped by a trained computer support person.

Hardware issues should be resolved as you work on compiling the EHR cost comparison. As you prepare the cost comparison, you will develop your hardware strategy and sources. The cost comparison will more closely reflect the final purchase costs and strategy.

COMPARING PRODUCT COSTS

Comparing costs of products is intentionally complex. Vendors do not want you to price shop their offering and products. Vendor pricing strategies and service levels vary widely. For example, one vendor quoted 175 hours of implementation support, while a competing vendor quoted almost 400 hours of support. Which vendor was right? Using the same hourly rate, was the 400-hour vendor more expensive?

To compare product costs, you should solicit a proposal based on the specific hardware, software and services needed to implement the EHR. At this point in your process, you should ask for the vendor's best and final quote. Otherwise, you will have to update your analysis each time the vendor updates its proposal. Many vendors calculate the number of users based on classifications of various staff types (e.g., doctors, mid-levels, nurses, technicians and non-clinical users). Other vendors have a single license fee for all users. Either way, the number of users will be an important issue for the vendor. The following information should be presented to the vendor to insure that you will receive an accurate and practical quote for your practice:

Number of Entities—If your practice operates under a number of corporate entities, you may have to pay a license fee for each entity. In some cases, you may also have to pay user fees for each staff person who may access the EHR. For example, if your practice is associated with a therapy group, optical shop or ASC that is a different corporation, you may have to pay additional fees for the second corporation. Additionally, you may have to pay a separate license fee for a staff member who may need to access information for both organizations (e.g., billing office staffers who work on the practice and the ASC).

Physicians and Providers—The number of physicians and providers should include all medical decision-makers. Many vendors will charge full provider licenses for any party that is billing under his own ID. If your practice uses part-time providers, mid-level providers who bill under a doctor's billing number and residents, don't forget these providers in your budget and your negotiations with the vendor. **ALERT:** A number of vendors charge license fees based on the number of providers but only allow for a specific number of users per provider. For example, you may be allowed only 5 users for each provider even though the license states that you are paying per provider. If you have a higher number of users per provider, you could have to pay additional fees.

Clinical Staff—Clinical staff includes technicians, nurses and other parties. These employees will need access to the EHR, and will count in the user total. **TIP**: Clinical staff may also need additional licenses to access the PMS system. Review the PMS access cost because an integrated system may not require such additional PMS licenses.

Other Users—A variety of administrative, billing and front-desk staff will need access to the EHR to interact with clinical staff and access medical records. The front desk staff may flag a patient who is ready for service as well as notify doctors of scanned medical information. Billing staff may access the medical record to support insurance claims and other functions. **TIP**: Ask for lower cost licenses for non-clinical users. Some vendors will do this. Other vendors include all users equally in the licensed user count.

Locations—The number of locations may affect certain hardware and software issues. Some EHR licenses include additional fees for each location. To support remote locations, you may need additional servers and licensed software. For example, some vendors charge a remote scanning license fee for any office that scans documents.

Hardware Specifications—To receive a realistic hardware configuration, you should specify your hardware requirements. The hardware requirements may include redundant components and fail safe options. For example, you may specify an uninterruptible power supply as well as hot swap disk configurations to mitigate the risk of a system stoppage. You may also ask for a full system proposal and a proposal that only includes the EHR server with all other hardware being supplied by your current hardware vendor. Be sure you consider your entire computer network and not just the vendor requirements. For example, you may use the new system backup for the PMS, document server and other systems, including the EHR. Similarly, you may need an additional server to manage the interface between your EHR and PMS.

Interfaces—The list of expected interfaces should be presented to the vendor. You may need interfaces for the PMS, diagnostic equipment and your lab information system. You may also need an interface for exchanges with hospitals and other practices. In addition to the interfaces you need now, you may also want to get information on any additional interfaces you may need. For example, the next time you are buying diagnostic equipment, consider products that are already interfaced with your EHR. Note that interfaces can require additional hardware. For example, the interface between a piece of diagnostic equipment and the EHR may require an additional workstation in the same room with the diagnostic equipment. **CAUTION**: You may need an interface server to manage the interfaces between the EHR and your PMS, or other devices.

Training and Services—You may include information on your training expectations and/or plan. Key items include the number of people to be trained and whether you will use a train-the-trainer plan. If you are comparing a vendor that uses a train-the-trainer approach versus full vendor training, consider any additional costs you may incur for overtime and/or replacement staff for your internal training effort. For example, you may need to hire your own trainer and set up a training facility. **TIP**: Many practices need more training services than the practice or the vendor anticipates. You should set aside some contingency money for additional training efforts. This will ensure you include the full cost of the training in your comparison. You may also include information on the onsite services you expect for the project. For example, you may have three sites that will require an onsite vendor representative on the Go Live date.

In some cases, vendors will present a single price for the system. However, you will need an unbundled price to compare the product with other proposals. In the event that the vendor will not provide a price breakdown, you may be able to break down the fixed price based on costs you have access to. For example, you may be able to get hardware quotes directly from the hardware vendors and back out services based on the vendor's hourly rate.

Once you have received the proposal or quote, you should compare the proposed systems in a table. A sample budget comparison table is included at the end of this chapter. Note that the table includes various components with a space for costs and maintenance fees. The comparison table also includes a space for contingencies. Vendor-specific contingencies may be based on a number of issues including hardware upgrades that may be needed and additional training services for a more complex technology.

The totals cover the acquisition cost and maintenance cost as well as a projected 5-year cost, including maintenance. The 5-year total expense will help you analyze the true cost of each product. For example, some EHR vendors have low license fees, but high maintenance costs. You can add projections for maintenance cost increases, equipment upgrades and replacements and an imputed interest rate to the cost comparison. You should also compute a monthly cost that can be used to analyze return-on-investment (ROI) and the payback from the projected savings and additional revenues.

Compiling the price comparison does require some analysis and creativity. Consider the following issues.

Scope—Each vendor may include different things in its proposals and costs. Vendors have a variety of methods to calculate charges and the scope of services could vary widely among practices. For example, some vendors omit subscription and acquisition costs for clinical content that may be needed from a third-party vendor. Other vendors may propose a basic system that will require a number of additional components and additional investment. In some cases, the vendor strategy may differ from your own. For example, some vendors provide training, but do not provide any advisory or practice management services. **CAUTION**: Additional services could spike your EHR costs. For example, customization of the EHR could represent a substantial cost that is not accounted for. At a minimum, the practice should allow for some contingency funds for customization. Other vendors include training in the base cost of the software license. Some vendors offer training at their offices while others may train at your office. Travel expenses may have to be weighed. Note that travel costs could be based on situations beyond your control. For example, a vendor may assign resources to your practice that is farther from your location that the vendor's nearest office.

Missing Items—If you have an item for one vendor and not others, then you need to determine if the item is needed or not. In some cases, the additional item is a requirement of the particular EHR. For example, some EHRs require a server to run email, while others have email built into their product. In other cases, the vendor has failed to address all you needs. For example, most practices will want a fax server or similar service to avoid scanning incoming faxes into the EHR. **ALERT:** Some vendors may fail to quote a remote terminal services server needed for remote users. If you have many remote users, and are concerned with performance, you may be able to minimize the communication requirements with a Windows terminal server and perhaps a Citrix metaframe. Note that ".NET" based products natively operate efficiently over the Internet. .NET based products do not need a remote terminal server. **CAUTION:** Some products are a mixture of .NET and technologies that will require a remote terminal server.

Cost Basis—Due to a wide variety of vendor strategies and issues, the EHR cost is frequently obscured. Many products are based on standard hardware infrastructures that are comparable. However, you will want to eliminate differences that you would address in any purchase agreement.

> **Better Hardware**—Hardware prices may vary due to more capacity or additional features to protect you from failure. For example, a $30,000 server may provide you a smaller chance of a complete hardware failure than a basic $10,000 server would. Do you consider the $30,000 server more expensive if it offered greater protection? If the hardware differences are due to better equipment then you should normalize the hardware items to the level of products that you expect to buy. For example, fully redundant disks, power supplies and fans should be included for any practice, but a cluster server (where two systems share a common set of storage devices) may be desired by a large practice. Similarly, a very basic workstation proposed by one vendor may be replaced with a better workstation that would be included in all vendor quotes.
>
> **Comprehensive Quotes**—Some vendors quote basic systems that you would not buy. For example, they may quote undersized hardware and exclude modules that you will need to buy (e.g., lab system interfaces). In some cases, the quote may not include items that depend upon implementation decisions. For example, if you decide to scan the old paper charts, you will need a lot more storage space. To make sure that you have all of the components you will need, verify the quote against your evaluation criteria as well as inventory the interfaces that you will need. In the event that a vendor does not include a component you know you will need, you can add the item to the vendor quote based on other cost information you may have. For example, you could plug in a tablet price based on a quote you can get from a hardware vendor. If the vendor does not include a price for training, you could apply the

vendor's training rate against the expected training hours you'll need from the other vendors.

Implementation Services—Implementation services are frequently quoted as a basket of hours to be used by the practice. However, you can find differences between the rates. Rates for services can range from $75-$250/hour or more depending on the level of staff and vendor rates. Make sure that the basket of hours proposed by the vendor would meet your requirements. If necessary, adjust the basket of hours to conform to your own implementation needs or the standard. Alternatively, you can assign all vendors the same level of hours and use the quoted vendor rate. Contingency allowances can also be used to permit for differences in the services' quote. For example, one vendor included a "reasonable" training program in the cost of the EHR. However, this estimate was based on a much larger number of hours than what was considered necessary. Note that some vendors limit the time when you can use purchased hours. For example, you may need to use the purchased hours within 12 months of the purchase. Make sure that you do not buy more hours than you can reasonably use during the implementation time limit.

Licenses—Using the number of users, providers and other counts, verify that the proposed license will meet your needs. A slight change in your license count could up the cost of the system. For example, some EHRs are licensed by provider, but only allow so many licenses for each provider. If you are above the users-per-provider count, you may have to pay additional fees. Note that you need to get the correct number of licenses in the analysis for each vendor. Otherwise, you could end up with incorrect figures and harm your comparison. For example, practices that use mid-level providers will want to be certain about how such providers are licensed. **TIP**: Some EHR vendors charge mid-level providers the same price as doctors, while others reduced the rate, sometimes even to nothing. Similarly, some vendors require EHR licenses for non-clinical users (Ex. Billers and appointment schedulers) while other vendors charge for each workstation. Thereby, you would have to pay additional fees for workstations that you may place to promote use of the EHR, but could not possibly be in use at once since your employee count is less than your number of workstations.

Functionality—The cost comparison should account for comparable functionality between the products. For example, one EHR vendor may offer an imaging product that allows for extensive indexing of scanned images. Another vendor may offer a more basic scanning product with the EHR, with an optional module that offers advanced indexing. You should include the more advanced scanning module for a more precise comparison.

Support Costs—Support costs are a major component of any EHR purchase. Support costs can range from 15%-33% of the original license cost on an annual basis. Support costs should include annual payments for clinical content, drug databases and other subscription items. Make sure the support costs account for any other adjustments you have made. Additional hardware and licenses could affect support costs. The support costs should be used to calculate a 5 year system cost. Such an analysis will help you determine the true cost of the system when the vendors use different support cost factors. **CAUTION:** Failure to correctly calculate support costs could distort your budget and costs. For example, some vendors include the first year of support costs in the purchase cost of the software. Additionally, the start date for support charges can be significant. For example, some vendors start support charges when the software is delivered, while other vendors start charging for support upon the completion of training.

Discounts—Some vendors will offer a system discount to compel you to buy the product. The offered discount should be included in the cost comparison. The discount line can be updated as you proceed with vendor negotiations. Note that discounts may be available for end-of-period purchases, combined EHR and PMS purchases and previous customers, among other offers.

Modularization of the Product—Vendors use a dizzying array of packaging techniques to sell their systems. Some EHRs are sold as a complete product with few options. Other vendors may sell a prescription module, transcription module and a clinical charting module. **CAUTION**: Some vendors charge for each area of medicine and/or clinical content package. To assure accuracy, verify that your evaluation requirements are covered by the proposed modules. Otherwise, you could be surprised to find out you need an additional area of medicine module. You should be especially careful for modules that are included in the companion PMS, but not the PMS that you will use with the EHR. For example, an appointment module may be needed to store appointment information in the EHR that is downloaded from your PMS.

Additional Upgrades—Depending on your situation, you should determine what, if any, additional modifications will be needed for the EHR. Upgrades to your existing network, and licensing current software versions may be necessary and should be included in your comparison. For example, one product may require licenses updates or even new workstations while another product may be able to work with the current system. **Warning:** You may need to move to an updated version of the PMS or the "next generation" PMS product to use the "companion" EHR product.

Clinical Content Development—Many EHR products have clinical content for selected specialties and clinical areas. The clinical content may consist of specific templates, system setups, pick lists and other tools to ease the implementation effort. Some vendors include clinical content assistance while others assume that the practice will perform all of the clinical content setup. Vendors may also offer a forum to access the clinical content setups that have been developed by other practices. Depending on your needs and analysis of the clinical content, you may want to allow for an appropriate level of clinical content support. If you are perfectly content with the current clinical content, then you may need minimal support. If you like the product but expect extensive clinical content changes, then you allow for a higher level of assistance. Note that clinical content development and enhancement can add substantial amounts to the cost of your EHR and lengthen your implementation timeline.

The completed cost comparison permits you to measure the incremental costs with the qualitative differences between the products you are considering.

FINAL DECISION

After collecting information on the capabilities of the product, impressions of staff, reference checks and site visits, you will have an extensive body of data that needs to be consolidated into a manageable and easy-to-understand form. The rest of the practice will not be in the position to review all of the data that you have uncovered.

When summarizing information, be concise. Of course, each of your conclusions will be backed up with the more detailed analyses. You may present a minimalist comparison of the products that merely rates features, support, services, references and cost. You may also provide another level of detail that addresses feature categories and/or cost components. In some cases, a ranking of the products in each category will help crystallize your final analysis. **TIP**: Rank the products as first, second and third in cost, support, features and references. Note that you may want to break down features in your summary into general areas, such as system support, workflow and clinical content.

Note that cost is a factor, but not *the* factor. In many cases, dramatic cost differences between products may be attributed to the different capabilities of the product or the target market. In many cases, you can negotiate away differences between comparable EHR products. However, you should seek a product that will work in your practice over a product that may be less expensive, but may require more labor on your part (e.g., clinical content development).

Feel free to try a couple of these summarization methods to identify the one or two top products for your practice. **TIP**: If you end up without a clear winner, don't panic. You may have been lucky enough to identify more than one product that could be successfully installed in your practice. That is you may have one or more good options that could satisfy your needs.

When presented with this situation, many practices will expend a significant amount of time and effort to arrive at the "best" decision. The lack of a "best" decision may result in no decision at all, but to continue to sap the time and resources in the decision-making process. If you cannot choose one option as the "best," then consider yourself fortunate and make a decision. In reality, you need to be careful to not exhaust yourself or the practice in making a decision, and then lack the energy to tackle the hard tasks associated with actual implementation.

Before you go any further, take a reality check. If necessary, call the top 1 or 2 vendors in for another demonstration. You need to be absolutely certain that the product can be effectively implemented and used in your practice. You should be planning the implementation of the product and visualizing the product in your practice to validate your final decision.

The actual presentation of your final recommendation should be carefully staged and prepared. Have your summaries, supporting documentation and list of vendors that you considered. Typically, the recommendation is made during a presentation to the management team, doctors, operations committee or some other group in the practice. The presentation should explain the EHR selection process, discuss options that were explored and then present concise summary information with your recommendation. The presentation should include the go-forward plan for the final decision, necessary negotiations and the implementation process.

As a matter of due diligence, the attendees will ask questions that should require going down a level or two into the details. The object of the meeting should be to pick one or two products and to proceed to the next step.

If you have made your choice or want to continue considering two products, you should feel comfortable if either choice would work for your practice. For the next steps, don't proceed with any product that you could not use.

To build support and enthusiasm for the chosen product or to make the final choice, you should schedule a drop-in day for the remaining vendor(s). The drop-in day is your opportunity to let your doctors and staff, see and touch the product. Don't present any product to the staff that could not realistically be purchased by the practice. The drop-in day should be scheduled to present the system to various groups of doctors and staff. You should schedule four or more sessions that will run through a script (similar to the script used for demonstrations) and allow employees to ask questions. This way, employees have several opportunities to see the product throughout the day and you can rekindle interest in the EHR project as well as jump start everyone on the daunting implementation task ahead.

If you have chosen the product, you can start work on contract negotiations before the drop-in day. If you're down to two final options, seek employee feedback to help you make the ultimate decision. Actively ask for their input. After choosing your EHR product, begin contract negotiations.

After making your final decision, you will hear from doctors and vendors about additional products, updates to products that you considered, and, in some cases, scare tactics to reopen your process. You should be prepared to address these issues in a methodical manner and seek to avoid any serious buyer's remorse. In many cases, the scare tactics are just that. Have enough confidence in your process and the analysis behind your decision to proceed with the selected EHR.

TABLE 8.1

EHR Cost Comparison	PRODUCT 1		PRODUCT 2	
	Cost	Maintenance	Cost	Maintenance
Servers				
EHR Application				
Remote Access				
Imaging				
Backup				
Fax Server				
System Software				
Software				
Wireless Network				
Firewall				
Printers				
Color				
Standard				
Scanners				
Front Desk Page				
Medium Volume				
High Volume				
Workstations/Tablets				
Workstation Upgrades				
Additional Workstations				
Tablets				
Network Upgrades				
Inter-Office				
Intra-Office				
Application Software				
EHR				
Imaging				
PMS Interfaces				
Lab Interfaces				
Diagnostic Interfaces				
Clinical Content				
Installation				

	PRODUCT 1		PRODUCT 2	
EHR Cost Comparison	**Cost**	**Maintenance**	**Cost**	**Maintenance**
Training				
Monthly Hosting Fees				
Less System Discount				
Totals				
Hardware Contingency				
Software Contingency				
Training Contingency				
Other Contingency				
Total with Contingencies				
5-Year Total Cost				
5-Year Monthly Cost				

Negotiating a Contract

By the time you have decided on a particular system, you may be so exhausted that you are in no position or mood to work your way through page after page of unreadable and less-than understandable contract text. Our first impulse is to rely on the vendor's agreement since "they do this all the time." However, the practice is clearly at a disadvantage since you will be depending on the capabilities and features of the EHR to service all of your patients. Your vendor is only at risk for the dissatisfaction of a single practice.

A contract is an agreement between two parties that establishes the rights and responsibilities of each party. What we think the vendor should do, and stand behind, is frequently very different from what most vendor contracts say. Consider some quick examples:

No Warranty—Many vendors exclude any warranty from your agreement. They will not contractually stand behind their product, services, hardware or software. In the event of a problem with the product, your practice may not have much contractual leverage.

Pay Before they do Anything—Many vendors want 50% of the cost when you sign the contract and another 50% when they drop the boxes of their product on your office floor (or in some cases when they ship the boxes from their plant). So, you have paid all your money out before you even see what's in the box.

Termination Clause—Most vendor contracts empower the vendor to terminate your ability to use the EHR on demand for a whole list of terrible actions including non-payment, letting non-employees see the system, making copies of their materials, moving the system and even buying additional equipment. Of course, the contract does not consider the irreparable harm and severe economic losses that would occur if the practice lost access to the EHR for even a few hours.

You need to be very clear about what you are and are not expecting from the EHR vendor. On the other side, vendors have certain things that they do, and certain things they do not do. Although, you should not buy an EHR or sign a contract with a vendor that you do not trust, you also should ensure that the contract protects your interests and effectively structures your relationship with the EHR vendor. A checklist is included at the end of this chapter to help frame your contract negotiating efforts.

Your initial contract effort should focus on the business deal and the relationship with the vendor. If you cannot work out the business points, then you should not waste your time trying to decipher the lengthy terms and conditions in the contract documents.

NEGOTIATING BUSINESS POINTS

To make the best use of your time, you need to identify the business relationship and the parties involved in the negotiations. Otherwise, you could spend a lot of time negotiating an agreement that you will never sign since the basic business agreement is not completed or acceptable. For example, you may not be able to get any support for a warranty from the vendor.

Key business points can be significantly affected by the contract terms and other aspects of your agreements with the chosen vendor. The key business points include:

Buy An EHR or an EHR Service

Many vendors offer an option to purchase their product on a system that will be installed in your office or as a service through an Application Service Provider (ASP) or Software as a Service (SaaS) offering. In the ASP/SaaS model, the Smaller practices may be attracted to the ASP/SaaS.

Vendor(s)

One of the more confusing aspects of negotiating contracts for the purchase of an EHR is who you are buying products from. Many EHR vendors are selling components from various vendors that are integral to making their system work. The EHR vendor may be selling software from one company, services from a second company and hardware from a third. In the event of a problem, you could end up in endless expensive discussions between two or more entities. For example, your EHR vendor may sell you software from another vendor to support voice recognition or faxing, but you may have to pay additional fees to the other software vendor to get support for any problems. **TIP:** Some of these situations include a second agreement from the EHR publisher that is presented at the last minute for signing. Make sure that you get copies of all of the agreements and paperwork that you will need to establish the relationship with the vendor and purchase the EHR.

The EHR vendor should take full responsibility for the EHR and the EHR working relationship with the various components regardless of where these components originate. In some cases, the vendor excludes any responsibility for third party software that, unknown to you, is a key component of the product you are buying. For example, your EHR may use a built-in imaging product from a vendor you have not heard of. If the EHR vendor does not take responsibility for working with these key third party components, then you need to identify the other software vendors that you may need to contact in the event of a problem between your EHR and these third party products.

Vendor and Practice Responsibilities

To produce a practical contract and successfully implement the EHR, the practice needs to clearly understand the vendor responsibilities as well as the responsibilities of the practice or other third parties. In most projects, the practice does not get a handle on these issues until the project is well under way. The delay in identifying these responsibilities can lead to a lot of confusion and additional costs.

Unfortunately, many vendors will not let you see their plan until you have purchased their system. Some vendors have extensive lists of tasks in a project management table, while others develop the project plan as you proceed. In most cases, you will need to create your own list of tasks to implement the EHR. Some key issues to understand in the context of the contract follow:

- What vendors are supplying what components?
- Has the EHR vendor verified the components and services purchased from other parties?
- Who will install the hardware?
- Who will install the software on the hardware and verify that the entire system is working?
- What documents will be presented to the practice to explain the hardware configuration?
- What are the training packages and timeframes for the training effort?
- What are the training responsibilities of the vendor and practice?
- What are the project and management responsibilities for the EHR vendor, other vendors and the practice?
- Who will represent the practice in dispute resolution with the EHR vendor?

For more information on managing the EHR implementation, see **Chapter 10—Implementing an EHR**. Make sure you clearly understand how the basic components of the project will be performed and who will be responsible for it.

Price

Many EHR systems use the same basic hardware setups. The pricing differences typically show up in the cost of the software, services and maintenance that the vendor provides to the practice. Some vendors will provide a discount on various components (e.g., discount licenses, lower the hourly service rate), while other vendors will offer a total system discount. Note that your comparison of price between two systems should include the maintenance fees over a certain evaluation period (e.g., 5 years). The key issue is the bottom price of the system (see **Chapter 8—Making a Final Decision**). To negotiate the price, you should have a detailed breakdown of the proposal, and insure that the "discount" is not based on cutting services or items that you will probably have to reinstate later. For example, one practice elected to have its training and implementation hours cut in half to "lower" the EHR cost. In another situation, a practice had to completely upgrade their hardware when they implemented the EHR under their combined PMS and EHR purchase.

Using the calculated delivered cost of the system (in **Chapter 8**), rework your estimate to account for the actual counts of users and the specifics of your situation. In some cases, you may need to contact the vendor to get specific details on the costs. For example, the software quote may contain several components for a fixed price or as a complete package. In some cases, vendors include a set number of hours in the software license cost. For example, a vendor may allow for up to 4 hours of training per license, but that may not be sufficient for a more complex organization.

Determine the differences between the final selection and the other products for which you calculated cost comparisons. Some EHR vendors have a single charge per user/provider while other vendors have a charge per module per user/provider. Unfortunately some EHR systems use a combination of charges. For example, they may charge per provider for the clinical content, per user for the EHR and per workstation for the scanning application. Verify the specific licenses you need to insure that you don't buy items you don't need. When in doubt, buy the lower quantity and include a clause in the contract that lets you buy additional licenses at the same price within a certain period of time. From a budgeting perspective, you should include the additional cost in a contingency fee.

In the pricing review, ensure that you consider the strategic plans and foreseeable events for your practice. For example, servicing another legal entity (e.g., therapy center, ASC) and adding providers could trigger unexpected charges that could substantially impact the price to the practice. After completing your working documents, consider the following issues:

- Is the package price hiding overpriced items?
- Are industry standard hardware and software items fairly priced?
- Does the hourly rate for various services favorably compare with other vendors?
- Were volume discounts received for a large numbers of licenses, service hours and workstations/tablets?
- Are maintenance and support charges discounted for the level of support directly provided by the practice?
- Was an additional discount available for purchasing or committing to purchase items that the practice may not need for a few months?

Warranties

A surprising number of EHR vendors provide little to no warranty. The typical contract states that the "Vendor provides NO WARRANTY." Vendors have a wide range of excuses for such terms, but your practice needs some assurance that the vendor will stand behind their product, solve you problems and allow you to rely on their EHR as the primary repository of patient information for your practice. Otherwise, you should find another EHR product.

Note that the promise to refund your money and de-install the system is not a practical resolution to a warranty issue. After you have started the implementation process, the cost of switching EHR products will dramatically increase for your practice. After the EHR is in use, switching to another EHR is extremely difficult (see Chapter 10—Implementing an EHR). The key to warranty issues remains the resolution of the problem to your satisfaction. The cost of backing out of the EHR for your practice may be too high for you to practically move to another product.

Warranties should cover a number of areas:

Software—The EHR Software should work with the hardware and within a functional standard. The functional standard should be easily referenced and reviewed. **ALERT:** Many EHR systems lack sufficient documentation to specify how the product works. Indeed, some areas of the product may be adequately documented and other features may lack any documentation.

Hardware—Hardware should work with the software and perform at a level that is needed by the practice. **ALERT:** If you are not buying the hardware from the EHR vendor, make sure that the hardware vendor is committed to the EHR requirements.

Standards Support—Whether you are planning on taking advantage of the Stimulus Incentives or not, the vendor should provide a warranty that they will maintain Certified EHR (Electronic Healthcare Record) status and support Meaningful Use standards. These two items will be needed to make sure that you have the option or ability to meet the Stimulus Qualifications, or, if you are not interested in Stimulus Payments, maintain the marketability of the product that you are committing to. Additionally, the vendor should warrant that the product has features to support HIPAA Privacy, Security, and Transaction standards.

Services—Services should be provided by competent staff and the practice should be able to rely on their advice. Services should be provided at a level that is responsive to the practice. **TIP:** This warranty is important to insure that you do not have to pay for poor services and pay again to get the appropriate services.

Support—The support should be provided on a timely basis considering the problem, and support should be provided for a reasonable time after the practice has installed the EHR. **ALERT:** Many EHR vendors reserve the right to terminate support in a timeframe (Ex. 30 days) that would irreparably harm you practice and put your access to the EHR patient records at risk.

Support

Your support needs will vary with your internal capabilities and the abilities of your staff. In the course of negotiating business points, the practice should ensure that the correct level of support is accounted for and included in the contract. The level of support should include appropriate levels of training, phone, onsite and consultations on issues and problems.

Before you will be able to negotiate support, you should determine how you will support your EHR users. You may have an internal support person who filters all user issues and resolves most problems before ever going to the vendor. Some practices completely rely on the EHR vendor to support all users. Your support strategy can significantly affect your support costs.

Negotiating contract terms is a time consuming process. Justify your effort by ensuring the following business issues are pretty much complete before you deal with contract terms and conditions (Table 9.1).

When you have agreed to the business points with the vendor, then you are ready to work on the specific contract terms that will reflect the business agreement that you have reached as well as ensure a results-oriented working arrangement with the EHR vendor. Check business issues against the contract terms as you conduct contract negotiations. Be careful to preserve the business deal and not include specific terms that undermine or change the basic arrangement with the software vendor. For example, you may negotiate a training plan that is directly contradicted by the standard contract terms.

NEGOTIATING CONTRACT TERMS

EHR contracts widely range in complexity and terms. Each vendor has a different focus and issues that will be conveyed in its contract language. Some vendors may provide you with several agreements. For example, you may have a software license, support agreement and hardware agreement to evaluate and sign to buy the vendor's product as well as a license from the owner of the EHR software. You need to carefully review each agreement to insure it consistently and appropriately meets your needs.

Guide your contracting efforts by the following principles:

The vendor contract was written for the vendor—Vendor contracts are written by the vendor's lawyers to protect the vendor from losses, and limit its exposure. In general, vendors have a legitimate concern that someone will steal their ideas and strategies, but the terms that they impose can cause serious operational problems or easily place the practice in technical violation of the contract. As you will see in Table 9.2, vendor contracts contain a wide range of terms and conditions that can make your life difficult and expose you to unnecessary risks.

Everything is negotiable—EHR software vendors want your business. The sales people will typically not want to walk away from a potential customer because you will not agree to little protection for you investment. The vast majority of EHR vendors will work with you to develop a workable agreement.

You are not the only person to have a problem with the contract—Some vendors will tell you that everyone signs his contracts as is, and that they fail to

TABLE 9.1

Business Point	Issue	Recommendation
License Costs	Vendors may license EHRs by server, practice, provider, location and/or user. Some vendors use complex combinations of these factors in the licensing and contract terms. For example, some vendors license by provider, but limit the number of users per provider. Other vendors require licenses for all workstations in your practice rather than licensing the users. A few vendors even require a separate licensing fee for each location. To measure the importance of the licensing costs, you need to develop a realistic projection of the number of providers and users. Once you determine the various doctors, clinical staff, billers, and administrative users that will access the EHR, make sure that the license costs support the user base. Note that some vendors differentiate between doctors, mid-level clinicians and non-clinical users. User classifications can have a substantial effect on the license costs. For example, PAs who support the doctors but do not bill for patient services under their own biller numbers may cost substantially less to license than PAs who bill for patient services. These license terms should be carefully evaluated in light of your strategic plans and options. For example, you may want to evaluate the impact of adding a location or a new modality to your practice.	Consider the size of your practice; negotiate a volume discount for the licenses. Negotiate a reduced license fee for part-time providers and mid-level staff. Negotiate terms to allow for an appropriate number of "fill-in" providers and staff. Negotiate price issues where the other products may have included an item that is a separate cost for the selected product. Accommodate your growth by allowing for future purchases at a preferred rate. Verify that the license will allow for the workstations, locations and users that will be needed to practically use the EHR in your practice.
Service Costs	EHR purchases include a variety of services: hardware installation, software installation, clinical content development, project management, training and consulting. Service costs may be quoted on an hourly or fixed cost basis. Your practice should have a clear understanding of the scope of the quoted services as well as the real level of services that will be needed to complete the EHR implementation. In some cases, vendor estimates are incorrect due to the lack of detailed knowledge of your practice or formulas that minimize hours to cut the purchase price. For example, practices without trained staff or effective EHR procedures may require more implementation and training services. Inject a dose of reality and develop an internal estimate that allows for adequate training and support for the practice and not just address an optimistic estimate. *TIP:* Make sure that you allow for sufficient internal support staff and time to fulfill your responsibilities for implementing the EHR. You should also review the level of services and allow for additional training and support services as the project proceeds. *TIP:* Monitor the level of available services and the estimate to complete to insure that you have allowed for sufficient vendor services.	Carefully review the scope of services to insure that the various tasks needed to support EHR implementation are included in the scope or accounted for by the practice. Lock in a favorable services rate for the duration of the EHR implementation. In the event that you need more services, the practice should not have to pay the standard (non-negotiated rate). Include a contingency cost in your internal EHR budget to allow for adequate services to complete the project.
Maintenance and Support Costs	Maintenance and support costs are typically based on a percentage of the hardware and software costs. Hardware maintenance includes troubleshooting problems and onsite maintenance of covered equipment. *ALERT:* Many warranties from hardware vendors do not allow for onsite services. Onsite services are typically available at an additional cost. Software maintenance includes updates (but not installation of updates or update training for staff), help desk support for selected members of your staff and technical support for problems.	Ensure that the hardware configuration minimizes risk of failures within your needs and expectations. Allow appropriate practice staff to contact the vendor for support. Include a response standard and competency standard for the vendor's help desk and support services.

Continued

Continued from previous page

Business Point	Issue	Recommendation
	In some cases, maintenance services include working with any member of your staff, while other vendors will only work with a limited number of key practice users. Many maintenance clauses include a variety of exclusions that may present problems. These exclusions could lead to problems or additional charges for maintenance services. For example, support outside of standard hours or support of third party software may not be included in the maintenance charges. Some support contracts exclude the interface with your PMS or diagnostic equipment. **ALERT:** In some cases, the EHR vendor will not support third party software even if the software was purchased with the EHR.	Negotiate a reduced rate based on the level of service that you are providing to your users. For example, if your practice has an internal help desk, you may be able to get a discount on the software maintenance services. Insure the EHR and/or hardware vendor stands behind the hardware.
Certified EHR	ARRA defined a process that established a Certified Electronic Healthcare Record (EHR). A Certified EHR meets a certain functional standard according to a published script. Even though an EHR may be certified does not mean that the product will be appropriate for a specific practice.	Vendor should clearly state that they will maintain a certified product. The warranty should include that the product will enable and support meaningful use to qualify for the Stimulus Payments.
Old EHR Data Conversion	If your practice has an existing EHR, then the data from the old EHR will have to be converted to the new EHR. The conversion of EHR data may be very difficult and time consuming. Since the practice is responsible for maintaining the patient's medical record, the contract should insure that the vendor and practice understands the source and destination of your patient information. (See Converting from One EHR to Another EHR in Chapter 10.)	Include a list of the EHR data to be converted from the old EHR to the new EHR. Define the conversion plan and strategy. Specify the conversion costs. Allow for a test and a separate Go Live conversion.
Tail Accommodations	In the event that your practice closes for any reason (retirement, or change in employment), you may be responsible for maintaining the patient medical record for a certain period of time according to state and federal laws. Similarly, if you merge your practice with another practice, you may want to maintain your current EHR to assure access to the original patient information. Since you will have a continuing need to produce the patient records, you need to define an accommodation that will not be overly expensive or difficult. **CAUTION:** Remember that you may need operating hardware and software to maintain access to the patient records.	Include a step down support level that allows access to the patient records but does not support active use of the EHR for a practice. Support a custodial phase where the vendor provides an ASP offering that supports access to the patient information. Convert patient information into a form that would allow the practice to meet the retention requirement without having the EHR. For example, producing an image file with all of the patient's chart contents.
Scope of Work	EHR implementation includes a wide range of efforts among many practice and outside resources (see **Chapter 10 – Implementing an EHR**). The practice should have a clear understanding of the specific work that is covered by the agreement and costs as well as the other necessary efforts by the practice or other vendors. Some vendors will provide a list of services that they will perform but fail to inform you of items that will be needed. In many cases, your responsibilities and vendor exclusions are buried in dense contract text.	Use Chapter 9 to verify the services that are provided by the vendor. Note that you may choose to eliminate vendor services based on your other vendors and internal staff. Verify that the practice can meet the performance requirements in the contract for services.

Continued

Continued from previous page

Business Point	Issue	Recommendation
	Before you buy into the scope of work with the vendor, ensure that you have identified the key tasks and who will be responsible for those tasks – otherwise you may get behind on your commitments and disrupt your EHR implementation. In some cases, client-based delays to the EHR implementation can lead to additional charges. **ALERT** – Many practices undertake EHR projects without selecting or identifying the practice resources that will be responsible for implementing the EHR. EHRs require active support and participation from the clinical and management staffs of the practice.	Itemize vendor service exclusions and identify practice resources and third party vendors that will be providing these resources. Allow for scheduled status meetings to monitor usage of services and progress.
Hardware Source	Your hardware purchase strategy should be accounted for in the business points. Since your vendor sells its software to many practices, it should be able to advise you on the hardware setup issues even if you are not buying the hardware from them. **TIP:** Some vendors have published hardware requirements for their systems. If your EHR vendor does not sell hardware, it should specify the hardware requirements for all components in your system. In some cases, the vendor specifies specific models. In any event, verify any hardware purchases with the software vendor. If your EHR vendor sells hardware, you should seriously consider buying at least the EHR server with the software. Thereby, the EHR vendor is fully responsible for the main system that contains the EHR and you are free to buy the other hardware from another party.	Include the hardware and communication requirements from the software vendor in the contract. Software vendor should warrant that the recommended hardware will handle the practice workload. Consider buying the EHR server from the vendor if you do not have an appropriate alternative source. If the software vendor is selling the hardware to the practice, the hardware and software purchase should be connected in the warranty, payment plan and implementation plan.
Electronic Clearinghouses	Electronic transactions and clearinghouses are an evolving issue for EHRs. Several HIPAA Transactions (Claim Information, Electronic Prescriptions, and Referral/ PreCertification/ PreAuthorization) and the Continuity of Care Transaction require an electronic link to a clearinghouse for the EHR. Although clearinghouse use is an evolving issue for EHRs, you should be informed of the requirements for such exchanges and what support may be needed for exchanges with your key business partners.	Ensure that the vendor is committed to supporting the transactions as needed by the practice. Verify that the vendor's clearinghouse or direct connections support exchanges with your key healthcare partners (payers, pharmacies, hospitals). Verify that electronic prescriptions feature and clearinghouse works with the local pharmacies.
Health Information Exchange (HIE)	In order to support the exchange of electronic information with your healthcare partners, you may need to support electronic relationships with a local HIE that exists today or may exist in the future.	Include a clause that obligates the vendor to support standard HIPAA and HL7 defined exchanges with the HIE or HIEs that your practice will need to support.
Timeline	EHR Vendors frequently want to defer any discussion on timelines until the contract is completed. Vendors do not want to commit their resources to a project that may not happen. However, you may have a pressing need to install the system by a certain time due to an office move, seasonal volume or some other obligation. On the other hand, the vendor may plan to implement the system in a timeframe that does not consider your needs and situation. If you have a tight schedule and have yet to complete the contract, consider negotiating a commitment letter with the vendor to get on the vendor's schedule.	Include key goal dates in the contract to insure the vendor will meet your scheduling needs and issues. Include a procedure for changing the goal dates at the practice's option. Compile an internal implementation plan to determine such dates and ensure that you have the resources to meet the goal dates.

Continued

Continued from previous page

Business Point	Issue	Recommendation
Clinical Content	Clinical content consists of the templates, documents, knowledgebase and/or forms that you will use with the EHR. In some cases, vendors provide a very specific set of clinical content. Other vendors include all of the clinical content in their product. Some vendors provide access to a library of clinical content developed by other practices or sell clinical content from other vendors. You should make sure that the purchase agreement includes the various clinical content areas that you need for your practice and expect in the EHR. You should be especially careful to include clinical content that you may have considered in your review of EHR products. For example, you may have seen clinical templates during a site visit or in the vendor's web site that was a significant contributor to the product decision. In some cases, the vendor will be developing the clinical content. For example, an EHR product may lack clinical content in your specialty and the vendor has offered to develop the clinical content with the understanding that it will add the content to its product. In the event that your practice is developing clinical content, you should have a clear understanding of the ownership of the clinical content and maintenance responsibilities. In some cases, vendors reserve the right to offer your clinical content to other practices. If you have a problem allowing other practices to use your templates, then the business arrangement should prevent the distribution of your templates.	Insure that the clinical content to be delivered with the product is included in the contract. For example, a primary care practice with cardiology specialists will need the cardiology content *and* the primary care content. **TIP:** For vendors that charge for clinical content, make sure that you arrange for your foreseeable needs. You are in a stronger negotiating and discount position when you are originally buying the EHR than when you try to add additional items later. If you will be developing clinical content, specify what assistance the vendor will provide as well as the disposition of the final clinical content. If the vendor is developing clinical content for your practice to enhance its own product, ensure that you have defined the scope of the clinical content, a timeline to meet your needs and a support commitment from the vendor. Itemize the clinical content that will be included in the purchase and/or sources of necessary clinical content.
Training Strategy	Depending on the size of your organization, you may have the vendor train selected staff and then have the selected staff train the rest of the practice or you may have the vendor train all of your staff. The training class location is also part of the training strategy. Training typically is split up into (1) setup training and (2) application training. Setup training addresses how you establish the various lists, shortcuts, templates and documents using the administrative and programming capabilities of the EHR. Application training focuses on the actual use of the EHR to track patients, chart visits and manage work. In some cases, vendors offer advanced training to teach additional features as well as programming of the clinical content. Vendors vary in their training strategies. Some vendors insist that you attend EHR training at their training centers. Others are just as committed to conducting training at your location. The training location should be determined during the contract negotiations to ensure that you contract for the services you need and that the contract accounts for the costs at the selected location. Training at vendor offices is typically based on a per day/student charge, while onsite training is based on a charge per day/per trainer. Several vendors offer web-based training and access to web training broadcasts. A combination of these training options will be used to complete the EHR effort.	Include the training plan and strategy in the contract. Select the venue for training. Allow for access to web-based training facilities for all staff and doctors. Identify the specific materials that will be provided to the practice in support of the training and implementation process.

TABLE 9.2

Contract Issues	Issue	Typical Contract Text	Mitigation Strategy
Access to the System	Many EHR contracts severely limit the types of people who can access your system. Contracts may limit access to your employees, employees who "need access," or some other measure. In some cases, the vendor demands that it be informed of who has access to the system and/or require people with access to sign an agreement with the vendor. Such a term is a severe impediment to your practice. Your practice may need to make the system available to consultants, contract physicians or prospective physicians and employees. You need to be able to pursue your practice's objectives without worrying about approvals from you EHR vendors or risking violating your contract. Note that many contacts with system access limitations will terminate your software licenses for failure to follow the procedures in its contracts.	Practice will provide system access solely to your employees Practice will provide system access to employees who have agreed to the conditions of this contract. Any party with access to the system will have signed the attached agreement.	Allow the practice to disclose information about the EHR system and provide access to the EHR system to pursue the business or service objectives of the practice. Permit the practice to provide screen shots and reports as needed to pursue patient service and business needs of the practice.
Additional Charges	Vendor contracts frequently specify a wide range of situations where additional charges may be incurred. Travel expenses are typically classified as additional charges. Off-hours support, questions from unauthorized staff (in the vendor's eyes, but necessary staff for your practice), excessive support according to the vendor, and information available from manuals may trigger additional charges. Some vendors even reserve the right to charge for support issues after they fix the problem. The practice needs to insure that additional charges are cost effective and authorized. For example, you may not want off-hours support for a non-critical issue that can be addressed during regular hours.	Vendor may charge for support services that it determines, in vendor's sole discretion, to be excessive. Support is limited to 2 hours of phone support per month. Additional time will be charged to the practice. Other charges will be billed when incurred. Bills for other charges are due upon receipt. Services must be provided by the Go Live date.	Include an estimate of additional charges that are expected for the project. Travel, communications, wiring expenses and other expenses not included in the contract should be estimated by the vendor. Require additional charges to be approved in writing by the practice. Manage the project to include periodic reviews of the remaining hours and an estimate of hours needed to complete the project. Insure that the contract allows you to switch unused hours from one category to another category as the project proceeds. Insure that additional charges are controlled and capped.
Assignment of License	Medical practices may merge or reorganize under another practice structure. Since the practice has already paid for the license, the inability to assign the license could lead to additional charges or a new license fee.	Non-assignable License License may not be assigned to any party.	Allow assignment of the license as part of a merger or reorganization of the practice without any additional charges. Assignment of the license should only require notification to and not approval of the vendor. Assignment of the license should allow for assignment of all rights for the software, support and other rights.

Continued

Continued from previous page

Contract Issues	Issue	Typical Contract Text	Mitigation Strategy
	Vendors claim that the clause prevents competitors from buying their product, but the practical effect is to expose the practice to additional charges or the loss of the license to use the EHR. For example, an unassignable license could not be assigned to an organization that acquires your practice or a spin off of your billing operation.		
Bill Payment	Most vendor contracts compel you to pay bills under the threat of losing your license or having support services withdrawn. Although you should pay justifiable bills, the lack of warranties in most contracts limits your power to compel the vendor to perform or seek redress for incorrect billing, and/or billing adjustments. In the absence of a dispute mechanism, your practice is at risk whenever you may dispute a charge. Unfortunately, problems with bills are fairly frequent and include early-support billing, billing for undelivered items and billing for unsatisfactory and unauthorized services. In many cases, vendors are difficult to work with on billing issues. They are impossible when the contract does not allow for billing disputes.	Failure to pay any bills is considered breach of the license. All bills are due upon receipt.	Establish a bill-dispute procedure to allow the practice to reasonably dispute bills without risking any problems or penalties. Establish a performance standard that allows the practice to dispute a bill in the event of unsatisfactory services. Allow for verification and acceptance of products and services in the contract. For example, you may pay the bill for the interface after you have tested the EHR interface with the PMS.
Business Associate Agreement	The Business Associate Agreement is a HIPAA Privacy issue that controls what the vendor needs to do to protect your health information in the EHR. **Beware:** Many vendors do not present the Business Associate Agreement until after the contract has been signed. Fortunately, many Business Associate Agreements are fairly compliant with the HIPAA Privacy requirements. Nonetheless, you should insure that the BA is acceptable and that the agreement is signed with the contract.	In many cases, the contract does not reference the Business Associate Agreement.	Contemporaneously review, negotiate and sign the Business Associate Agreement with the EHR purchase contract.
Clinical Content	Many EHR systems offer clinical content, templates and documents for your area of practice and specialty (See Business Points Above.) However, some vendors are presenting clinical content that is not included, sold by another entity or not operational.	EHR is sold as is. No mention of clinical content in the contract. Practice can use (unspecified) clinical content available on the vendor website.	Insure that the specified clinical content is included in the contract. For example, the contract may specify a content package or clinical area that will be included in the purchase.

Continued

Continued from previous page

Contract Issues	Issue	Typical Contract Text	Mitigation Strategy
	Many contracts address the ownership and support for the clinical content. Options range from vendors that provide a complete panel of clinical content to vendors that provide a toolkit that allows you to develop your own clinical content using their toolkit. Some vendors provide only access to clinical content that have been developed by other practices. The clinical content from other practices can be downloaded to your system and installed in your EHR. If the EHR vendor develops content for you, the vendor frequently reserves the right to provide or sell the templates to other practices.	Templates and documents developed by the vendor or practice can be sold or provided to other practices without compensation to the practice.	If the clinical content is a key requirement, you may want to itemize the clinical content that is included in the purchase as well as a delivery and installation mechanism for your purchase. Allow for access and use of additional clinical content based on additional services provided by the practice. Include updates to clinical content as part of the support agreement. If desired, limit use of templates, documents and other clinical content developed by or for your practice as confidential information. Limits on distribution may be especially important for practices that develop specific clinical content to support a proprietary process that is important to your practice.
Communication Requirements	EHRs will generate more data exchanges with remote offices than anything you have done to date. EHRs collect more information for a visit that a PMS and the use of images will push the level of communications far beyond your current connection. The vendor should indicate the bandwidth level needed to support the number of workstations and necessary connections at each location. The Practice should be especially careful with the communication requirements needed to support scanning of documents on a day-to-day basis as well as the volume of scanning for legacy paper charts. **TIP:** Due to the lead time for communication upgrades, your should make sure that your order the communication services in time to meet your EHR implementation plan.	Practice is responsible for adequate communications between remote sites and the server. Practice must provide adequate communication access to the EHR server for the vendor.	Include specifications for necessary communications between the practice locations. Specify what, if any, communications will be necessary for vendor access. Insure that the delivery of communications will be in time to support other vendor activities, such as testing and training. Review the image scanning and management requirements for the EHR. For example, some EHRs burst the images, which may require a higher bandwidth.
Confidential Information	Confidential information consists of the policies, procedures, processes, forms and practices of your practice. In many EHR contracts, you are obligated to protect the EHR vendor's confidential information, but most vendors do not have a reciprocal obligation to protect your confidential information. A vendor could take materials from your practice and provide those materials to other vendor customers. If you have a specific workflow process or clinical content that you consider proprietary, you will want to limit the distribution of these materials.	All vendor information including documentation, flowcharts, screen shots and documents are considered confidential information. Practice may not provide confidential information to any party except authorized practice employees.	Limit vendor use of any and all information related to practices' procedures, business practices, clinical strategies, contractual relationships and any patient information. Prevent distribution of any practice information that could help a competitor. For example, promotional strategies and marketing channels, as well as suppliers may be proprietary information.

Continued

Continued from previous page

Contract Issues	Issue	Typical Contract Text	Mitigation Strategy
	Depending on the importance of the policies, procedures and other confidential information, you may want to restrict their use by the vendor.		
Customization	Some EHRs include customization services. Customization services may include adding clinical content or the development of an entire set of screens to support a specialty that the vendor currently lacks. If a lot of customization is required, you should consider an initial project to specify the changes before you buy the product. The vendor can show you mock-ups or initial screens of the EHR before you buy. And the vendor will be able to specify the costs of the effort as well as the delivery time. EHR customization should be subject to an acceptance and testing process. The process may include testing of actual patient information as well as a warranty period to cover the initial EHR use. **ALERT:** In some cases, you may implement adjustments to the vendor's clinical content to meet your needs. Those changes may have to be reinstalled to future vendor releases, or you may have to forgo use of the vendor's standard clinical content.	Vendor will develop clinical templates for the practice on a time and materials basis. Vendor provides NO WARRANTY.	Specify the scope of the customization effort. Scope documents may include lists of functions, screen mockups and descriptions. A standard of performance or functionality should be included in the Agreement. Include a cost estimate or fixed price. Define a testing and acceptance process for the customization effort. The testing process should include documenting patient visits from existing patient charts, as well as live shadowing of patient encounters. Include support for customized components (e.g., interfaces, and clinical content) in vendor support responsibilities.
Documentation	Most EHR contracts limit the use of the documentation in the same manner that the access to the system is controlled. You may not be able to copy the documentation or present the documentation to people who are not authorized users. You may want to make extensive use of the documentation. You may need to provide documentation on the system to outside clinical chart review consultants and quality assurance staff from a key payer. You may need to use the documentation to develop the procedures and processes that are required under the HIPAA Privacy and Security standards.	Cannot copy documentation for any reason. Documentation cannot be provided to anyone who is not an employee of the practice.	Allow the practice to copy, store, duplicate, and use the documentation to pursue the business purpose of the practice. Permit use of copies of documentation in procedure manuals and other practice operational materials. After the practice stops using the system, the documentation should be retained by the practice to assure continuity of medical record information and access to the purchased EHR.

Continued

Continued from previous page

Contract Issues	Issue	Typical Contract Text	Mitigation Strategy
Electronic Data Interchange	Electronic data interchange (EDI) involves the exchange of electronic data between various healthcare organizations. Currently, EHRs may send electronic prescriptions to selected pharmacies. In the future, EDI will support the exchange of information on patient treatment, clinical records and the Continuity of Care Record (CCR.) The key issue is the ability of the system to support the sending and receiving of transactions and the mode of transmission (e.g., clearinghouse, direct). Although many EHR systems do not support these capabilities currently, the practice should have a clear understanding of its options.	Vendor supports EDI with the ABC Clearinghouse. All electronic transactions are router to the vendor's clearinghouse.	Insure that the vendor supports current transactions including electronic pre-scriptions. Include a clause that commits to the support of industry standard transactions such as the Continuity of Care Record, and the Additional Claim Information HIPAA Transaction. Commit vendor to supporting exchanges with key payers, hospitals and providers. Note that some vendors will specify the HL-7 transaction format for the electronic exchange of information with other parties. Such a standard is a reasonable approach for electronic exchanges.
EHR Support	Typically, EHR support consists of problem-solving resources as well as the right to receive future updates. However, some vendors charge additional fees for future updates. For example, the vendor may reserve the right to add a surcharge for future updates, or split the product into modules which must be purchased by the practice to continue to have access to current functionality. Some EHR vendors require that you upgrade to the newest version of their product within a certain calendar period or until a specific number of new versions have been released. Support terms frequently control who can contact the vendor, what the vendor will do and the obligations of the practice. For example, some vendors exclude support for third-party products that may be an integral part of your EHR. For example, the EHR may use a third-party drawing tool that is built into the EHR. If the vendor runs into a problem with the third-party software, you may have to cope with reduced functionality or performance problems. Other vendors may only authorize a specific employee to contact the vendor support staff.	Support services consist of phone support to designated users and distributions of updates to the EHR that the vendor may release from time to time at its sole discretion. EHR support fees may be increased with 60-days notice. Phone support provided to designated users. EHR updates may be released at vendor's discretion. Practice will update its EHR to the current version of the software within 30 days of software version release. Vendor will only support the current release of the EHR software.	Insure continuous vendor support of the EHR product for at least 5 years after the practice installs the EHR. Vendors should not be able to terminate support for any reason during that period. Notice of support termination should be provided by the EHR vendor at least 18 months before support ceases. This gives your practice time to move to another EHR product. Limit support fee increases to a specific percentage or standard (e.g., CPI or consumer price index). Establish a support performance standard. The standard should include a response requirement for critical problems and system failures. Installation of the current version of the product can be delayed by the practice for a reasonable period of time. Support for the previous version or two previous versions of the EHR software will be provided by the vendor for a period of time that would allow the practice to review and test the new EHR software version.

Continued

Continued from previous page

Contract Issues	Issue	Typical Contract Text	Mitigation Strategy
	In some cases, EHR support is a requirement for continuing use of the EHR. If you terminate support, the vendor terminates your license. As a practical matter, you may terminate EHR support when you stop using the EHR but the practice may still need to access old EHR records for years after the switch. If you have to continue support to get access to the EHR and patient records after you stop using the software, your practice may have to pay thousands of dollars a year for an indefinite period of time.		
Entity	The contracting entity may be a significant issue for the contract. If you are a single corporation, LLC or other entity, the contracting entity is the practice. If you have several entities, including a clinical practice and other entities (e.g., ASC, optical shop, physical therapy), then you need to insure that the various entities are included in the contract.	EHR may only be used to serve the customer. Exclusive agreement between the customer and vendor.	Include all relevant practice entities in the contract term. Add a term to allow the practice to use the EHR with its related entities. List the related entities that will use the EHR in the contract.
Environment	Many vendors stipulate general requirements for the computer location and support. Vendors may include power, air conditioning and access requirements. Note that the environmental issues may be impacted by your hardware vendor source. For example, the EHR server may be installed in a rack provided by your normal hardware vendor. To insure continuity of operations and reliable access to your EHR, you should follow the appropriate vendor guidelines but add in an additional standard to mitigate the risk of an EHR failure (**see Chapter 10 – Implementing an EHR**).	Practice must maintain the computer equipment in an appropriate space with adequate utilities and ventilation. Vendor must be able to access the system at any time without impediment.	Include the vendor's standards in the contract. Then you may have recourse for a performance or sizing problem. Insure that the vendor agrees to your equipment and hardware setup. Verify that you are in compliance with the vendor's specified standards. Analyze the vendor standards in light of the HIPAA Security standards. If necessary, negotiate down issues that exceed the HIPAA Security Requirements.
Error Definition	Most vendor contracts address errors that your practice may encounter. Unfortunately, many contracts provide wide latitude to the vendor in acknowledging an error. Some contracts require a reporting window, while others exclude problems as a result of data "entered" by the practice. It is difficult to image that an error would not be triggered by practice data.	Vendor will fix errors that the vendor determines is not consistent with the operation of the system. Vendor will not fix problems that are caused by practice data.	Include a clause that establishes a reference standard for the operation of the software. Potential standards could include the manual or what a user could "reasonably expect" from the system. If the performance standard is online documentation, make sure that you print the supporting documentation in support of any errors. In some cases, conflicting documentation has disappeared or the vendor has "fixed the documentation."

Continued

Continued from previous page

Contract Issues	Issue	Typical Contract Text	Mitigation Strategy
	The best strategy is to include a defined standard against which errors will be measured. The standard may include documentation, industry practices or a "reasonable" expectation.	Vendor may fix the error or amend the documentation.	Note that some EHR product documentation generally lacks the specific performance or description that would support your practice in a dispute. Make sure that you fully understand the quality of the documentation and how it may be used to support any functionality and performance issues.
			Error correction should be performed on a best-effort basis for errors that effect the day-to-day operations of the practice.
			Require written-practice approval for error correction charges by the vendor. Such a process should allow for a testing phase before using the corrected software in your live database.
Exit Strategy	Vendor contracts are written to describe the early stages of your project and the implementation effort. In the event of a license problem, contract dispute, product obsolescence or your decision to move to a new EHR in the future, your practice needs to allow for a smooth transition to another EHR. Your practice will also need continued access to the existing EHR for reference purposes.	Practice may terminate the use of the software with X days notice.	Insure that the vendor will support the conversion of practice EHR data, when and if the practice moves to another EHR.
		The practice will discontinue use of the software and destroy all copies of the software.	Regardless of the reason for moving to another EHR, allow continuous practice access to the EHR system and data for as long as the practice needs. Such access may be needed to check the original medical record data that was brought over from the old EHR. The ability to access the old EHR should be available for as long as the practice deems necessary.
	If you were to move to another EHR, you will have to deal with a project that is many times more complex and demanding than any PMS conversion. To understand the magnitude of the problem, you should note that many PMS vendors will not accommodate conversion of patient ledger details. Will your practice be able to function without your prescription list, or procedure list from the "old" EHR? Imagine the difficulty you would have if you could not access or had EHR information split among two EHR systems. Such a situation may prevent you from maintaining the "Designated Record Set" mandated by the HIPAA Privacy Standards.		Access to the old data should not be contingent on paying continuing support costs.
Hardware Support	A hardware failure could be a localized issue or a complete shutdown of your facility. The best strategy for hardware support is to invest in hardware that minimizes potential failure.	Hardware support will be provided by vendor through a third party organization of the vendor's choosing.	Support will be provided by the EHR vendor to assist in the analysis of hardware issues on a best effort basis.

Continued

Continued from previous page

Contract Issues	Issue	Typical Contract Text	Mitigation Strategy
	Cost effective options should be considered in light of your risk of loss and operational issues (see **Chapter 8 – Making a Final Decision**). Some practices have no tolerance for an EHR loss and other practices can tolerate a brief loss of the EHR system. A number of cost effective hardware investments include a high availability cluster server(s) with redundant disk arrays, power supplies, fans and other components. Additional system redundancies can be purchased to control the risk of a complete system failure. Nonetheless, you should insure that the hardware support accommodates a level of risk that you can live with. For example, if you purchase a system with several redundant components, an 8-hour response may be acceptable. But another practice may seek a 2-hour response and/or invest in more system redundancy.	Onsite hardware support will be provided within one business day of the support call. Hardware calls should be placed to the practice hardware vendor. The EHR vendor support line will address only software issues.	Provide onsite hardware support services within 4 hours of a hardware support call or some other response rate that meets the practice's needs. Allow for additional EHR vendor hardware support outside of standard business hours as needed. Specify onsite hardware sparing requirements to shorten recovery time.
HIPAA Compliance	If your Practice is a covered entity, then you need to comply with the HIPAA Privacy, Security and Transaction standards. Many vendor contracts are silent on the support of HIPAA standards. Practices will be under increasing pressure to support electronic interfaces with other healthcare organizations. Many of these exchanges will be based on the HIPAA Transaction Set. HIPAA Transactions include several exchanges that will require an EHR. The practice should insure that the vendor will support appropriate HIPAA transactions. The HIPAA Privacy standard specifies tracking disclosures and the paperwork needed to support such disclosures. Since many disclosure of Protected Health Information will come from the EHR, the EHR should support tracking and managing disclosures.	Software product will be maintained to meet applicable state and federal laws.	Maintain the Software product to meet the current HIPAA Privacy, Security and Transaction Requirements. Insure that vendor warrants that the software will enable the practice to comply with the HIPAA Privacy Standards, HIPAA Security Standards and use the relevant HIPAA Transaction Sets. Insure that Vendor will supply appropriate communication and transaction processing facilities to allow practice to use the EHR to formulate and process appropriate HIPAA Transactions.
Interfaces – Diagnostic	Interfaces support the exchange of information with other software products or systems. An EHR may need to interface with the PMS, lab system, reference labs, diagnostic equipment and other provider systems. For example, the practice may have an EKG machine that produces electronic images.	Many contracts are silent on these interfaces. Interfaces may be included in the purchase order.	Compile a list of the diagnostic equipment in your practice. Verify the electronic interface between the diagnostic equipment and the EHR. Identify the strategy and components needed to get the diagnostic information into the EHR.

Continued

Continued from previous page

Contract Issues	Issue	Typical Contract Text	Mitigation Strategy
	Some diagnostic equipment supports direct interfaces with other systems. For example, the diagnostic equipment may produce an image that can be accepted into the EHR.		Include diagnostic equipment interface products, and, if necessary, custom interfaces in the purchase order. Include services needed from the vendor to get the interfaces to work with your equipment.
Interfaces – Lab	EHRs accept lab orders during the patient visit. Depending on the capabilities of the EHR, the lab orders may be electronically transmitted to selected reference labs, and the results returned electronically to the EHR. Note that some reference labs subsidize the purchase of the lab interface.	EHR includes an interface with reference labs specified in the purchase order.	Verify that the lab interface works with the local office of your key reference labs. Insure that the purchase order allows for the lab interface module as well as the services to test, use and support the lab interface.
Interfaces – PMS	If you are buying an integrated system, you have no interface issues. If you have an existing PMS that you will be integrating with your EHR, the contract should include a commitment to support and maintain the interface with the PMS. **ALERT:** Even if you are buying the EHR from your PMS vendor, you may need to insure that the product interface will continue to be maintained. If you are interfacing your EHR with your PMS, you want to insure that you have such an option in the future. If you plan to replace your PMS at a future date, the EHR contract should accommodate the purchase and implementation of the future interface.	EHR does not include interfaces with any products. Interfaces are the responsibility of the practice	Itemize the interfaces supported by the PMS interface (e.g., demographics, appointments, charges) with the EHR. Include the interface software as well as a warranty and support arrangement for the interface. If the PMS interface is not a standard product, include a warranty and defined standard for the operation and speed of the interface. For example, the EHR should post demographic and appointment information from the PMS within 5 seconds of receipt of an interface transaction. If no PMS interface is being implemented, include a term that allows for such an interface in the future. The item may even include selected products or interface standards (e.g., HL7).
Key Contacts	Before the contract is signed, you will be working with the sales team. After the contract is signed, most vendors turn the practice over to the implementation team. In many cases, you have not met the implementation staff. If possible, try to meet the implementation manager and key trainer *before* signing the contract. Otherwise, reserve the right to approve the key staff and insure that adequate warranties are in place to assure competency.	Vendor will staff the contract with qualified employees and/or third party resources.	Identify the vendor project manager and other key people for the EHR implementation. Reserve the right to approve the project manager after an initial interview. In the event of a change in key vendor personnel on the project, reserve the right to interview replacement vendor staff. If the change was driven by the vendor, the practice should not have to pay additional money to get the new staff member up to speed on the project.

Continued

Continued from previous page

Contract Issues	Issue	Typical Contract Text	Mitigation Strategy
Licenses	Vendors may offer a license to use the EHR for a set period of time (say, 5 years) or subject its use to other conditions, including locations and placement of the server. As a practical matter, the practice should be certain that the license does not include limitations that are not practical, or may be overlooked as the practice pursues its objectives. Be especially careful to avoid license terms that require additional payment and unexpected approvals from the EHR Vendor.	Practice is buying a non-exclusive license to use the software for X years. Practice may use the software for as long as the practice pays monthly support fees.	Insure that licenses for a set period clearly state the renewal terms and conditions. In the event of license termination or non-renewal, the vendor must support the exit strategy.
Patents and Copyrights	Vendor contracts include terms to protect their intellectual property rights over the design, interface and other EHR aspects. Most vendor contracts include terms that protect the vendor in the event of a competing copyright or patent claim. Typically, the vendor will try to reach a licensing agreement, change the EHR product or remove the offending software/feature. Removal of the software/feature is an unacceptable outcome since your practice may depend on the eliminated item. Even a refund of a portion of the license fees is unacceptable. The vendor should address the legal issue without affecting your practice's EHR capability.	In the event of a ruling against the vendor, the vendor may pay a license fee to the patent holder, change the feature to remove the infringement or remove the feature from the software.	Insure vendor uses its best efforts to make sure the practice has continued access to the feature or EHR. Prevent vendor from avoiding the problem by paying a portion of the license fees back to the practice. Verify changes to comply with copyright claims do not increase the complexity of using the product or the feature.
Payment Schedule	Vendors typically seek to get a substantial payment upfront and the rest of the money before you have a chance to see the EHR. Indeed, some contracts have you paying remaining charges upon the delivery of boxes containing your EHR components. Unfortunately, you cannot go too far with a box of components. Ideally, the vendor should be paid based on performance and your receipt of value. Key payment triggers to consider are when the hardware and software are available for use, completion of training, and Go Live of the EHR. If the purchase includes customization services, then some payment may be appropriate after you have tested and accepted the changes.	Practice will pay 50% of the total contract at the signing of the contract and the remaining 50% when the products are shipped from the vendor's office.	Minimize the payment at contract signing. Pay a portion of the fee at delivery defined as the software is available for use and working with your workstations and tablets. This term may require coordination with your hardware vendor. Pay for time and expense charges as the charges are incurred. Allow for fixed price or volume buy services to be used beyond the Go Live date.

Continued

Continued from previous page

Contract Issues	Issue	Typical Contract Text	Mitigation Strategy
Performance Standards	A wide variety of variables can impact the performance of the system and the software. The capacity of the communication lines, your hardware base, network setup and other user activities can effect how quickly the system responds to a user. Nonetheless, you should seek to establish a base performance level to set your expectation as well as to commit the vendor to work with you on any performance issues. Performance issues will be based on the hardware and software setup recommendations of the Vendor, as well as what other users are doing with the system.	Vendor makes NO WARRANTIES.	The recommended hardware and software should produce a response time to a workstation request of no more than X seconds.
Providers	Many vendors base license charges on a provider. However, many practices employ various "providers" – such as nurse practitioners and physician assistants – who exclusively assist the doctor and part-time providers. Paying a full license amount for all providers could result in substantial fee to the practice. The definition of a provider is an important factor to consider. The practice should seriously review the current list of providers as well as future plans to insure that you do not pay for provider licenses for those providers who work less than full time or under supervision.	A provider is anyone involved in clinical decision making for patients. A provider is a doctor, nurse, LPN or other licensed healthcare professional.	Define a provider considering your clinical staff. The contract should itemize special situations including supporting PA/LPN/RN, technicians and other clinicians who provide limited independent patient services. Allow for licenses to be shared by providers who are not full-time providers or may fill in for the doctors. For example, the practice may employ fill-in providers on an as-needed basis. The practice should be able to give access to fill-in providers without paying a full license fee for each provider. Allow for a reporting and authorization process that is not difficult and can respond to the practice's need to provide quick access to fill-in doctors/staff.
Services Purchased	An EHR contract may include a variety of services based on different charge methods. Services may be based on a time-and-expenses basis or a fixed-price basis. Service charges may vary by method (e.g., onsite, offsite, phone, Internet). Note that many service proposals look like fixed- price proposals, when they're really time and materials agreements. You should verify that the contract services are sufficient and appropriate for the practice.	Full payment will be made when the system is delivered. Services will be provided by vendor staff or third parties as needed. Services include training, implementation, project management and other efforts in support of the practice.	Services should be paid as incurred. Carefully review the scope of work to manage the use of hours and fixed price exclusions. Include an option to purchase additional services at a negotiated project rate. Insure that the mix of services is reasonable for the practice. Include a periodic review process to track the services provided by the vendor and the progress of the project. Allow for swapping services among the various areas as needed during the project. For example, leftover training hours could be used to purchase more practice management services.

Continued

Continued from previous page

Contract Issues	Issue	Typical Contract Text	Mitigation Strategy
Software Requirements	In some cases, practices have some critical EHR functionality that is an absolute necessity for success. In the course of demonstrations, the Practice may have the impression that the EHR product meets the requirement. Unfortunately, some practices find out that they didn't buy what they saw or the product demonstration showed an impractical workaround. If the product has the critical item currently, you may want to highlight the requirement in the contract. If the product lacks the function and the vendor has promised to add the capability, or do some custom work, then the strategy and function should be specified in the contract with a completion or delivery date.	Product is sold as is without any representation that the software will meet the practice's needs. Practice understands the specific capabilities of the EHR Product. Practice is solely responsible for determining that the EHR product meets the practice's needs.	Itemize the critical functionality and/or feature as a primary reason for the purchase of the EHR. The itemization should include a description of the capability sufficient to understand the requirement and process. Verify that the product handles the issue to the practice's satisfaction or itemize the changes and delivery schedule for the enhancement.
Source Code Escrow	The EHR program is based on source code that is owned by the software publisher. The source code normally is not stored on your system. However, source code is needed to make changes and fix bugs. Some vendors have an established escrow agreement that gives you access to the source code in the event of bankruptcy or business failure. Note that access to source may not be as comforting as you think, since the source code would have to be studied by trained programmers before they could help you make changes or fix problems.	Source code is the property of the vendor. Source code is not included in the purchase of the software.	Insure that the vendor supports an escrow program with an established agent (setting your own escrow facility up is a more expensive and complex task). Determine the frequency and currency of the escrow program in light of the EHR product releases. Participate in the vendor's escrow program.
System Activation	System activation or "Go Live" drives a variety of issues and services. Vendors may turn the support over to the vendor's support team, require the start of support payments and/or stop project management services. In the case of EHRs, you may spend several months setting up the system to be used while the vendor may consider the system activated when the system is delivered in boxes or when the EHR server has been connected to your computer network. In other cases, you may actually be using the system to scan old charts and track patient messages, but be months away from the charting of patient visits by doctor. You need to make sure that you have continuing support to carry you through to actual use of the EHR.	System will be considered activated or Go Live when the purchased items are delivered. Practice will pay in full when the EHR is available for use.	Activation should be defined as the point in time when your practice is using the system for productive work. For example, activation could be defined when the staff has been trained and doctors are using the system to chart patient services. Activation can trigger payments as well as the start of EHR support from the vendor. Activation may consist of several steps: scanning charts, routing messages, managing patient flow, tracking orders, charting services and sending charges to the PMS.

Continued

Continued from previous page

Contract Issues	Issue	Typical Contract Text	Mitigation Strategy
Third Party Vendor Exclusions	EHR contracts typically exclude third party products from the obligations of the EHR vendors. The key problem is that many of these third party products were specifically selected by the EHR vendor. Although, the EHR vendor cannot vouch for all third party products, the EHR vendor should guarantee that its product will work with the specified hardware and software products that it indicates in its documentation.	Vendor is not responsible for any and all third party software or hardware products.	Practice will be provided with 12 month notice of changes to hardware and software standards for the EHR. The EHR vendor should insure that third-party software needed to support functionality of the EHR will continue to work with the EHR.
Users	A number of products are licensed by user. Users may be defined as someone on the system at any given time or on a workstation with EHR access. Users may be differentiated from those who chart patient information (e.g., doctors, nurses, PAs) and those who may access information (e.g., billing staff). Note that the definition of a user can have a substantial effect on your cost and cost comparison. For example, licensing by workstation may be more expensive that licensing by user and licensing by concurrent user. Licensing by workstation requires a license for all workstations whether they are in use or not. Similarly, licensing by user requires a license for each registered user even if not all users are using the EHR at the same time. Licensing by concurrent user requires a payment for the highest maximum number of users at any given time.	A user is anyone who accesses the software at any time.	Negotiate a reduced fee for the number of users that will be using the system. Include adequate users per provider license for vendors that license by provider. Insure that you are not paying for idle workstations and users to get the right to use the EHR.
Warranty	Many vendors fail to warrant the system, software, services or hardware. Vendors typically back off of any warranty for a variety of reasons including risk, payment and financial reporting (e.g., Sarbanes-Oxley). A practice can get caught when a vendor fails to perform but the practice is committed to continuing use of the EHR due to the difficulty of changing EHR systems.	Vendor makes no warranties, including fitness for specific purpose, for any of the software, hardware, products or services. Practice is responsible for making all decisions on the use of the software. Vendor is not responsible for how the software is used by the practice.	Include vendor warranty that the EHR software will enable the practice to comply with the applicable HIPAA Privacy and Security Standards Allow the practice to use the relevant HIPAA Transaction Sets. Insure vendor warrants that the software will support the practice in complying with the HIPAA Privacy Standards and HIPAA Security Standards.

Continued

Continued from previous page

Contract Issues	Issue	Typical Contract Text	Mitigation Strategy
	The lack of a warranty creates a number of problems for the practice. The lack of a software warranty leaves any software problem resolution at the discretion of the vendor. Having no hardware warranty leaves little recourse in the event of performance or sizing problem with the workstations or server. Unwarranted services could result in additional expenses to pay for training or implementation support that was not done the first time. You may have to struggle with incorrect guidance and information from the vendor. One of the key challenges is establishing a warranty standard. In the absence of a standard, the practice may end up in an intractable argument on the specific way the product works in a specific situation. The contract language should allow for a standard upon which the products and services will be based. The key remedy is for the vendor to correct the problem and allow your practice to go forward. Restarting the EHR implementation or switching EHR products is a costly and time-consuming effort that you should avoid.		Verify that the Vendor will offer additional enhancements to support HIPAA Transactions that may be released under the HIPAA Transaction Set requiring EHR information. Warrant that training and support services will be provided by qualified personnel and in a professional matter. The services will comply with the system requirements and include advice, instruction and services that will be an effective way to use the system. Warrant that support services will include maintenance of the product to allow the practice to meet general industry requirements as well as advice that the practice can rely on. Warrant that the EHR will be Certified under the ARRA Stimulus requirements and will support the Meaningful Use standard.

understand what the problem is. However, you are often dealing with a company that is not local, and your practice could pay the price for a delay or disruption in the implementation or use of an EHR. Whether anyone else has a problem or not is not the issue: you are the one who will have to work within the terms of the contract.

Remember that you will have to live with the contract structure for as long as you use its EHR. As such, you need to establish a results-oriented relationship that will provide you with the structure to establish and manage a continuing relationship with the vendor. The following table itemizes the key contract issues and presents a mitigation strategy for these key issues. Note that EHR contracts may contain a number of other issues that you will have to address, too (see Table 9.2).

WORKING ON THE FINAL AGREEMENT

As you negotiate the contract with the vendor, you will go through several iterations of text. Some vendors will add the changes into the body of the contract, while others will create an addendum that will be attached to the basic contract. Changes in words, concepts and terms throughout the contracting process could affect other areas. To manage the contracting process, compile a list of issues.

To keep things simple, make sure that all changes are tracked and be on guard for unexpected additions and changes. For example, one vendor added contract items that contradicted other contract terms. Another vendor unilaterally made changes to a final copy of the contract to "clean up the language." In both cases, the changes would have substantially changed the nature of the contract and the agreement. Successfully manage the negotiations by considering the following:

Maintain an Issues List—When the contract is initially reviewed, compile a list of issues and your desired outcome. The issues list should be used to track your progress and outstanding items. Make sure you identify which items are negotiable versus items that you view as less important. You do not want to spend a lot of time and effort addressing a minor issue and then have to compromise on a more important item. Note that you should include your business points in the issues list. Frequently, a contract change will undermine or change a business point that has already been addressed. For example, the vendor may introduce a new term to deal with your problem, but creates ambiguous language in other sections of the contract. When your contract issue is to align the contract with the business point, vendors are typically more accommodating.

Track Changes—Use a markup copy of the contract in a document file. Verify that no additional changes have been made by using the document compare feature of the word-processing program. Be sure to challenge any unexpected changes. A series of unexpected changes could create some unanticipated problems or lengthen the contracting process. For example, one contract version changed the nature of the license for the entity, but created problems with the provider count that require user licenses.

Total Agreement—Constantly check the entire agreement to insure that problems and inconsistencies are addressed. Be especially careful with attachments and appendices. For example, a negotiated payment schedule in the contract may conflict with the purchase order attachment. In another case, the contract referenced Terms and Conditions on the Website that completely invalidated the negotiated terms and conditions. Consistency is especially important since the staff that administers the contract is frequently not the sales staff. **ALERT:** The EHR accounts payable department may base their billing on the standard contract when you have negotiated alternative payment terms. A consistent contract will effectively communicate your needs and expectations. For example, one contract included the original wording for support payments in one place and a negotiated change in another. The vendor's billing department took months to determine the correct billing and render a correct bill.

Once you have completed the contract, perform a final reading to verify that the contract and attachments are correct. Once you have completed the final reading, make sure that the reviewed document is the contract that you sign. With the best of intentions, there have been mix-ups at the final signing when vendor staff used an older contract version to print the contract for signature.

LIVING WITH THE FINAL AGREEMENT

Once you have signed the contract, you still need to insure that the project proceeds according to the contract. Deviations occur for a number of reasons, including the vendor going by the standard (and *not* your negotiated) contract, and billing errors. For example . . .

> **EXAMPLE**: A project was seriously delayed due to the failure to transition from the contract to implementation on a timely basis. The contract included a timeline that was not communicated to the implementation staff.

> **EXAMPLE**: One vendor issued a combined bill for the hardware, software and support upon delivery, when the contract clearly stated that the support fees did not have to be paid until go live.

> **EXAMPLE**: A vendor rendered a bill for an upgrade to the new product version when the upgrade was included in the negotiated contract.

> **EXAMPLE**: A change order upgrade included language that superseded the original agreement.

> **EXAMPLE**: An "updated" final contract was submitted for signature that didn't include any of the agreed-upon changes.

To insure that you get the full benefits of your negotiated agreements, the contract should be the starting point for the development of supporting materials for your EHR implementation project. Transition to the implementation effort by using the negotiated agreement for the following transition tasks:

- Meet with the vendor sales and implementation team toward the end of contract negotiations or immediately after contract signing to properly structure the project and insure that all participants understand the relevant issues of the negotiated contract.

- Create a contract abstract of key information and terms as a reference tool for the project. In situations where the standard contract is supplemented by an appendix or addendum, ensure that you note the affected standard terms in the standard contract with a reference to the appendix change.

- When you compile your implementation plan, include key dates from the contract and any key issues that may effect the implementation.

The completed contract and agreement for the purchase of your EHR should be used to establish a results-oriented relationship with your EHR vendor. Your practice will have a tool to guide your implementation effort as well as structure an effective working relationship with your EHR vendor long after your have completed the initial EHR implementation.

TABLE 9.3

Negotiation Issue	Status	Assigned To	Comment
Business Terms—Establish the following business terms before attempting to work out the contract details.			
1. Licensing Issues—			
a. Does the license accommodate the practice structure?			
b. What are the types of licenses and user counts?			
c. What additional licenses are needed for other items such as clinical content and interfaces?			
2. Product Costs			
a. What is the net cost of the product after volume discounts?			
b. What are the costs of services?			
c. Are the quoted services sufficient for installing the EHR for the practice?			
3. Continuing Costs			
a. What are the continuing support costs?			
b. When does the practice start paying continuing support costs?			
c. What are the annual software and content support costs?			
d. What annual hardware support costs are needed to maintain the level of response and support the practice has chosen?			
4. Interfaces			
a. What are the interfaces needed to work with the PMS?			
b. What interfaces are needed to exchange orders and results with labs?			
c. What interfaces are needed to exchange information with diagnostic equipment?			
5. Timeline			
a. What are the implementation stages of the project?			
b. What are the due dates for the various implementation stages?			
c. What are the connections between the dues dates and payments?			
Key Contract Terms—The following contract terms should be understood and handled to the practice's satisfaction. Note that every vendor contract has different structures and terms that could affect your relationship with the vendor and your project.			
6. Responsibilities			
a. What are the vendor responsibilities in the contract?			
b. What are not vendor responsibilities that could cause problems or delay the project?			
c. What are the practice's responsibilities in the contract?			

Continued

Continued from previous page

Negotiation Issue	Status	Assigned To	Comment
d. What additional responsibilities doe the practice have to assume to succeed with the EHR?			
7. Warranties			
a. What is the feature standard under which the product will reasonably perform?			
b. What areas of medicine does the vendor warrant for the clinical content?			
c. What is the standard of performance for services provided by the vendor?			
d. What is the standard of performance for the recommended hardware and system software?			
e. What obligations does the vendor assume for compliance with HIPAA Security and Privacy standards?			
f. How long are the warranties valid and when do the warranties start?			
g. How does the vendor resolve warranty issues?			
8. Software Support			
a. What services are provided with Software Support?			
b. Do the service hours cover the practice's needs?			
c. Does the software response commitment satisfy the practice's needs?			
d. Is the software support guaranteed for a sufficient period of time?			
9. Hardware Support			
a. What is the response commitment for serious problems?			
b. How does the vendor monitor hardware to mitigate the chance of a serious failure?			
10. Payment Terms			
a. Are payment terms adequately tied to the project plan and vendor performance?			
b. Do payment terms include a dispute resolution process?			
c. Are payment triggers clearly defined?			
11. Termination			
a. Are termination triggers appropriate to the problem?			
b. Do termination triggers allow for a resolution period to avoid termination?			
c. Does the termination process allow for sufficient time and support for an exit from the EHR that will support continuing operations and a transition to a new EHR?			

Implementing an EHR

To guide and manage your implementation effort, you need a plan and a workflow design. Practices that do not plan ahead will be working on the fly and may make a number of decisions that will doom the project to failure or, worst yet, succeed in the implementation but fail in the clinic. For example, many practices do not set up the computerized chart to facilitate access to the chart contents. Other practices only partially implement the EHR and end up with a hybrid system that is more difficult to use. For example, a number of practices have an EHR that is used by a few doctors, but the rest of the doctors use the paper chart. Such practices must spend additional monies to maintain both methods and exchange information between the paper chart and EHR. In another situation, the EHR was used by doctors for messaging, but the paper chart was used for everything else. Such a strategy could lead to confusion and complicate maintaining the HIPAA mandated designated record set.

Vendors commonly include "project management services" in their purchase orders. What many vendors mean by project management, and what you mean/need are often very different. Typically, vendor project management services include working with your project manager on the implementation of the system. The vendor project manager will coordinate the vendor's services, keep in touch with the vendor's hardware and technical people and act as your contact point for the project. Vendor project managers will not normally manage your internal resources, third party suppliers of hardware and communications, or make decisions about how the EHR will be used in the practice. Indeed, vendors typically defer decisions to the practice which may not be in a position to make key decisions since they have never used an EHR.

Some vendors have implementation plans that describe their responsibilities but do not necessarily guide a practice through implementation. For example, one detailed vendor implementation plan had detailed step by step tasks for the vendor effort but trivialized the practice's responsibilities (e.g., practice will set up master templates). Such documents do not adequately define the scope of the project for the practice or properly quantify the practice staff and resources that will be needed to successfully deploy and activate the EHR.

Practice items are normally more numerous and complex than the EHR vendor's plan. For example, upgrading various workstations may be the responsibility of the current hardware vendor, and coordinated by your practice. Your practice may be facing a number of policy, staffing and workflow decisions that will require substantial study and research. For example, the practice may need to establish a standard for charting selected patient conditions as well as a mechanism to insure that the doctors are using the mechanism. Otherwise, the practice may not be able to determine and measure their compliance with pay for performance standards or attain Meaningful Use. Dealing with the current medical record requires detailed analysis of the current records and discussions with doctors that vendors may not support. For example, the doctors will need to decide on the electronic "tabs" that will be used to organize the EHR contents.

If you are using a PMS interface, your practice will be responsible for buying and installing the PMS interface as well as organizing testing between the EHR and PMS. The EHR vendor may limit its responsibilities to the receipt of PMS data. You may find it difficult to adjudicate communications and performance problems with the EHR and PMS interfaces. The EHR vendor may only focus on when the practice will be ready for training, but not necessarily the various tasks that are needed to prepare your network for the installation of the EHR server. For example, establishing work priority and the appropriate codes to flag users may require a detailed analysis of current issues and clinical practices.

Understanding practice implementation responsibilities is especially significant since the EHR vendor does not make EHR setup decisions: **your practice will need to decide how and when the EHR will be used**. You may have someone who can make these decisions or you may use a third party to help you through the process (consultant, e.g.). In either case, your project manager will be the point person for the project. In the final analysis, the EHR vendor project manager is one resource available to your practice but few vendors provide the project leadership needed to complete EHR implementation.

Dozens of strategies may be used to structure the EHR implementation. This chapter structures the EHR implementation into the following areas (Table 10.1):

CLINICAL STANDARDS

The clinical record setup defines how the EHR will be used. Clinical record setup includes practice preferences, information choices and display options. Many vendors like to point out that EHRs allow each physician to record whatever information they want

TABLE 10.1

Area	General Tasks	Resource Types	Time Frame
Clinical Standards	Establish Clinical Standards Strategy	CMO Doctors Clinical staff	Start immediately and work throughout the project.
Policy	Establish practice policies to support the EHR. Assure compliance with HIPAA and other regulatory standards. Provide a practice governance structure to support and advance EHR implementation.	Practice Management Project Manager	Mostly at beginning of project.
Project Management	Track Progress Manage Project Plan and Resources Make Decisions on Issues Address Contract Issues Resolve Problems and Issues	Project Manager Practice Manager Physician EHR Champion	Throughout the project.
Workflow and Procedures	Develop EHR Workflow Identify Use and Setup Issues to Support Workflow	Department Supervisor CMO	Created early in the project and updated as needed.
Facilities Management	Establish Secure Computer Room Adjust Offices to Accommodate EHR	Contractors	Start of Project
Technology Base	Manage Server Installation Identify Changes to Existing Hardware Identify Changes to Existing Communications Select Tablets and Other Hardware Verify Installation	Technical Support Hardware Vendors	Heavy at beginning of the project.
Software Setup	Translate Workflow Concepts to the EHR Make Setup Decisions Verify Clinical Content Develop Interface with PMS Develop Interface with Diagnostic Equipment	EHR Project Team Key Clinical Users	After Hardware Installation and Before End-User Training
Data Conversion	Develop a Scanning and Information Retrieval/Entry Strategy for Paper Charts Execute the Scanning Strategy Execute the Retrieval of Required Information from the Paper Chart and Entry into the EHR Convert data from PMS	Medical Record Staff Clinical Staff Technical Support PMS Vendor Hardware Vendor	Through EHR Go Live date
Training	Setup Training Plan Identify Training Packages Train Super Users Develop Focused Training Materials Train Staff	EHR Project Team Practice Super Users	From hardware installation to Go Live
Continuing Support	Transition to Supporting the EHR on a Day to Day Basis Establish a Maintenance Strategy	EHR Project Team	From Go Live Onward

regardless of what other physicians are doing. In the paper world, this situation is analogous to having a different intake form and/or unique clinical flow-sheet for each doctor in the practice, even if they are providing the same services. The staff has to adjust to each form and the process for each doctor. Although an EHR does not technically eliminate these differences, the practice needs to discuss the implications of these differences, and what, if any, value the differences bring to patient service, physician effectiveness, practice operations and practice performance.

In an EHR, different clinical setups and documentation standards have several implications:

Implementation Costs—If each doctor creates a different solution to the same problem, then the practice will absorb the cost of setting up the system multiple ways for the same clinical purpose. For example, some practices invest time and resources to change the order of EHR template items to match the current paper form or the preferences of one or more doctors. The practice will have to maintain multiple setups or templates for the same chief complaint or problem. As important, the doctors will each have to take their time to design the specific screens that they want. A single clinical standard will allow one doctor to work on the standard that will be used by several doctors. A single standard will *cost less* to maintain and setup.

Workflow Differences—In some cases, the clinical content reflects and/or dictates the flow of patients and issues in the practice. Different clinical chart standards may require different clinical workflows. For example, serious issues could be flagged in one manner by one doctor and another doctor may expect staff to note problems through the use of key words. The diversity of workflows could cause differences in a variety of setups and EHR uses. For example, one doctor may use a task feature to manage patient services while another doctor may use a chart note which is more difficult to manage for workflow purposes. A single standard will lead to shared workflows and enable the practice managers to use the EHR to track performance on an hourly or daily basis. For example, EHRs with workflow tools may allow the manager to quickly identify patients that have been waiting for a return call on an urgent clinical matter past a certain time limit.

Clinical Documentation—The use of different standards and rating scales could complicate the use of the EHR among the doctors and staff. Although the lack of consistency is common in paper medical records, EHRs offer more flexibility in operations by allowing many staff members to view a medical record instantaneously. By having to adjust to different reporting and documentation standards, the staff may not be as efficient. For example, one doctor may use a number to flag serious issues while another doctor may use a text note. Staff would have to be trained on the different documentation methods for each doctor.

Reporting Limitations—Using different measures, standards and record structures may complicate your ability to produce reports. For example, different doctors may use different scales, data items or information to classify patient conditions and status. Reporting would be complicated since the different scales and strategies would require complex normalization programming to produce summary statistics, or list patients with a specific condition. For example, two physicians may use different sets of adjectives to describe the same situation. The report options would have to be programmed to insure that "High" for one doctor is the same as 8 to 10 for another doctor, and "Severe" for a third doctor. The reporting situation may be further complicated when different doctors collect information that is not easily related in the EHR. For example, one doctor may collect three pieces of information that are summarized in another doctor's chart note. Complicated programming will be needed for a report containing patients from both doctors that meet a certain selection criteria. Reporting limitations are especially significant for practices that are facing pay for performance standards. If a practice cannot easily and reliably identify patients requiring a service, at risk, or with an outstanding treatment program, then the practice will not be able to effectively allocate clinical and administrative resources to ensure that patients are managed within Meaningful Use and pay for performance guidelines. Additionally, inconsistent entry and information access could complicate your ability to support interoperability standards that are needed to maintain electronic relationships with other healthcare providers. For example, you may have difficulty building a transaction with specific information if the transaction has to be built from one set of information for one doctor and a different set of information for another doctor.

Support Costs—Maintaining the EHR clinical content and training staff will be more expensive with multiple standards for a single clinical condition. If a change is required for a clinical standard, that change would have to be programmed for each template and reported separately. Your support investment will produce a better return by focusing on refinements that allow the practice to capitalize on economies of scale instead of paying multiple times to solve the same problem in each template.

Many doctors are concerned with the loss of independence and the inability to customize their clinical records. For example, a patient chief complaint may not fit in a checklist designed by the vendor or practice. Similarly, the EHR may not allow for the textual richness that the physician uses to describe a patient condition. However, most EHR products allow physicians to insert an ad hoc note into the clinical record. Judicious use of specific notes and appropriate clinical standards will allow most practices to maintain a balance between the benefits of clinical standards and documenting unusual situations.

TIP: If the practice decides to use a single clinical standard for each clinical condition, the physicians and medical practices committee should set up a process to insure that the standard is used and evolves to meet the changing needs of the patients and physicians. The development process should include a review by the doctors that addresses the specific documentation needs of each physician and meets patient service objectives. In these situations, each change should be analyzed and reviewed to insure that the continuity of the medical record information is preserved and that the practice workflow is modified to take advantage of the change. Otherwise, the practice could encounter serious problems analyzing clinical results for pay for performance and Meaningful Use if different documentation protocols are used in a span of time.

POLICIES

Under appropriate practice governance, the practice management team needs to establish policies to support the EHR implementation and its use.

Although a number of factors will affect the particular policies you choose, one of the more challenging issues is managing and maintaining the "Designated Record Set." The HIPAA Privacy Standard defined the designated record set as:

(1) A group of records maintained by or for a covered entity that is:
   (i) The medical records and billing records about individuals maintained by or for a covered health care provider;
   (ii) The enrollment, payment, claims adjudication, and case or medical management record systems maintained by or for a health plan; or
   (iii) Used, in whole or in part, by or for the covered entity to make decisions about individuals.
(2) For purposes of this paragraph, the term *record* means any item, collection, or grouping of information that includes protected health information and is maintained, collected, used, or disseminated by or for a covered entity.

The designated record set affects your policies, transition strategy and support. The implications of the designated record set are extensive since you will be completely changing the nature, composition and usage of your medical information from a paper chart to the EHR.

Practices that include several entities (e.g., practice, therapy center, pain center and ASC) will face a challenge maintaining an individual medical record for each entity. The EHR setup, as well as the EHR features, will affect your ability to meet these requirements. For example, the EHR audit and security features may allow you to maintain separate records in the system but the separate records may be difficult to access across the entities. If you have one database for the practice and another database for the therapy center, then you will need to have a mechanism to communicate information from the clinic to the therapy center and vice versa. Otherwise, you could be in the ironic situation where the staff prints out information from the ASC's EHR to scan into the practice EHR.

The EHR implementation effort must address the transition from a paper-based medical record to an EHR. These policies help you manage patient treatment continuity and maintain the contents of the paper chart as part of your designated record set. Your practice policies must be maintained to govern the transition while making sure that you comply with the HIPAA standards. See additional information on medical record composition issues in other sections of this chapter.

Additional policy issues include:

EHR Project Management—The implementation of an EHR will affect all employees, doctors and aspects of the practice. The practice management should establish enabling policies and support for the EHR. Such policies should include support for the project and project team as well as an escalation policy to get management involved in resolving any problems. For example, an approved workflow strategy to establish a triage line for patients must be backed up by management support for the change to insure that the service is used and that individuals will not be able to bypass the practice's decision. The EHR project must have adequate resources and management support to achieve the goals of the project within the timeline established and approved by practice management.

EHR Clinical Content Management—The practice needs to formally empower the EHR Implementation Team to establish the appropriate clinical standards for the practice and implement the EHR features to support those standards. In many cases, practice clinical standards are a foreign concept. The lack of standards do not necessarily affect the other doctors in the practice. For example, the use of different intake sheet for the same condition may not be a factor if doctors typically do not collaborate on patient care. However, with the EHR, the lack of standards could inhibit the ability of the practice to capitalize on the EHR for workflow improvement, compliance, treatment management and patient care. For example, differences in EHR documentation could inhibit tracking of outstanding patient care plans and tasks. In the final analysis, the doctors are the key to clinical content management. However, the EHR Project Team needs to establish a process that guides the doctors through the approval process and insures that the doctor's decisions are implemented on a consistent basis throughout the practice. The responsibility rests with the doctors to develop a standard within the EHR and set up the EHR to take advantage of the standard. This effort may include a comprehensive analysis of the EHR clinical content, identification of issues based on the practice's needs, and development of solutions to any clinical problems or issues. The solutions should be vigorously tested and then rolled out to the clinical staff and doctors in a standardized fashion.

Establish Privacy and Security Officers—The HIPAA Privacy and Security Standards require the appointment of a Privacy Officer and a Security Officer for covered entities. If your practice is a covered entity, the EHR will dramatically empower these positions to comply with the HIPAA requirements. For example, role-based security in an EHR will allow you to comply with the HIPAA Privacy requirements. The audit trail will allow you to monitor medical record access and track disclosures. However, these features must be backed up with policies and procedures that insure timely review as well as supporting personnel policies to assure compliance. For example, the existence of an audit trail is ineffective unless the Privacy and Security Officers check for compliance with practice standards and compliance is reported to management on a periodic basis. Similarly, your policies will not be effective if user access rights are not maintained on a timely basis for new employees, and former employees, as well as changes to job responsibilities and roles for continuing employees.

Audit Policies—Most EHR systems maintain audit trails of medical record changes, additions and accesses. The practice should establish audit and access policies to guide the enforcement and tracking mechanisms. The audit policies will determine when the audit trails will be analyzed and where the audit will focus. Audit focus may be driven by policy changes or previous analysis of audit issues. For example, you may conduct periodic audit trail review of medical record for patients in the public eye that is backed up by stringent personnel policies. Note that audit reports to management should be based on a reporting period and not purely driven by exceptions and problems.

Security Policies—Security policies should address the physical, administrative and technical security safeguards mandated by the HIPAA Security Standards. The policies should recognize a security standard for the practice, as well as a process to review security issues and vulnerabilities on a periodic basis. You could let incidents trigger a security review (e.g., hardware changes or software installation), or conduct the reviews every six months or once annually. Security policies should cover a wide range of issues including the maintenance of offsite backups, backup standards, computer room access, authorization standards for doctors and employees, training standards and reporting protocols. The security policies should also include an appropriate report to the Security Officer and practice management on the current compliance status of the practice. This way the practice will meet the HIPAA requirements as well as maintain appropriate controls over the EHR system and data. This process should include items that may be "behind the scenes" of your system, such as firewalls, virus software and general access to your computer systems. Indeed, many problems can be traced back to a series of violations that lead to a significant problem. For more information on HIPAA Security Standards, contact the Office of HIPAA Standards at CMS.

Notice of Privacy Practices—The HIPAA Privacy standards mandate that covered entities have a Notice of Privacy Practices. A new consent or acknowledgement of the notice is required for any substantive changes to the Notice of Privacy Practices. The Notice of Privacy Practices may require changes to accommodate the EHR. For example, the EHR may affect the tracking of disclosures, availability of medical records and nature of medical records that can be provided to the patient. The practice should consult with legal counsel to determine if the current Notice of Privacy Practices will require changes to accommodate the EHR. In any event, your EHR will effect how you manage privacy issues and meet the release of information needs of patients. Note that you need to verify that privacy information is easily accessible to EHR users to assure compliance with patient limitations and issues. For example, some EHRs allow for an alert message that is displayed when a patient record is accessed. You could note any privacy issues on the alert message.

Personal Use—An EHR significantly increases the risk of loss from a system failure or problem. Practice policies may be created to significantly limit or prohibit the personal use of practice computers. Personal computer use has exposed practices to viruses and other damaging corruptions. For example, downloading freeware into a practice-based computer exposed a network of 100 workstations to a 2-day stoppage due to a virus that overloaded the mail server. In other cases, loading a game onto a workstation created a conflict with critical software needed to run the EHR. The more control you assert over system use, the less chance of a problem for your system.

Clinical Data Access—When an employee looks at a paper chart, the paper chart does not make a record of the access. An EHR allows instantaneous access to any medical record subject to security constraints. Some EHRs allow you to limit access by type of clinical information, and even to a list of selected patients. Depending on the capability of your EHR, you may be able to limit EHR access based on patient type, location and a number of other options. However, the EHR makes a record of every employee action for future reference and review. The practice may want to define a specific policy and review standard to limit employee access to the need-to-know standard of the HIPAA Privacy Standards. Such a process should consider the retention strategy for these access logs. For example, you will want to keep adequate logs online to look back and review problems even though such logs may consume a fair amount of disk space. In some cases, these policies may affect other relationships. For example, one practice could not dismiss employees for inappropriate access to the medical records due to a union agreement.

Role-Based Access—The HIPAA Privacy Standards require the use of a role-based access strategy. Ideally, the practice should design and establish an access policy based on the definition of roles. Each role would have a defined access and edit capability. The policy should allow for exceptions to be approved by the Security and/or Privacy Officer with appropriate reporting to practice management. Note that exceptions to the role-based security strategy should be reviewed and approved by appropriate practice supervisors and/or management. For example, some EHRs allow the user to violate security access in an emergency. Typically, the EHR records the unauthorized access in a special audit log. However, someone needs to check the log to verify the emergency access.

Paper Record Retention—Practices pursuing paperless medical records will need paper retention policies to support the EHR. A paper retention policy will be needed for existing paper charts that are scanned into the EHR as well as paper documents received from the Go Live date going forward. The paper retention policy should be developed in consultation with your legal counsel and malpractice insurance carrier. For example, your legal counsel may not have a problem shredding the documents when scanned, but your malpractice carrier may require retention for a year. For example, some states recognize the EHR chart as a valid and legal replacement for the paper chart from the day the EHR chart is available. Typically, the paper charts are retained for a certain period after scanning of the chart. Miscellaneous paper documents scanned after EHR Go Live are typically retained for a certain period after the document is scanned. Note that some practices shred the charts and paper documents as soon as the information is scanned. If you keep the documents, make sure that you have a strategy to locate a document in the unlikely event that you need to get the original. For example, you may file the scanned documents by date and user.

Implementation Policies—EHR implementation is a strategic move by a practice. Practices need to consider what, if any inducements or penalties will be used to insure that the EHR is adopted by the physicians and employees. If some physicians are using the EHR, and others are not, then the practice will have to maintain the paper records as well as pay for the EHR. Some physician practices establish policies that insure the paper records will be eliminated. For example, the EHR implementation is based on a strict guideline and timeframe. Policy options include establishing a clinical standard for the practice and terminating availability and access to the paper records after a certain date. On the financial side, physicians who continue to use dictation and paper medical records could be charged for paper medical records and the EHR computer system in their compensation formula.

Practice policies are key tools to convey management support for the EHR implementation. The right polices will avoid a myriad of implementation challenges and insure that the EHR project is adequately supported. This way, the implementation effort can focus on a successful implementation and not get sidetracked with the question of whether the practice should have an EHR. For example, one practice implemented an EHR which was not adequately supported by management. The project went through many sudden changes and was significantly delayed.

PROJECT MANAGEMENT

Managing an EHR implementation project encompasses a number of tasks and issues. Unfortunately, few practices are fully aware of the scope of managing an EHR project due to the lack of clarity in the EHR vendor relationship. Typically, vendors do not expand upon practice responsibilities and process. Vendor project meetings frequently monitor your progress in preparing for the next vendor step, but do not necessarily specify the types of tasks you need to manage. For example, an EHR vendor may say that you need to set up the scanning system, but it will not walk you through standardizing your document descriptions, capturing scanned images or the disposition of the scanned documents.

To succeed, the practice needs to manage resources for the EHR project. Some practices use internal resources, although few practices have internal expertise in EHR implementation. Some practices use vendor resources at an additional charge, and other practices use independent consultants. Vendor EHR expertise may be offset by the independence of an external consultant. In some situations, vendor staff may not be able to act as an advocate on the practice's behalf in the event of problems and misunderstandings. For example, an error may not be as vigorously pursued by a vendor's employee. In other situations, vendor conversion errors may by corrected by the practice staff rather than the vendor redoing the work correctly.

Regardless of your strategy, the project should be guided by a formal management process as well as management tools:

Project Plan—A project plan is a running list of the various EHR to-do items. The project plan is used to monitor project steps and includes administrative, technical, workflow and other implementation issues. Project plans may be managed through a spreadsheet, project management product or a word-processing table. The project plan should be initially compiled with as much detail as possible. The actual items will evolve as the project proceeds, so you can respond and focus on evolving issues. For example, an initial project plan may specify that the current workstations need to be reviewed to meet the minimum EHR requirements. As the project proceeds, specific tasks may be defined to upgrade various workstations. **ALERT:** Two sample project plans are included at the back of this chapter one for a small practice and a second for a larger practice.

Key Issues—A variety of problems and issues will arise as the project proceeds. From getting a policy decision on record retention to scheduling staff and doctors for training, problems and issues must be tracked and managed. In some cases, the issues may affect progress and, in other cases, issues may involve evolving issues. For example, EHR reports may require review by a clinical practices committee that has yet to be formed. In another case, you may want to set up sessions with key referring practices to train them on the changes to your procedures and outgoing reports. A sample key issues table follows (see Table 10.2), and another sample can be found at the end of this chapter.

TABLE 10.2

Area	Issues	Status	Assigned	Start	Due	Comment

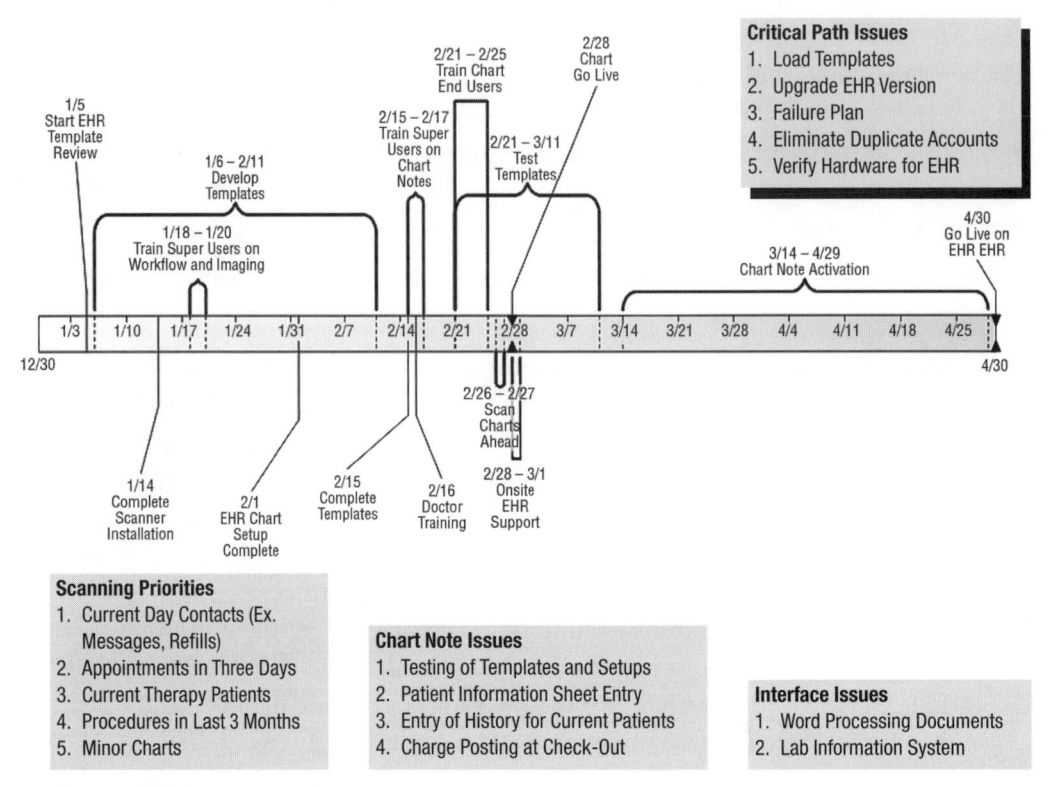

FIGURE 10.1

Timeline annotations:
- 1/5 Start EHR Template Review
- 1/6 – 2/11 Develop Templates
- 1/18 – 1/20 Train Super Users on Workflow and Imaging
- 2/15 – 2/17 Train Super Users on Chart Notes
- 2/21 – 2/25 Train Chart End Users
- 2/21 – 3/11 Test Templates
- 2/28 Chart Go Live
- 3/14 – 4/29 Chart Note Activation
- 4/30 Go Live on EHR EHR
- 1/14 Complete Scanner Installation
- 2/1 EHR Chart Setup Complete
- 2/15 Complete Templates
- 2/16 Doctor Training
- 2/26 – 2/27 Scan Charts Ahead
- 2/28 – 3/1 Onsite EHR Support

Critical Path Issues
1. Load Templates
2. Upgrade EHR Version
3. Failure Plan
4. Eliminate Duplicate Accounts
5. Verify Hardware for EHR

Scanning Priorities
1. Current Day Contacts (Ex. Messages, Refills)
2. Appointments in Three Days
3. Current Therapy Patients
4. Procedures in Last 3 Months
5. Minor Charts

Chart Note Issues
1. Testing of Templates and Setups
2. Patient Information Sheet Entry
3. Entry of History for Current Patients
4. Charge Posting at Check-Out

Interface Issues
1. Word Processing Documents
2. Lab Information System

Timeline—Project plans are great tools for managing a project, but they may not be the best tools to communicate with the project team. Project plans can consist of 100s of implementation items spread across a couple dozen pages. However, most people involved in EHR implementation will not be able to understand the complete project plan or dig through the details that they need to know. You should consider supplementing the project plan with a project timeline. The project timeline presents key events and issues affecting the EHR project. While the project manager is responsible for the detailed plan and issues, the rest of the project team needs a tool to understand the context of the project and evolving issues. A timeline can focus on the more immediate issues and additional details added as the project proceeds. The timeline can be annotated with important information for the project. For example, you can highlight key critical path issues and important strategies. A one page document presents a concise view of the project and will help your group understand the big picture. A sample timeline is shown in Figure 10.1.

Critical Path Diagram—Another useful project management tool is the critical path plan. The critical path plan graphically shows the relationship and sequence of items by category. The critical path plan will help highlight the key tasks and status as the plan progresses. For example, the critical path plan may

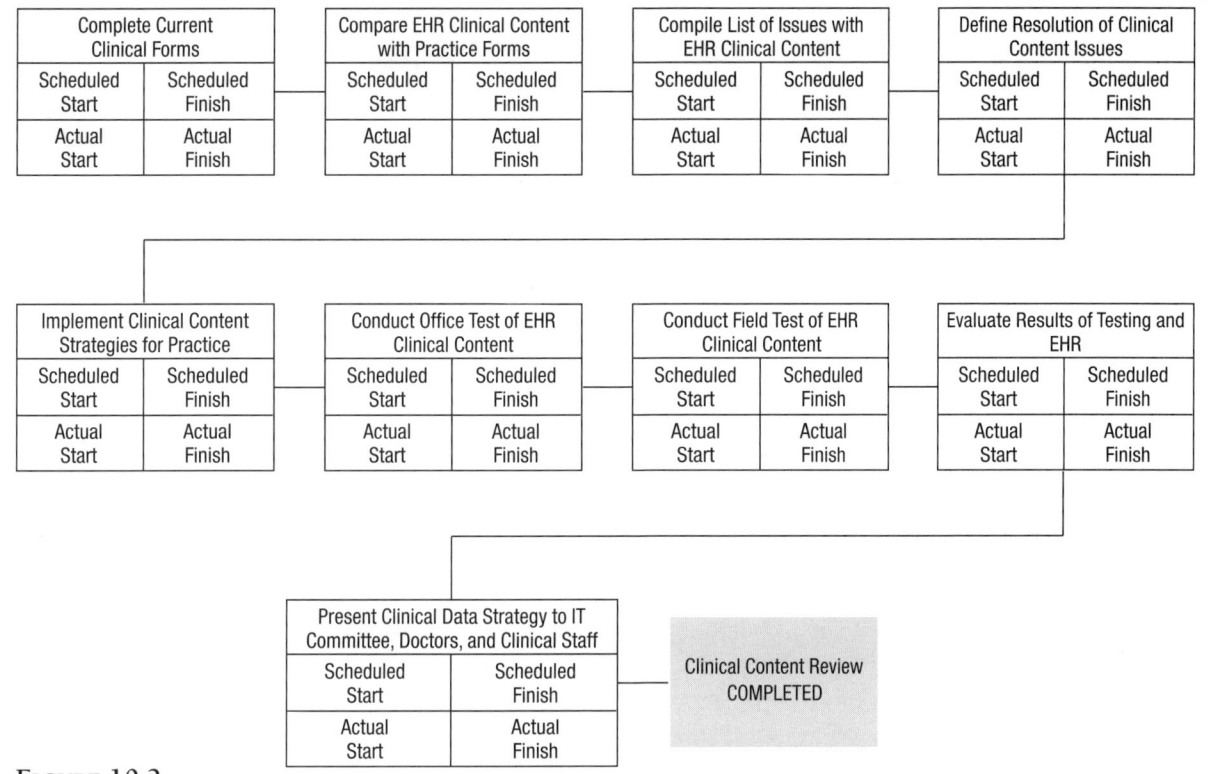

FIGURE 10.2

show the relationship between hardware installation and the start of training. A sample critical path diagram is shown in Figure 10.2.

Clinical Content Tracking—EHR projects that include clinical content changes or development should use a separate table to manage the clinical content. The clinical content items should be listed for the practice, and the various steps should be tracked and monitored. In general, clinical content efforts take the most time and require the most limited resources: doctors and clinicians. At a minimum, your staff should verify the clinical content, to define any changes and enhancements. Depending on your EHR strategy and tools, you may want to hold off on implementing any changes until you have verified that there is not a viable workaround. In the absence of an alternative handling of the clinical situation, any changes should be tested and approved by the appropriate doctors and clinicians. A sample clinical content tracking table is shown in Table 10.3.

A single document or tool will not help you to communicate with all of the various internal parties involved in the project. Using a combination of project plan, timelines and, if appropriate, critical path diagrams will insure that the details as well as the big picture project issues can be effectively planned, communicated and coordinated according to the various needs and interests of the EHR project team.

TABLE 10.3

Clinical Area	Assign to	Review EHR Content	Inventory Issues/ Changes	Design Changes/ Setup	Program Changes/ Setup	Unit Test Changes/ Setup	Field Test	Present to Drs/ Staff
Internal Medicine								
OB/GYN								
Cardiology								
Nurse Triage								
Advice Line								

Possessing the tools of the project is very different from managing the project. Managing the project includes assigning tasks, organizing resources and coordinating the effort of various parties. As soon as you have chosen your product, you should identify an EHR project team for the practice. The internal project team will not necessarily include an EHR vendor representative. As a practical matter, the vendor representative should not be privy to a number of project issues including strategies for dealing with issues and managing other vendors. Additionally, the practice may need to undertake extensive discussions of policy, strategy, and operational issues that are avoided by many vendors. The project team should consist of the following resources:

Project Manager—The project manager is the guide and architect of your EHR effort. Depending on the internal resources and expertise, the project manager may be an internal or external resource. The key role of the project manager is to set expectations, track progress and address issues. The project manager will be responsible for working with internal resources to get everyone up to speed and focus efforts on the implementation effort. The project manager role should include helping the practice arrive at decisions on using the EHR as well as compelling doctors and staff to support the EHR project. Such efforts may include one-on-one discussions and dealing with key needs of a particular doctor or staff person. For example, a doctor may be concerned about how they will be able to access information that their nurses record on a log that is kept on the doctor's desk. If the EHR contains the information, the project manager may arrange for a special report or screen view to be made available to the doctor.

Technical Resource—In the final analysis, the practice will need a key person to address technical issues and problems. The EHR is too important to leave all support to an outside party. You do not necessarily want a high-level technical person, but rather someone who can work with staff on common problems and issues as well as coordinate the resolution of more complex issues with the EHR vendor or hardware vendor. Ideally, the internal person should be able to help staff address day-to-day issues and needs. For a once a month or a once a year issue, you may decide to use an outside resource such as a systems integrator or a local network management team. The technical resource should be knowledgeable of your current technology base and work with the appropriate vendors on upgrades to support the EHR.

Clinical Resource(s)—Depending on the nature and size of the practice, clinical resources may include doctors and nurses. At a minimum, clinical resources should *include a subject matter expert in each clinical area* covered by the practice. In many cases, more than one clinical resource will be needed. Primary care practices may have too broad a set of clinical areas to be managed by one person, and specialty practices may need support in sub-specialty areas. Scribes and technicians may also serve as clinical resources. Practices in which doctors do their own documentation will want to use doctors as clinical resources. The clinical resources are charged with verifying the clinical content and practice setup. They also become the defacto resident experts to the staff as the EHR is activated. Therefore, you need people who have the time, skills and will to help the other people in your practice use the EHR. The clinical resources will review the clinical content and make adjustments as needed. However, any adjustments should be carefully reviewed to determine that the adjustment is effective and appropriate as well as not already handled by the EHR. For example, some practices have developed a strategy outside of the standard product to perform a function that is built into the EHR product. The clinical resources will coordinate testing, perform training and support other implementation efforts. A key challenge will be to manage patient services while the EHR effort proceeds. The implementation schedule should allow adequate time for the doctors and other clinicians to work the EHR efforts into their schedules. You need one or more doctors who are willing to put in the time to verify that the EHR clinical content will support your practice, and spend the time to become familiar enough and confident enough to move forward with using the EHR.

Medical Records Resource—The medical records resource should be the manager or supervisor of the Medical Records Department. The medical records resource will be responsible for formulating, testing and executing the conversion strategy for paper charts as well as supporting the flow of electronic healthcare record information. A survey of current paper medical records as well as testing of various scanning and paper management strategies may be necessary. The paper medical record strategy and supporting policy drives this effort. However, the real challenge is the conversion of the paper records to the EHR. Depending on your go live strategy and scanning decision, the handing of the existing paper record in the conversion effort is a massive undertaking. Whether you are scanning selected pieces of the paper chart or entering key information into the EHR (Ex. Previous procedures, and immunizations), the medical records resource will need excellent management skills and be in a position to manage this important aspect of the conversion effort. For example, you may need a medical assistant or nurse to support your paper record strategy if analysis of medical information is part of the conversion effort.

Business Office Resource—The business office uses information from the EHR to justify claims as well as dispute claim payment with payers. Front desk staff will scan clinical information into the EHR and trigger the tracking of patient office flow in the EHR. The daily reconciliation process will be redesigned to reconcile charge posting from the EHR to the PMS. Additional procedures may verify task completion standards. For example, the Business Office may verify that all tasks are completed on a daily basis. Otherwise, the number of outstanding tasks will become unmanageable. The business office resource must work on insuring the continuing billing process in the absence of a paper chart and even without a fee slip. For example, your business office may require different audit procedures since there are no fee tickets when charges are recorded in the EHR. This effort may be made all the more difficult for practices that replace their PMS before implementing the EHR.

To manage the project on a daily basis, the project manager must maintain contact with the appropriate working teams to monitor progress and address issues. Several forums can be used to maintain project momentum:

Ad-Hoc Discussions—The quantity and complexity of issues is a major problem for managing an EHR project. The number and variety of issues that arise can be daunting. EHR issues could include who gets a tablet, verifying the medical record generated by the EHR, training staff and deciding on changes to clinical workflow. The parties that can resolve and address any pending issues need to have the flexibility to pull away for meetings on appropriate matters. Some practices have experienced serious delays due to scheduling issues. For example, one practice had to wait two weeks to hold a meeting with managers on medical record scanning. Flexibility and quick response to evolving EHR issues will insure that you maintain project momentum and continuity. This situation is especially challenging during the initial rollout of the EHR when adjustments may be needed on a real time basis.

Vendor Project Meetings—Most vendors use project management meetings to coordinate the vendor resources. Vendor project manager meetings frequently address the expected services and activities of the vendor in light of the current practice efforts. Typically, vendors do not see their role as making the decision on what to do, but offer the practice options on what is possible with the product. The vendor meetings may be held with the entire practice EHR project team or key representatives from your EHR project team. ***TIP:*** Make sure that you are prepared to take the initiative and effectively manage the vendor. In a number of cases, vendors defer to the practice on issues that the practice staff is not prepared to address. The outstanding issues can lead to delays and even additional costs. In order to avoid such problems, the practice should keep track of all issues and insure that the vendor provides an agenda for project meetings. In the absence of a comprehensive agenda, you may not be able to meet your meeting objectives or even have the practice staff needed to arrive at a decision.

Internal Project Meetings—Internal project meetings are used to coordinate the efforts of staff and monitor progress. The internal meetings may be held every week or two depending on the project stage and activities. The project meetings should be based on an agenda and notes of key decisions should be published and shared after the meeting. In some cases, project meetings will result in changes to the other project management tools. Internal project meetings should involve the entire EHR project team, but not necessarily the vendor. The internal project team may be discussing issues that are not relevant or appropriate for the vendor. In some cases, the internal project meetings may include a changing set of participants. For example, initially you may include the PMS vendor to deal with interface issues, or the manager of the first office to go live with the EHR.

The key project goal is maintaining the pace of work, and keeping the team up-to-date on evolving issues. Many EHR projects get sidetracked due to competing priorities and lack of progress. The implementation of an EHR involves a complete set of work in addition to the continuing operations of the practice. If you do not have additional resources to support the EHR effort, you risk delays in implementation or failures due to a lack of focus.

Before you proceed, make sure that you have a workable plan and you feel confident in the capabilities of the software and the project team. For example, one practice scanned more than 30,000 medical records into its EHR. After the scanning process, the practice discovered that the EHR enhancements would not work for the practice and it moved to another product. The conversion of the images from the "old" EHR was difficult due to technology problems. In another situation, an EHR project was undertaken by a single clinician without the support of the practice or staff. The goal of the project was to "try" a medical record, but the project was merely a waste of time and money.

Project plans dramatically differ among practices due the differences in the various implementation areas. For example, an EHR project that includes extensive clinical content efforts will differ from a project that takes clinical content "out of the box." To formulate the implementation plan that is right for you, consider the issues outlined in Table 10.4.

After designing the project plan, the plan should be maintained as needed to track the project and problems. The project manager should feel free to edit, delete, split and combine items to keep the plan current and useful. For example, you may have expected to develop an interface that is available from a third party. Once the go forward decision is made, the plan should be updated. Note that the practice (not the EHR vendor) EHR implementation plan can run to several dozen pages, but the use of timelines and plan summaries will help you highlight the important issues that the project team should focus on.

In the course of the EHR project, you will encounter problems. The problems may be self inflicted or a function of how certain components work together. For example, you may

TABLE 10.4

Area	PROJECT MANAGEMENT ISSUES TO CONSIDER
General	What are the key project task areas and what are the resources needed for each area? What are the current critical path items and who is responsible for addressing them? How much time can the EHR Team members practically dedicate to the project on a daily basis? How much time can "champion" doctors practically commit to the EHR project? What addition resources will be needed and for how long?
Clinical Standards	What are the clinical content areas that require verification? What clinical content areas require substantial development? Who are the key physicians and other clinical staff in each clinical area that could work on EHR implementation? What is the verification process? What is the development and modification strategy? What is the testing strategy? What is the deployment and activation strategy?
Policy	What are the practice policies that need approval from the practice management team? What policies require legal counsel and/or risk manager advice? What policies are needed to address risk management issues that are unique to the EHR product? What policies are needed to address risk management issues associated with the way the practice uses the EHR? What policies are needed to prevent acceptance problems and issues? What is the escalation policy to insure quick resolution to problems and resistance? What is the governance structure that will represent practice management for the EHR implementation?
Project Management	What are the resources that will be available to support the EHR project? What staffing strategies will be used to maintain continuity during the project? What are the reporting and management lines for the EHR project? How often will meetings be held for the practice EHR project team? How often will management meetings be held with the vendor?
Workflow and Procedures	Who are the key people who understand current operations? What workflow packages are needed to guide the EHR project? How will reasonable access to patient records be maintained during the various transitions to EHR? How will workflow change as new EHR functions are added? How will workflow changes be approved and implemented? What are the organizational changes needed to support workflow changes? How will the departments be reorganized to capitalize on the EHR? What process will be used to reassign and redesign staff positions?
Facilities Management	Where can the computer room be placed? What other facility accommodations are needed for the EHR? What level of security does the practice need to reasonably reduce risks? What physical areas are available to support medical record scanning? Where should printers, scanners, and workstations be placed to support continuing access to the patient record and workflow information? Where can tablets be placed when patients are being examined or procedures are being performed?
Technology Base	What are the current technologies that may need further review? What are the hardware investments needed to mitigate the risk of EHR failure within the practice's budget? What are the communication requirements needed to accommodate the increase in users and the larger amounts of information needed to support the EHR? What hardware will be support an effective server base for the EHR? What workstation and tablet models will be used by the practice? What are the scanning, and printing requirements of the various departments and locations? What verification process is needed to validate the delivery and installation of equipment? What verification process is needed to check the interoperability of system components?

Area	PROJECT MANAGEMENT ISSUES TO CONSIDER
Software Setup	What current information is needed to support EHR setup? How will expected changes to the practice effect EHR use? What policies are needed to support software setup? What testing is needed for interfaces to the PMS and diagnostic equipment? What is the timing of the initial download of patient demographic and appointment information into the EHR?
Data Conversion	What process will be used to determine the disposition of paper medical records? What resources will be needed to prepare and process information from the paper records into the EHR? What information will be preloaded into the EHR for a patient? What strategy will be used for converting existing electronic data to the EHR? What hardware, facility and staffing resources will be needed to support the EHR? How will the data conversion process assure quality and avoid duplication of information?
Training	What training materials will be needed to support the project? How will the practice train doctors and support doctors in their initial use of the EHR? What training tasks will be done by practice staff? How will training be broken down into manageable pieces for users? How will super-user training differ from regular-user training? What materials will be needed to deal with cross-vendor training related to hardware and interfaces? What supplemental training plans will be used to develop staff knowledge and flexibility? What programs and procedures will be needed to assure adequate support for users and super users?

find that an expected interface is not available, or that the condition of the medical records precludes certain conversion strategies. In any event, you need to insure that you can get the relevant project team resources organized to address the problem, adjust the plan, and move forward.

WORKFLOW AND PROCEDURES

From the initial call on a patient problem to the office visit and follow-up tracking, the EHR will change the way you record, use and access information. How you manage and prepare for this change will affect your entire effort.

Given that these massive changes will occur, you need a strategy to practically manage, guide and deal with the EHR. Some practices wait until the system is installed to "see what happens." Other practices look to the vendor to guide the changes. If you wait until the system is installed, you may corrupt your EHR effort with constant changes. If you look to your vendor, you may not get a solution that best fits your practice. The time between signing your contract and the installation of the hardware can be used to formulate your EHR vision.

To put the issues into perspective, look at how you would go about the design of a new office. Would you go to a hardware store and buy the materials without a blueprint? Would you leave the design decisions to the construction crew? The approach of most practices to EHR implementation is analogous to building an office without an architect or a general contractor. One way to avoid such a problem is to develop a workflow model that will serve as your blueprint for the EHR implementation.

The workflow effort will help you cope with the real effects of an EHR. Key changes to consider include:

Staff Interactions and Use—EHRs with workflow features will enable staff to interact on patient service issues. The workflow model supports the entry and tracking of patient tasks. For example, a task can be sent to a doctor on a patient issue and forwarded to another staff person for follow-up. The EHR simplifies the use of staff by physicians and provides a tracking tool to manage patient issues. As important, an alternative view of the pending tasks will help supervisors identify problems and proactively address patient needs.

Instantaneous Access—EHR supports immediate access to patient medical records. EHRs eliminate the problems with co-locating patient issues, the medical chart and the provider. For example, some practices use a message center or phone message service to take patient messages with the prospect of a return call to the patient. If the EHR provides instantaneous access, should your practice have a nurse line and address specific problems immediately? For those practices with nurse lines, the EHR will empower the nurses to more effectively address and document patient issues. Indeed, you may be able to address a patient issue during the call. Such a response will reduce patient anxiety and make better use of staff and doctors. Thereby, doctors could have more time to deal with the more serious issues and problems.

Information Velocity—By storing and routing images, lab results, faxes and other items, EHRs significantly speed up the flow of information. For example, an interfaced diagnostic test may cut several steps from patient test ordering and results access. The speed could change the way the practice manages patient services as well as how staff coordinates care with the doctors. For example, an EHR interface with a diagnostic tool cut intake processing time in half for a specialty practice. The faster intake cut wait times and resulted in less wait time for the doctors and patients. As important, you may be able to serve more patients with the same diagnostic equipment.

Before you start considering the effect of the changes and set up your workflow "blueprint," gather some important information on your current status and the tools you will be working with:

Cataloging Current Clinical Data—Some practices have no clinical forms and do everything in free form notes, and/or transcription. Other practices have a wide range of clinical documentation tools and forms. Intake forms, clinical forms and treatment plans are examples of existing clinical data.

Initially, the practice should gather copies of every form used in the clinical areas. Clinical forms may include patient intake forms, check-off sheets for specific diseases or chief complaints, order forms for services and therapy and surgery scheduling request documents. **TIP**: If you have multiple offices or departments, make sure that your get copies of the different forms used at different locations and even forms used by different doctors.

For each form, you should document the source of the form, situations the form is used for and the relevant staff or doctors. You should carefully note any special or unclear information on the form as well as any special usage issues. For example, a form may include a coding system that is unique to the doctor. In some situations, the practice may use the form for a unique case, perhaps because there is no other form available or the form has never been updated.

Document Current Procedures—To get a clear picture of your situation, review your current procedures. Current procedures may be documented in a manual, written notes held by staff members or other informal documentation. The current procedure documentation will facilitate the design of new procedures and workflow with the EHR.

If you have a current procedure manual, the manual should be verified with the actual office operation. The procedure review process should identify the actual procedures that are used as well as key nuances and exceptions. Even if you have a procedures manual, verify the current procedures and clinical processes.

Some practices have no written procedures and rely on a key person or the staff to know how to function. However, the HIPAA standards require a written procedure that establishes the operational standard for the practice. At the end of the EHR implementation process, you will be well positioned to create such a document. However, you will need current procedure information to guide the EHR project. In these cases, you should invest the time briefly to document the current procedures. The documentation does not have to be formal, but the information is necessary to guide your EHR workflow design process.

In either case, the practice should gather information on the actual patient service and clinical management processes. Be especially careful to document hand-offs among staff and doctors as well as the information that is communicated among the various departments. For example, some procedure manuals mention the doctor passing the patient onto diagnostic services, when the patient actually was served by diagnostic services at the direction of mid-level staff. These details will guide the EHR team in designing the workflow that establishes the use of the software and the assignment of hardware to staff.

Include the nuances that will be significant to the EHR project. For example, some locations may use different procedures since they offer other services, feature other staff or have unique equipment. In some cases, different procedures are not based on any clinical or organizational issue; no one ever tried to standardize procedures across all locations.

Compile a List of Key EHR Features—A list of key EHR features will help you determine the effect of the EHR on your processes. The key features can be derived from the EHR analysis. Key features include scanning, tasking, templates, clinical orders, clinical content and patient routing. Surgical scheduling, transcription and patient surveys should also be documented. The key features document should include a few brief observations on the feature, as well as the general implications of the feature for the practice. You may even include a screen sample to clarify the EHR option. For **EXAMPLE**,

> A description can be assigned to a scanned image. The user, date and time are automatically assigned to the scanned image. The description should be structured to consistently identify the key image information.
>
> Tasks may have a due date and priority that can affect clinical standards. Performance standards may be established for responding to tasks with a certain priority. A management function may be established to monitor overdue tasks as well as retrospectively analyze performance and response.
>
> Patient flow may be tracked through the appointment schedule that notes patient status and location. The practice standards would define when the status or location is changed and the significance of status codes.

The information on current clinical issues and the product highlights are your reference point for the development of a new workflow model. After gathering the current information, you should consider establishing the optimal workflow model for the practice. You may be wondering how you can create a new model without getting specific EHR training. However, you should have a general idea of what the system does from your decision-making process. After compiling a list of requirements, attending demonstrations, analyzing various products and visiting a site, you should have a good idea of what the EHR can do for you. If necessary, conduct another demonstration with the vendor as a kick-off to you effort. The next question to answer is how the EHR should operate in your practice.

The workflow design itemizes your expectations and vision. This document will be a blueprint or reference point for the rest of your effort. Thereby, you have a tool to guide you in working with the vendor as well as help you evaluate the effect of various decisions and strategies on your practice. Without such a tool, you will be constantly reacting to the collateral effects of every change and issue. The workflow strategy allows you to look at the situation and issues before your get absorbed in the intensity of EHR implementation. Practices that make it up as they go along frequently end up with partial EHR implementations that do not fully capitalize on their EHR investment.

In support of your workflow design, you need a workflow design facilitator. The facilitator can be an internal or external resource. External facilitators may be useful since they are not tied to your current problems and processes. External facilitators may also have experience implementing EHRs and knowledge of technical issues that may be lacking in your practice. An internal facilitator may be useful since they have a deep understanding of your operation and patients. You may also consider EHR vendor facilitators. However, many EHR vendors do not provide such services and some vendors may impose a model that is not the best solution for your practice. A non-vendor facilitator will help you explore all of your options and help you think creatively. For example, one vendor facilitator tried to impose an operational model that was successful in an orthopedic practice on an ophthalmology practice with an optical shop. The hand-off to the optical shop was not fully developed and the shop was not fully integrated into the EHR. The optical shop continued to use its paper-based forms and logs outside of the EHR. Therefore, the optical shop staff was recording prescription information on a form that was printed by their EHR system in the same office.

You can document the workflow in several different formats. You can document the workflow using written procedures and/or a flowchart (see below). The purpose of the workflow design is not to document every keystroke and patient interaction. **The workflow design should define the movement and handling of information in the practice.** You can start with general workflow concepts and add details as you proceed. Going forward, you will catalog issues that you uncover, key system features that will be used and setup requirements. See the example on the next page.

Documenting the key EHR functions needed for the relevant area will help you plan training as well as insure that you consider all of the effected areas when you design your EHR setup. For example, immunization order tracking and fulfillment may affect patient scheduling, patient intake and patient routing in a pediatric practice. A pediatric practice would want immunizations to be considered in the patient routing steps and orders as well as the recall strategy (see Figure 10.3).

To work with manageable areas, break the workflow into the various areas of your practice. The workflow documentation will become the basis for the setup of the EHR, your detailed procedures and even hardware placement. Workflow design even affects your training plan and strategy. The following table gives you some issues to consider in your workflow effort (see Table 10.5).

By mapping the EHR workflow upfront, you will create a structure and standard for the implementation effort as well as catalogue issues that will be addressed during implementation. Workflow documents allow you to map something you know about (your current clinical processes) with a vision based on your general knowledge of the EHR product. For example, you know the types of outside documents that are received by the practice and added to the paper record. However, such documents are not currently tracked or managed. If those documents could be tracked, what would you want to know about their status, who would be responsible for managing the flow and how would the documents be organized? The answers to these questions would determine a number of setups in any EHR product. The workflow will be refined and detailed as you move forward. The workflow document will facilitate a closer match of the product to your practice.

The workflow document establishes the reference point for your further EHR efforts. The workflow document will affect your hardware setups, software options, training

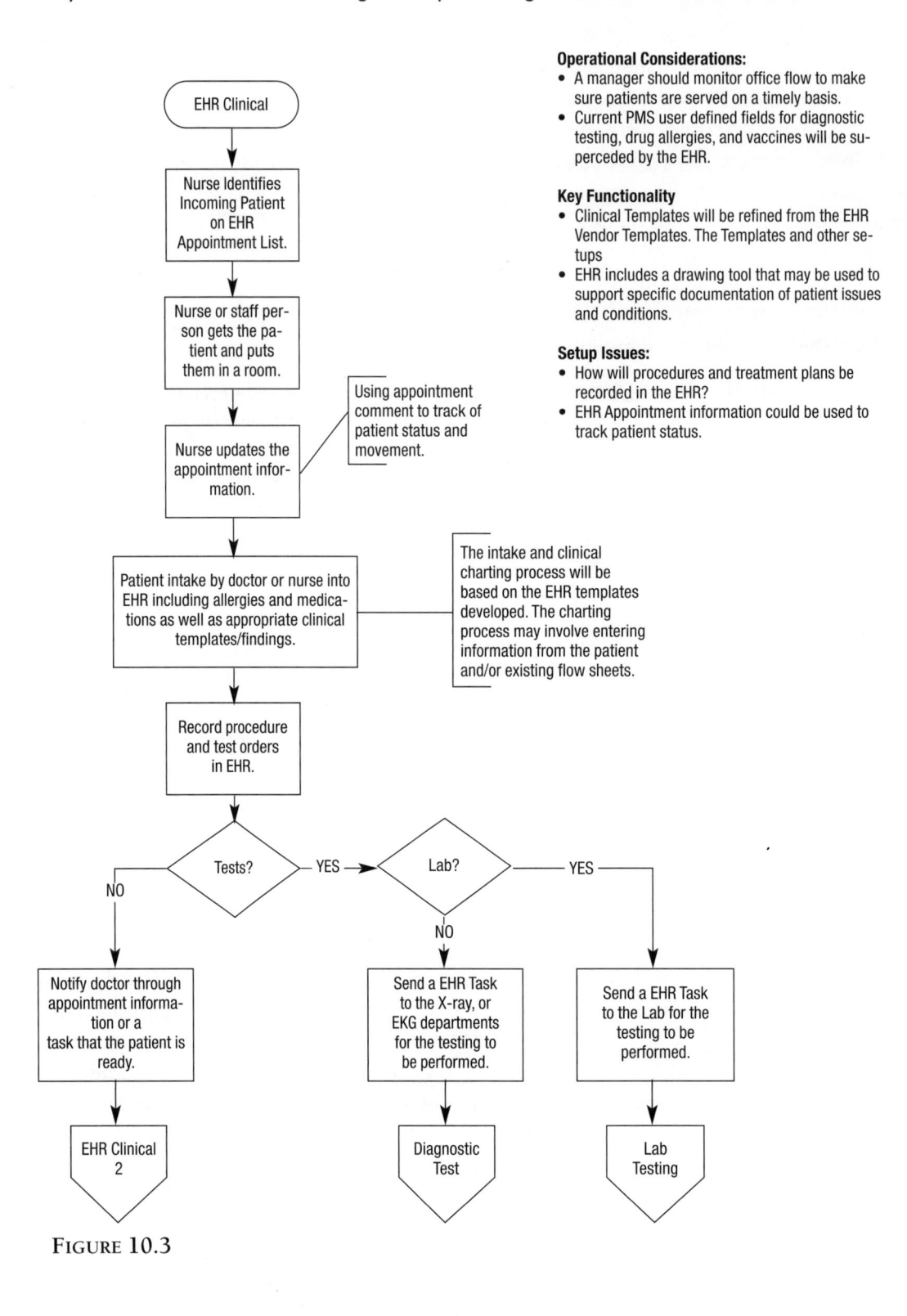

200   Keys to EMR/EHR Success: Selecting and Implementing an Electronic Medical Record

Operational Considerations:
- A manager should monitor office flow to make sure patients are served on a timely basis.
- Current PMS user defined fields for diagnostic testing, drug allergies, and vaccines will be superceded by the EHR.

Key Functionality
- Clinical Templates will be refined from the EHR Vendor Templates. The Templates and other setups
- EHR includes a drawing tool that may be used to support specific documentation of patient issues and conditions.

Setup Issues:
- How will procedures and treatment plans be recorded in the EHR?
- EHR Appointment information could be used to track patient status.

```
EHR Clinical
   │
   ▼
Nurse Identifies Incoming Patient on EHR Appointment List.
   │
   ▼
Nurse or staff person gets the patient and puts them in a room.
   │
   ▼
Nurse updates the appointment information. ──── Using appointment comment to track of patient status and movement.
   │
   ▼
Patient intake by doctor or nurse into EHR including allergies and medications as well as appropriate clinical templates/findings. ──── The intake and clinical charting process will be based on the EHR templates developed. The charting process may involve entering information from the patient and/or existing flow sheets.
   │
   ▼
Record procedure and test orders in EHR.
   │
   ▼
Tests? ──YES──▶ Lab? ──YES──▶ Send a EHR Task to the Lab for the testing to be performed. ──▶ Lab Testing
   │              │
   NO             NO
   │              │
   ▼              ▼
Notify doctor    Send a EHR Task to the X-ray, or EKG departments for the testing to be performed. ──▶ Diagnostic Test
through appointment
information or a
task that the patient
is ready.
   │
   ▼
EHR Clinical 2
```

FIGURE 10.3

TABLE 10.5

Area	WORKFLOW ISSUES TO CONSIDER
General	What overlapping functionality exists in the EHR and PMS systems? Which product (EHR or PMS) will be relied upon to address the overlapping issues? What are the key features of the EHR that should be considered in the new workflow? How does the EHR impact the allocation of employees to the various practice areas and locations? How can the EHR improve the organization of the practice by modality, doctor, pod and/or department? How will the velocity of information flow affect the working styles and workload of clinical staff and doctors? Where does the EHR effect the utilization of administrative staff by clinical operations?
Appointment Scheduling	How can the appointment scheduler access information on pending patient services to more effectively schedule appointments? How will clinical staff trigger appointment scheduling activities? How can the appointment scheduler track expected test results in working with patients on upcoming visits? What connection is maintained between outstanding services, recalls and appointment scheduling?
Patient Portal	How will the practice register patients for access to the patient portal? What supporting EHR features are needed before the patient portal can be activated? What patient portal features will be rolled out and in what order? How will patients access the patient portal from the practice offices? What staff and processes will be used to keep track of patient services items coming in through the patient portal? Who will be able to accept patient information from the patient portal into the EHR?
Medical Records	What are the scanning strategies and standards for the current paper chart? What events will trigger the scanning of the patient's paper chart into the EHR? What are the response requirements for chart-scanning tasks? How will Medical Records prioritize scanning of charts for same day visits, as well as messages, prescription refills and other priorities? How will scanned patient charts be indicated in the EHR and PMS? How will Medical Records produce outgoing medical information including referral letters and medical record releases? What is the initial, transitional and final EHR staffing strategies for the practice? How will Medical Records maintain disclosure logs in the EHR? How will release of information requests be logged and tracked in the EHR? How will ROI activities and disclosures be logged in the EHR?
Phone Triage	What are the priorities for the various phone messages received by the practice? What are the treatment and clinical advice guidelines for patients calling in for service or advice? What is the routing strategy by message types to the appropriate clinical staff? What routing options could the practice use to make better use of clinical resources? How does message routing affect clinical staff utilization? What are the escalation strategies that are possible with the EHR? How will non-patient messages be managed? Who will monitor messages to assure that patient services items are completed in a reasonable time? Should a central call center be used by the practice? What performance tracking measures will the practice want to use for phone triage calls?
Check-In	What PMS based information is needed in the EHR? How will the information be recorded in the EHR? What will be done with clinical documents delivered to the check-in desk by the patient? How will the information be routed? How will the appropriate clinical staff be notified? How will the clinical area be notified of patient arrivals through the EHR? What clinical information is needed to be entered before check-in? What patient clinical information will be captured at check-in? How? What is the assumption/requirement for information transfer from the PMS to the EHR for clinical treatment?

Area	WORKFLOW ISSUES TO CONSIDER
Initial Intake	How does the EHR effect the assignment of intake staff to doctors and patients? What information should be gathered at intake to smooth the clinical process? To what extent should pending patient orders be managed at patient intake? How will the intake staff identify patients ready for service? What documentation requirements will be fulfilled at the initial intake? What services should be performed or triggered before the patient is seen by the doctor? What, if any, historical data should be entered into the EHR during the first patient visit after EHR Go Live? What are the care triggers to enter historical clinical information into a patient's record? How will the intake staff notify the clinical staff on the patient status?
Clinical Treatment	What is the effect of the EHR on the departmental organization of the clinical areas? What is the workflow standard for clinical services in the practice? What clinical workflow variations are needed to accommodate subspecialties or location (e.g., equipment, services) differences? What are the doctor sign-off standards for patient services provided by mid-level staff? How should additional services be verified for payer coverage and/or referral requirements? Does the process affect the entry of an order into the EHR? How are orders for ancillary, lab and diagnostic services recorded and communicated to the appropriate department? What are the treatment plans and follow-up standards for key clinical conditions? Where and how will prescriptions be presented to the patient? Where and how will patient education be presented to the patient? Where and how will information on procedures be presented to the patient? How are follow-up treatment plan items recorded and managed? What is the time line for treatment plans prescribed by the doctors? Who will monitor unsigned notes?
Diagnostic Studies	How will the technicians track pending study orders? What process will be used to assimilate the diagnostic images into the EHR? How will the EHR be used to track the status of diagnostic studies: ordered, completed, reviewed and accepted? What is the routing protocol for diagnostic study orders? What are the performance tolerances for diagnostic studies? Who will monitor outstanding studies and follow through with the patient and/or ordering doctor?
Lab	How will the lab track pending lab orders? How is the performing lab selected for a patient? How will EHR lab orders be entered into the Lab Information System? What mechanism will transfer the lab results to the EHR?
Ancillary Services	What are the priorities for services and how are those priorities indicated? How can the practice smooth the conversion of the patient from the clinic to ancillary services? How are ancillary service orders managed? What status information should be maintained for patients receiving ancillary services? What documentation standards should be used to simplify the reporting of patient status to the doctor? How are product orders (e.g., DME, hearing aids, contacts) managed and tracked?
Check-Out	Is there any EHR information that needs to be reflected in the PMS? How? What, if any, editing of charges from the EHR will be necessary before posting to the PMS? What can the check-out staff do to charge information from the EHR? What will be the audit procedures to insure that all charges from the EHR are posted to the PMS for billing?

Area	WORKFLOW ISSUES TO CONSIDER
Transcription	How does the EHR track dictation that is to be added to the patient's EHR record? How will transcription tasks be tracked in the practice? What effect does the EHR have on outside transcription services? How long will transcription support continue? How will the EHR support the review and distribution of transcribed documents? How will transcription documents get into the EHR? What will be the acceptance procedures for incoming transcription?
Surgery Scheduling	How will the surgical scheduler be informed of pending patient surgeries? How will the surgery scheduler manage the various clinical and administrative issues associated with surgery scheduling? Where will the patient forms and information print for the patient? What status information on pending surgeries will be available to practice staff and doctors? Where will signed patient forms be kept and how will the forms be organized? What information will be saved in the PMS and EHR? How will the information in the two systems be kept current?
Billing	How will posted charges be reconciled between the EHR and PMS systems? What process will verify the coding of charges? How will coded changes be reflected in the EHR? How will the billing department identify PMS claims requiring EHR documentation? Where will the billing department locate and access reports and documentation needed for claims submission?
Recall	What recall standards will be established for key diseases and conditions? How will recalls information be coordinated between the EHR and PMS? What is the purpose of PMS recalls and EHR treatment plan items for the practice?
Collections	What EHR information does the payer collections staff need access to? What format and information will be generated from the EHR system to substantiate submitted claims? What are the transmission options and standards for sending clinical information from the EHR to the payer?
Incoming Documents	How will incoming faxes and other incoming documents be added to the patient medical record? What tools are available to support physician signoff and management of incoming documents? What is the routing protocol for incoming EHR documents? How will non-patient documents and faxes (e.g., Medicare EOBs) be stored in the imaging feature of the EHR?
Quality Assurance	What are the daily procedures to insure the maintenance of medical records on a timely basis? What are the documentation requirements for various chief complaints and diseases? What are the clinical end of day procedures? What are the verification items for clinical end of day? How will the practice monitor outstanding issues and completion of overdue items?
Practice Management	What are the performance and operational standards that should be monitored during the working day? How should overdue tasks and orders be handled? How will PQRI compliance be monitored? How will fulfillment of Meaningful Use be monitored and tracked? How will management evaluate the performance of the practice on a retrospective basis?

and data conversion strategies. Indeed, the workflow document will ultimately be used to create the detailed written procedures that are your key to compliance with the HIPAA Privacy and Security standards. As important, the written procedures will establish the processes that you need to meet the Meaningful Use standards.

FACILITIES MANAGEMENT

EHRs require facility accommodations to protect your investment as well as practically support the EHR.

The first priority should be securing the EHR servers and other key equipment. The typical PMS system is kept any place the practice has room. Practices keep their PMS systems and network servers in employee offices, medical file rooms, hallways, lunch rooms and just about any other place in the practice. If you are using an Application Services Provider. the focus will shift from the server hardware to establishing appropriate communication facilities with your ASP provider.

On the regulatory side, the HIPAA Security Standards include physical security guidelines that should be considered for your practice. You should seriously consider how to protect your EHR from an accident that could damage you equipment or allow inappropriate disclosures. In addition to the HIPAA standards, you want to avoid an incident that could disrupt operations and impact patient service. EHR based facility issues include:

> **Secured Computer Room**—Due to the mission critical nature of the EHR, your practice should protect the system from physical and environmental risks. Your computer room should be separated from areas frequented by staff and patients. The room should not include printers and workstations that increase traffic. The computer room should include a solid core door with a lock and be large enough to allow for quick access to the equipment. In some cases, practices squeeze the EHR systems into the small room that currently hosts the PMS. You should seriously consider improvements that mitigate the risk of problems from environmental factors:
>
>> **Security Alarm**—The computer room should be protected with a security alarm system. Depending on office access issues, you may connect the alarm to the general office access controls.
>>
>> **Limited Access**—Computer room access should be limited to a few select and trained supervisors and managers. The computer room should not contain any equipment (e.g., printers, scanners, workstations) that would require regular access and use by others.
>>
>> **Fire Protection**—Computers can be damaged by water from fire sprinklers. To avoid damage from water, the practice should consider a waterless fire suppression system ($7,000-$10,000).
>>
>> **Air Conditioning**—Servers and other computer equipment can generate enough heat to cause equipment problems and automatic shutdown. The computer room may need supplemental air conditioning to compensate for the equipment. Supplemental air conditioning may be supplied by an extra vent or an additional unit. **ALERT:** Adequate air flow

is an important consideration for any air conditioning evaluation. You need to insure that the cabinets are not positioned to cause "hot spots" that could damage your equipment.

Direct Circuits—Power outlets should use direct circuits to prevent power disruptions from other equipment on the same circuit. Even with power conditioning equipment such as uninterruptible power supplies, many practices should use a direct circuit to mitigate many variables on a cost effective basis.

Uninterruptible Power Supplies (UPS)—UPSs mitigate the possibility of power disruptions to system operations. Depending on the reliability of power in your facility, you may seek a 15 minute or more power supply. The UPS must be powerful enough to support the complete operation of the system. For example, you may need power for a router and a workstation to access the system as well. *TIP:* UPSs have significant limitations since they cannot reasonably run the air conditioning in the room. For example, buying 4 hours of UPS services will not be very useful if the room will become too hot for the equipment 30 minutes after the power fails. Some practices connect to a UPS backed up by an on demand generator to insure the system is still operational for a long period of time even if the building loses power.

Backup Communications—Remote offices may connect to the EHR over a fast line to service all users. The practice may choose to use a backup communications channel that provides a lower level of service, but supports continued operations. For example, you may suspend scanning during a communications problem with the primary communications line and switch to a slower DSL line. *TIP:* The backup communications line should be through a different service that the line you are backing up. Otherwise, a single point of failure could cut off both lines: you would have paid for a service with the same risk factors.

Offsite Server Hosting—In some cases, you may move the computer servers to a hosting site that provides the various safeguards that are listed above. Your servers would be hosted at the site for a monthly fee. Note that you may incur additional communication expenses for the high speed line between your office and the host site.

Training Room—Regardless of your setup and training plan, you will need to have an onsite training room for your staff. The room will be used for the initial training as well as teaching of new employees and continuing training needed for your employees. You may choose to set aside a conference room or other location. Bigger practices with several large locations may establish more than one training room. The training room should feature the equipment in use with the EHR. Sufficient workstations and tablet access, as well as scanners and printers, should be available. Note that the training room can also be used as a staging area for the initial entry of information and/or scanning.

Clinical Office—EHR users require appropriate workspace. **TIP**: Account for practical places to put tablets in the exam rooms as well as surfaces to work in the hallways. You should also validate the location of workstations according to workflow and user viewing needs. For example, some practices install a workstation at the clinical working areas even if all staff use tablets. The workstation with a larger screen may be used to view diagnostic images. Don't forget a convenient location for printers to be used by staff as well as adequate locations for workstations. Note that the current locations and shelving used for medical record storage may be useful for the EHR equipment. For example, you may be able to place a printer at a clinical desk that is currently stacked with medical records. Patients may need to see a screen to view patient education aides when the doctor is explaining a condition or procedure.

Front desk—Incoming documents from patients will be scanned at the front desk into the EHR. In many situations, space at the front desk is at a premium. However, each front desk station will require a scanner to capture incoming documents. Note that the entire front desk setup should be reviewed since additional patient service work will be performed there. For example, patients may be providing completed forms that will be scanned into the EHR in support of the office visit. If the front desk can not accommodate scanning, then you may need to perform front desk scanning elsewhere in the office. However, you need to insure that the incoming documents can be scanned before the patient is seen.

Reception Area—The practice should consider installing one or more workstations in the reception area for patients. The workstations could be used by patients to access information on the practice, as well as information on various clinical conditions. For example, online patient education for various procedures could be accessed. Some EHR systems support patient information entry into the EHR. Typically, the patient is given a unique number, and accesses a Web Site to enter information and answer questions. Web-based information entry may allow for changes to demographics, appointment requests, refill requests, communications with doctors and staff, as well as viewing lab results and recall issues. Patient information is held for review by the doctor before acceptance into the EHR. In order to support the entry of information, the practice may need workstations in a private area for patients.

Medical records—If your practice will scan the patient charts into the EHR, the medical records area will need a major redesign. Most medical record areas lack adequate space for scanning. **CAUTION:** Depending on your strategy, medical record scanning could be very intense for at least 6 months after EHR Go Live. Medical record scanning requires preparing the chart for scanning, the scanning of the chart, connecting the chart to the patient and preparing the scanned chart for storage or destruction. Considering that a substantial number of charts will be partially or completely scanned daily, you need to insure that sufficient space is available. You will need space to pull charts several days in advance as well as to hold charts that have been prepared for scanning, but need to be scanned. A major problem for many practices is storing the scanned charts and preventing further access after scanning. Unfortunately, you will need to allow for extra space for these functions before shelf space is freed up to support the scanning process. Note that areas and surfaces used to organize charts for refiling and the entire filing process will change with an EHR. **TIP:** Some practices use a conference room, or temporarily rent space from another practice to support chart scanning.

Office facilities are part of the infrastructure needed to support you EHR effort. Some of these facilities will be driven by HIPAA standards.

TECHNOLOGY BASE

EHR installation triggers a dramatic expansion and upgrade to the practice technology base. To support an EHR, you will certainly add new servers, workstations and tablets as well as the network and peripherals needed to support clinical workflow. You will also make hardware investments to "harden" your system and insure continued access to the medical records in case of a variety of system problems and/or failures. The following issues should be noted as you work on your technology base:

Server Availability—You should closely examine your server and network setup for the weakest link and review the possibility of a problem. Even if you have invested a substantial amount of money in the EHR server, your entire system could be at risk for the failure due to a relatively inexpensive component. For example, one practice suffered a system crash due to a failure in the Active Directory Server, which could have been prevented by a small investment. Alternatively, those practices that are using an Application Services Provider will want to assure the reliability and capacity of the communication facilities from each office.

Communications—An EHR will generate much more computer traffic between your sites and the location of the EHR Server(s.) Additional traffic is due to more users, more use of the EHR by each user and the use of images. Communication changes typically have the longest lead times of any of the hardware areas. Changes can take at least 30 days without accounting for the labyrinth of vendors you may have to deal with. Unfortunately, you may lack any quantitative information until the system has been installed. However, a careful review of the vendor's recommendation and monitoring use as the EHR is activated will help you anticipate a problem before your practice is affected. For example, some vendors recommend a certain amount of communication bandwidth for each user at a remote site. You should verify that your communication plan allows for the requisite service. **ALERT:** Some communication services can be quickly upgraded from a remote location, while new services can take up to 90 days to install. Make sure that communication orders are properly placed on the critical path for the EHR project.

Workstations and Tablets—Virtually everyone in the practice will need access to the EHR. Many employees will need access to both EHR and PMS. For example, clinical staff may schedule patients for procedures as well as work with the medical record. Workstations and wireless tablets offer users different access options according to their needs. In general, desktop workstations are appropriate for doctors and staff that primarily work in a specific location. Wireless tablets are useful for doctors and staff who move around the facility. **ALERT:** The appropriateness of the device can be effected by the EHR software. For example, some EHR products are easier to use with a stylus or touchscreen than with a mouse. Selected EHR products are designed to let a nurse record information, and turn over the workstation at the current step in the record to a doctor. When looking at a specific user, the practice needs to examine the user's role. Of course, the user has to be comfortable with his situation. For example, a desktop station in an exam room may be difficult for a user who moves from room-to-room with different patients. In other situations, a mid-level nurse, PA and/or tech may actually document the patient visit as the doctor is working with the patient. This user may be more comfortable with a workstation. Note that maintaining confidentiality for workstations requires users secure the workstation from access by unauthorized users before they leave the exam room. In some cases, you can enforce security standards by automatically shutting down the user after a period of inactivity (e.g., 5 minutes or 30 minutes).

Scanners—The key benefit and objective of an EHR is the paperless office. Even if you succeed in establishing a paperless office, your patients, trading partners and other organizations will continue to send you an avalanche of paper (e.g., ER reports, consulting doctor reports, diagnostic test results) and demand paper from you. Initially, you will need scanner capacity to scan paper medical records as well as scan relevant paper received by your practice. A fax server allows you to receive faxes and load the fax image into the EHR without printing a fax or the need to scan it. However, you will need to have scanners available to capture paper documents and enter the information into the patient record.

The installation of hardware and system software will evolve over the course of the project. Although you can expect few changes to your EHR servers, other items will depend on the EHR workflow and user preferences. For example, most products will print a consent form that is signed by the patient and scanned into the EHR. You would need a scanner that could be conveniently used to scan the consent form or a computer signing pad to record signed consents. The key factors affecting the technology include the lead time for items, final hardware decisions and the general implementation plan for the practice. If you are using more than one vendor for hardware, the technology effort will be more complex, since you will have to coordinate the two or more vendors and insure that all of the purchased products work together. **TIP:** Make sure that orders from multiple vendors are properly coordinated by an appropriate IT coordinator to insure that the products are correctly installed.

During the contracting process, the EHR vendor supplied hardware specifications for its system. If hardware is being purchased from another source, you should have verified the items purchased with the EHR vendor. As you proceed to finalize your technology base, you should consider the issues listed in Table 10.6.

Installation of the hardware is a complex affair due to the number of changes and EHR setup issues. For example, some EHRs have a special piece of software that must be installed in each workstation and tablet. If you are buying all equipment from the EHR vendor, then you don't have too much to worry about. If you are buying the components from multiple vendors, then you need to plan the sequence of the installation to insure that you do not cause work stoppages or penalties from other vendors. The hardware installation plan should account for the following:

1. The primary network, workstation and tablet vendor should install enough hardware to test connectivity with the EHR Server before the EHR Server is installed on your network. The primary hardware vendor should allow for a resource to work with the EHR vendor when the EHR Server is installed.

2. Insure that your internal technical support person works with the EHR vendor on the installation of the EHR Server. Your internal technical support person should understand the general setup of the EHR server and the requirements for the various devices that access the EHR. **TIP:** Most practices need a higher level support person on call to address any issues that cannot be resolved by the internal resource.

3. The internal technical support person and your primary hardware vendor should understand the various tasks needed to stage, prepare and configure a device to access or use the EHR.

The final proof of the hardware setup is when the entire system is hooked together. When the EHR Server(s) and infrastructure are available for use, your practice should verify the delivery and operability of the EHR system using your own staff as shown in Table 10.7.

After confirmation of the hardware installation, written documentation on installation of equipment and maintenance issues should be developed for the EHR. The documentation should include instructions on the hardware requirements, software installation and connectivity setups. Make sure you also compile information on system backup and recovery. You should also compile a list of key contact numbers, vendors and names to help staff in the event of a system problem.

SOFTWARE SETUP

Software setup involves selecting from a variety of EHR options and classification tools to customize the EHR for your practice. Although system features and setup options vary, several options are available on most EHR products:

TABLE 10.6

Area	TECHNOLOGY ISSUES TO CONSIDER
Policies	Does the practice have a policy on upgrades and changes to the technology base? What is the technology replacement strategy, and policy for the practice? What is the strategy for accessing the EHR? What hardware components are needed to support the policy? What are the lines of responsibility for the installation and support of the EHR hardware?
Servers	What additional servers are needed for the EHR besides the equipment being purchased from the EHR vendor? Are current network servers (e.g., active directory server, print and file server, email server) adequate for the EHR and the anticipated larger user-base? Do the number of users warrant additional facilities for remote users, communications, printing services, and availability of workstations/tablets? If using a communications server (e.g., Windows Terminal Server or Citrix), which workstations and tablets will work through the communications server to the EHR? Does the backup device capacity and strategy account for all of the servers on the practice network? What is the strategy to protect the servers and workstations from virus, spyware and other intrusive software? For ASP users, what is the specific bandwidth needs for each office based on the larger number of EHR users?
PMS	Does the PMS system require an upgrade before the EHR is installed? What, if any, equipment is needed to support the EHR interface? What is the working relationship between the PMS and EHR systems and vendors? Do the code sets and master files used by the PMS require changes before the PMS is interfaced with the EHR? Do the triggers for sending data between the EHR and PMS systems adequately support the use of both systems for patients in the office?
Communications	Are the communication links between offices sufficient for the EHR? Are adequate protections in place to prevent intrusion or disruptions from outside sources? Is there adequate network protection through firewalls and internal security? Do the internal network facilities in each location have the capacity to support an EHR? What are the security features of the network to protect against unauthorized access? What are the wireless network issues in each location? Is there any existing equipment that may interfere with the wireless network?
Workstations	What, if any, upgrades are required to meet the minimum EHR standards? What additional workstations are needed to support the EHR? What screens will provide the best view of EHR data and images? What other initiatives (Ex. PACS, new diagnostic equipment, access to hospital information) could affect the number and placement of workstations?
Tablets	What criterion determines tablet use by a user? What is the deployment plan for tablet distribution? How will doctors and staff who work in multiple locations use tablets? What is needed to provide adequate wireless access to the users in the office and related areas (e.g., lunch room)?
Scanners	Where will scanners be needed to scan incoming documents into the EHR? What scanning devices will be needed in medical records for old paper charts? What is the planned scanning throughput that will be available for medical record scanning? How will the scanners fit in the medical records department and other areas?
Printers	Where will patient materials be printed? What printers will be needed to support EHR printing requirements?

TABLE 10.7

Area	VERIFYING TECHNOLOGY INSTALLATION
General	All equipment should be verified against the list of equipment ordered from each vendor. Verify that: • Each server, workstation and tablet contains the ordered memory, disks, and other features. • Each scanner and printer is the ordered model and/or meets the order specifications. • Interfaces with diagnostic equipment are properly connected and working. • Servers can be backed up with the back-up equipment and the backup is valid.
Servers	Verify the ordered equipment and operability of high availability options, such as dual power supplies, dual fans and hot swap disk arrays. Verify that all servers are communicating with the network at the expected speed. Verify that all servers can access other servers as needed (e.g., PMS and EHR servers). Verify that the PMS and EHR systems exchange information on a timely basis through the purchased interface. For ASP users, verify the connection bandwidth and response times from each location with the ASP location.
PMS	Insure that the appropriate EHR workstations can still access the PMS system as needed. Verify the interface between the PMS and EHR system for appointments, demographics and charges.
Communications	Verify interoffice communication links operate at the expected speeds. Verify network speeds in offices support use of the EHR.
Workstations	Check that upgraded workstations can operate with the EHR. Verify that the EHR and PMS products can be run simultaneously on workstations that will require simultaneous access to both applications. Test printing to appropriate printers for each workstation. Verify viewing of EHR information and images.
Tablets	Verify wireless access and operation of the EHR on each tablet. Test printing to appropriate printers for each tablet.
Scanners	Test the ability to scan a document into the EHR. Verify the quality of scanning and the stored image in the EHR meet the clarity and precision needs of the practice.
Printers	Verify printing reports from the EHR to selected printers. Check the default printer for the user as well as the availability of appropriate network printing resources.

Security—The security setup can be derived from the workflow document. The workflow document lays out what each person in each area will be doing. The workflow document can be used to define roles, which are included in the security setup. Some EHRs allow restrictions based on record types, locations, patient types and doctors. Security restrictions at these levels should be based on practice policies and the recommendation of your security officer. ***TIP:*** The practice should have a formal document that defines access rights for each type of employee as well as a formal process to give selected employees specific rights or additional capabilities. ***ALERT:*** Securing access to particular components of the patient record (Ex. Mental Health) may be needed to comply with a variety of confidentiality issues.

Imaging—Imaging modules support scanned images from paper records, incoming documents and diagnostic images. To keep track of the various images, you can define image types. To organize image types, you should compile a list of the types of images that you want to be able to select immediately from the patient EHR chart (e.g., office notes by date, diagnostic reports by problem). At a minimum, you need image types for the old medical record (e.g., old office notes, old lab results), incoming reports, letters from physicians (such as referral letters) and letters from patients. You may also define image types for audiograms, patient information sheets, radiology reports and ER documents. To compile a report list, scan through your paper medical record and note the types of documents that you would want to be able to immediately access. You may also have non-clinical documents among the EHR images. For example, a referral authorization from an insurer or a scanned image of the insurance card may be stored in an EHR. Some imaging products allow for a free form description. The practice should establish a standard format for the description (e.g., "Shoulder X-ray—Central Radiology"). Other imaging modules allow you to define a specific set of data items for each image type. For example, you could enter the hospital name and date of service for an ER report and the optical lab and due date for a custom optical product.

Tasks—Tasks record "to do" items in an EHR. Tasks may be assigned to one or more people and labeled according to a priority. These classify tasks to allow the recipient to immediately identify the nature of the task as well as allow management to print reports by task type. Task types may address incoming documents (e.g., "Review a Lab Report"), clinical communications ("Approve a Mid-Level Note"), patient service ("Refill Request") and patient treatment ("Perform Lab Test," "Schedule Surgery Request," "Waiting for an X-Ray," etc.). Make sure that the list addresses ancillary services, and the vast array of interactions on patient issues. The list should be organized into groups to keep the number of task types to a manageable number. **ALERT:** Some products have multiple options to flag tasks that are needed by larger practices. For example, you may be able to assign a priority, department, and type to a task. If a product only allows for a short description line, then a larger practice may have difficulty tracking patients.

Department Areas and Locations—EHR setup should reflect your department and location setup. However, you should consider the operational departments that would facilitate use of the EHR. For example, you may have a diagnostic pod that contains lab, radiology and ultrasound, but in your operational analysis, you may be better off making them separate EHR departments. **TIP:** The use of departments may not be fully developed in the EHR. For example, if you can assign departments, but cannot view patients and tasks by department, then department will not be as useful. If you can view patients, tasks, documents, and other items by department, the EHR will support more effective management tools for the practice.

Appointment Tracking—Some EHRs include patient flow features within the EHR appointment scheduler. You may be able to enter a patient status, room number and/or comment. Complile a list of meaningful statuses that reflects the possible situations a patient may encounter in your facility (e.g., "Roomed," "Technician Intake," "Waiting for Doctor," "Procedure Pending." etc.). Use statuses that apply across several departments. For example, a general status of waiting for a test that could apply to the lab and radiology is preferable to a separate "waiting for test" status for each department. The department should be communicated through the assigned area and/or room assignment. **ALERT:** You may want to consider how you identify and classify the various departments of your practice. For example, if each room in each office is separately listed in the EHR, then you may be faced with a long list of rooms when you want to record a patient move in the EHR. However, if the EHR tracks the location and pod of the patient, you may be able to use a shorter list of room numbers that are standardized across all practice locations.

Plan Items—When a doctor is recording a plan for a patient, she may select procedures, tests, patient education, recall appointments and other actions to support patient care. These plan items should be compiled from existing records to speed the EHR setup process. Plan items may include lab tests, radiology studies and treatments. Plan items lists may be assigned to diseases and/or physicians depending on the EHR. The plan items should be standardized across all doctors to ease management of patient care. For example, support staff needs to be able to easily identify pending treatment items without having to deal with different coding systems for the same plan item. Note that plan items should relate to or be associated with the evolving care standards that may be used in your area. You will be better positioned to track and manage the evolving quality of care and pay-for-performance initiatives.

Software interfaces will require appropriate setups and testing. Setup may include programming the various interfaces as well as compiling translation tables to support interfaces. The interfaces should be mostly managed by the EHR, PMS and diagnostic equipment vendors. The EHR project manager will be mostly responsible for coordinating the various parties on the following interfaces:

PMS Interface—The PMS system should send patient demographic and appointment information to the EHR. The EHR should send charge information to the PMS. The software interface should work fast enough to allow a patient at check-in to be properly reflected in the EHR system as well as transfer a charge from the EHR to the PMS in time for patient checkout.

Diagnostic Equipment Interfaces—Diagnostic equipment interfaces with the EHR should allow downloading of the results to the EHR or viewing the diagnostic results from the EHR in time to support review by the doctor. Note that many EHRs do not necessarily save the diagnostic image, but store a pointer to the diagnostic image on the diagnostic equipment. When you select the diagnostic image from the EHR, the EHR invokes the diagnostic image viewer and the user is now viewing the patient image through the diagnostic equipment tools. **ALERT:** Such connections mean that the results on the diagnostic equipment are de facto extensions of the EHR. However, you need to adequately backup the images on the diagnostic equipment to maintain the integrity of the patient's medical record. In some cases, your EHR can send the order information with the patient identification to the diagnostic equipment to eliminate duplicate information entry. **TIP:** Insure that you purchase diagnostic equipment interfaces with your EHR and future purchases of diagnostic equipment should include the interface needed for the EHR.

The clinical content should be carefully reviewed to avoid problems during the training and deployment effort. Clinical content review and acceptance requires active involvement of doctors and clinical staff. The medical staff dedicated to the EHR implementation effort should lead the following effort:

Review the Current Clinical Content—Super user doctors and other clinical staff should review the EHR clinical content for their designated area. The clinical content review should cover the applicability of the clinical content to the practice as well as nuances that may be required. For example, a patient population that is at a high risk for a particular disease may require some additional information in the EHR. Similarly, a subspecialist needs to review the content in the EHR for his area. As the review is conducted, the user should take notes on enhancements and changes needed to meet practice requirements. Enhancements should be noted between those items that are a necessity and those items that would be useful, but are not needed immediately. For example, the resulting note may not be exactly how the doctor would have transcribed the issue, but may correctly reflect the patient's situation. **CAUTION:** Many practices start off customizing the clinical content without fully understanding the "out of the box" clinical content. You could end up customizing the clinical content for something that already exists. Before you invest time and resources in any custom content, make sure you understand what the purchased system does and evaluate whether it would work for you. **TIP:** Note that the clinical content may work, but may be different from how you would do it yourself. If the clinical content accurately documents the patient condition and treatment, you may save a lot of time and effort accepting the standard, instead of customizing the EHR content to reflect how you would have designed or set up the EHR.

Design Changes—If changes and enhancements are needed, describe the list of enhancements in as much detail as possible to avoid problems and mistakes. For example, you may request that a flag for diabetes be added between the heart problem and arthritis questions instead of stating that "diabetes is not included on the problem list."

Implement Changes or Setups—The vendor and/or trained practice staff will program the changes into the EHR clinical content. Be careful to monitor the effect that multiple requests may have on a screen or clinical content list to avoid redoing work. For example, some practices rework areas several times (at additional cost) before arriving at a workable solution. The implementation of the change should have a specific delivery date, and you should have a specific test to verify the change. For example, you may include an example of what the resulting screen and document will look like. **TIP:** Most practices will need an internal resource that understands how to customize and enhance the clinical content. However, those changes should be carefully designed and evaluated by the clinical users, before the practice invests time in changes that may already be available in the EHR, or may not add much to EHR utility. For example, a user may want to see a particular piece of information in a certain place in a selected screen even though the information can be viewed on another screen within the EHR.

Test Changes—After setting up the various clinical content system options or customizations, the doctors should test the EHR to validate the handling of clinical issues. The testing will allow the physician to verify the content, and gain confidence in the EHR. The testing should include a variety of key clinical areas. Several testing strategies should be considered:

> **Retrospective Records**—Previously documented encounters will be entered into the EHR to verify the ability to document a visit. The resulting report will be reviewed by the doctor to analyze the result in light of the actual chart note. Know that the new system will not necessarily produce the exact note, but an accurate and correct document.
>
> **Role Playing**—A medical exam will be conducted in a conference room setting with a doctor or clinician recording the information being presented by another practice clinician. The purpose of role playing is to test the flow of the EHR in an interactive environment with the ability to backtrack and rework the "exam" with the EHR.
>
> **Patient Shadowing**—An actual patient visit is shadowed with the EHR. The user will record the patient information in the EHR at the same time other records are kept by the doctor performing the services. The resulting record is reviewed to verify that the note and record are acceptable to the practice.
>
> **Document Production**—If the clinical charting is working well in testing, the practice may try documenting patient visits using the EHR. The EHR will be used to produce the report that will be saved in the paper chart until the practice moves to the EHR. This strategy maintains the integrity of the designated record set.

EHR software setup is particularly sensitive due to the importance of the clinical content. The effort involved in verifying and testing the clinical content with the practice's clinical information and treatment strategies will mitigate the chance of a failure as the practice moves forward with the activation of the EHR.

DATA CONVERSION

EHR Data conversion is more complicated that anything that you may have encountered with a practice management system (PMS). The implementation of a new PMS system involves the manual or electronic conversion of information from the old PMS to the new PMS. The old PMS has a patient demographic record and so does the new PMS. Indeed, the new PMS data structures and items are generally analogous to the old PMS.

Current medical record information primarily consists of paper patient charts. Some practices may also have electronic patient information in a number of places. For example, you may have transcription files, test results in lab information systems and various images in selected diagnostic testing devices. Additionally, a number of first time EHR users are moving to new EHR systems for a variety of reasons including obsolete products and products that cannot be certified under the ARRA HITECH standards. Conversions of data between EHR products may be the most difficult conversion of all. Converting to an EHR will be difficult and complex. You need to carefully review the options and understand what you will have at the end of the effort.

Initially, the practice should determine what information you need to move to the EHR and where the information is currently stored. As a practical matter, the current information could consist of the following:

Paper Record Conversion—Conversion of paper records is covered in a separate section below.

EHR Conversion—EHR conversions from an existing legacy EHR product to a new product is a complex and challenging process. This effort is covered in a separate section below.

Transcription Files—Some practices have transcribed word processing files that may go back several years. Ideally, these records should be a valuable basis of information that could be loaded as a starting point into the EHR. However, many practices have procedures that could undermine the utility of these saved files.

Editing and Side Notes—If the electronic document could differ in any way from the patient chart document, the conversion of the electronic document could cause inconsistencies in the EHR and expose the practice to problems. Practices where the doctor may edit the final chart document by hand, or note additional information on the chart document should be wary of any electronic conversion. Similarly, doctors who record supplemental notes, phone calls and other information on the bottom of the transcripted note may not be able to rely on the electronic version of the note as the most current patient information.

Certainty of the Document—Word processing documents are not secured from access or change in the vast majority of practices. Indeed, small changes could be introduced in a variety of scenarios that created differences between the electronic document and the document in the patient chart. For example, some practices maintain a single file for a patient and append new dictation to the end of the document. However, there is no mechanism to prevent changes to information that is already in the word processing file.

Document Organization—Some practices use a single file to store all doctor dictation in a day or on a tape. If the separation between patients is not clearly indicated and consistent, the separation of the documents may be complicated or produce inconsistent results. Indeed, some vendors cannot support electronic conversion of transcription files unless a file only contains a single document for a single date of service for an easily identified patient.

Patient Identification—To support computerized loading of transcription files into an EHR, patient identification must be clear and certain. Patient name alone will not be sufficient. The patient name, medical record number, sex and date of birth in a consistent place will enable the electronic loading of the word processing files into the EHR. Most practices do not include a complete complement of patient information in each transcripted document.

In the final analysis, any differences between the saved transcription files and the patient paper chart could lead to problems. If your practice does not save transcription files that could be electronically converted, you should consider changing procedures to insure the reliability and accuracy of future electronic documents. You may be able to electronically convert the transcription files from the point of the changes with confidence in the reliability of the document.

Lab Information System (LIS)—Practice-owned LISs contain lab results that predate the EHR. If previous results could be loaded into the EHR, then doctors could use the graphing tools to review trends, as well as look at previous lab results in the lab flow-sheets. With an interface that links LIS results to your EHR, the old results from the LIS could be downloaded into the EHR. The loading would add a considerable amount of patient information as well as test the LIS interface. However, the EHR must be able to accept lab results for tests that were not ordered through the EHR.

Diagnostic Equipment—Some diagnostic equipment store information and images from previous tests. Diagnostic equipment in the typical practice may support an electronic interface with an EHR, or support a workaround strategy that creates an image file that can be loaded into an EHR. In some cases, the diagnostic equipment cannot support any interface. Diagnostic equipment with interfaces to the EHR could be used to download previous results into the EHR. Otherwise, the previous results must be printed or exported to a computer file for transfer to the new EHR.

Master Files—In many cases, EHR master files must be manually established and maintained. EHR Master Files may include procedures, diagnoses, doctors, locations and insurance companies. Some EHR vendors may load selected PMS Master File information, such as insurance company, diagnoses and procedures, into the EHR at installation. Note that even when PMS systems update the EHR master files, the scheduling may cause problems. For example, some vendors update the records on a daily or even a weekly basis. If the additional information is needed sooner, the EHR may just ignore the unknown master file code. For example, a new payer added to the master file would not connect the patient with the correct medication formulary if the payer and formulary in the EHR is not updated on a continual basis.

Demographic Information—Some EHRs have an independent demographic information database that can be maintained through the EHR. A limited number of products rely exclusively on the PMS interface for demographic information. With an interfaced EHR, all current PMS patient information must be loaded into the EHR. Otherwise, patients who have not been seen since the EHR's implementation will not be accessible through the EHR. Phone messages, incoming results and other information could not be entered into the EHR prior to the patient's first post-EHR Go Live visit. Note that integrated PMS and EHR products share the same demographic and master files. Information entered in either area is immediately accessible to the other EHR components. **ALERT:** Most EHR interfaces do not send demographic updates to the EHR. However, EHR users may update EHR demographic information but not remember that the updates will not be passed to the PMS. This problem is especially troublesome when EHR users frequently access the EHR demographics and may even add information to the EHR demographics as part of using the EHR. For example, you may go into the EHR to maintain an alert message or add information that is not even contained in the PMS (Ex. Preferred pharmacy.) While updating the EHR demographic information, the user could accidentally update some information (Ex. Address or contact phone) that should be posted to the PMS. Another related problem can be exposed when the triage staff answers a patient call and gets a new phone number for the patient. The new number has to be associated with the patient message in the EHR, but the new number has to be separately posted to the PMS.

Appointment Information—With an interfaced EHR, the current appointments should be sent to the EHR. After the initial appointments, changes to the appointment schedule will trigger the maintenance of the EHR appointments for each PMS appointment change. The appointment schedule enables patient workflow management through the EHR. Note that the key issue for any interface is the trigger mechanism. In some cases, changes to some appointment information may not necessarily trigger an update to the EHR appointment schedule. For example, an update to the appointment time will certainly trigger an update to the EHR, but the entry of a note may not be sent to the EHR from the PMS. *TIP:* In most cases, PMS systems do not track patient progress through the office and at the most only know that the patient has presented for service. PMS products that support check-in will send the check-in information to the EHR. However, PMS systems that do not support patient check-in are more challenging. If the PMS does not support check-in, then the front desk staff will have to access the appointment information in the EHR to check the patient in. The EHR check-in status indicates to the clinical staff that the patient is ready to be seen.

Depending on the ability to convert this information, you could start off with some significant EHR patient data on EHR Go Live. However, the practice needs to plan ahead to enable the conversion of data into the EHR.

PAPER CHARTS AND THE EHR

EHR structures and data collection strategies are completely different from the current paper-based methods. For example, many EHRs maintain separate lists of medications, diagnoses, procedures, allergies and other key patient information. This information is typically buried in various places in the paper record. Even practices that maintain separate logs of medications and key patient information (Ex. Immunization, Previous Surgery) cannot be absolutely sure that the paper chart contains information that has not been entered in the logs. Indeed, some practices have procedures to check the records to make the logs are complete before the patient is seen. The maintenance of such logs is often inconsistent and prone to errors. For example, an obsolete medications' log may present a misleading view of the patient situation and risks, if staff fails to update the log after the last visit. In many cases, you cannot even tell the last time such logs were checked or verified.

Converting paper medical charts requires a complex and time consuming effort. The key issue to consider is what information you need from the current paper charts, and what effort will be invested to get the information into the EHR. Information from paper charts are entered into the EHR as a scanned image of the paper records, and/or as discrete information from the paper records (e.g., medications). For example, a practice may decide to scan the medical chart into the EHR, but also review the EHR to enter the patient's medical history into the chart. In some cases, the practice will not really have a choice about entering specific information into the EHR. For example, a pediatric practice must enter the patient immunization information into the EHR. Otherwise, the health maintenance rules may flag patients who "need" immunization shots as far as the EHR knows, but could be up to date according to the patient paper record.

Virtually no practice sets up their paper records to facilitate or support scanning. For example, paper charts lack consistent patient identifiers on the individual chart pages. The organization of the paper chart may complicate scanning. For example, practices may keep paper records in the order received and not by visit, condition or type of document. In some cases, practices maintain family charts where patient information is commingled with information from other family members. Other practices may maintain "case" charts for each patient problem. As a practical matter, a number of practices maintain separate charts in each office for each patient seen in each office. If a patient is seen in more than one office, they could end up with more than one chart. The paper medical record poses a number of challenges to scanning including:

A variety of paper sizes—Paper size differences can slow the scanning process or leave awkward images. For example, a limited number of legal-sized pages may have to be separately scanned from the rest of the chart or regular-sized images may appear to have empty space at the bottom of each page. Undersized prescriptions, tapes from diagnostic equipment and other undersized documents may have to be taped to a more scanner friendly form.

Two-sided images—Some charts contain information on both sides of some pages. To scan information on both sides of the page the staff may copy the second side, or use a dual-sided scanner to scan both sides of a page in one pass. However, with dual scanning, blank second sides may also end up in the scanned record. Some scanners include software that will identify blank pages according to a specific standard or tolerance. In other cases, a "blank" second side may be a form that does not contain information but will not be considered empty by the scanning software. An additional complication may occur when the second side is upside down to simplify review of paper charts. In the scanned image, the second page will be scanned upside down with dual-sided scanning. An EHR user will have to rotate the image to see the image right side up.

Unnecessary Information—Many practices have charts with duplicate information and obsolete data that has never been removed. For example, the chart may contain patient information and insurance cards from years ago, or various reports that were superseded by interim or final reports. In some cases, practices make copies of medical chart contents for Release of Information and return copies of all information sent in the paper chart. Other charts contain copies of chart pages that were scanned or faxed to other offices and returned to the paper chart. The additional images may complicate locating the information needed in much the same way that the doctor has to leaf through the extraneous documents in a paper chart.

Information on the file folder—Many practices record key patient information on the front, back and/or inside covers of the medical chart. Key medical issues, procedure history, allergies and prescription stickers are some of the items placed on medical chart folders. Unfortunately, the chart folder is difficult to scan. The chart must be placed on a flat-bed scanner and scanned a surface at a time.

Loose documents/forms—Some paper charts contain loose pages that are in the middle of the chart. The appropriate place for the loose pages is not always certain. In other cases, the patient chart is a collection of unsecured pages. The practice may have a clinical staff person "prepare" the chart for each visit by reorganizing some of the loose pages into an order the doctor prefers. Note that the staff may be continually reorganizing the chart for each patient visit and as new information is collected in the chart.

Curled papers—Over time, chart papers can curl, bend or become worn. Such pages will require more time to prepare for scanning since the paper feed is sensitive to paper quality. Ultimately, more paper feeding problems may be encountered as the documents are scanned.

Stapled documents—Staples and paper clips must be removed from documents when scanning. You may be able to save some prep time by tearing off the stapled corner of a document instead of removing a staple.

Poor copies—Paper medical records commonly include poor or aged documents that are difficult to read. Examples include faxed images of EKGs, copies of documents in poor condition, and old thermal paper images. Carbon pages may be of poor quality and difficult to read. Such documents may not scan well.

Color images—Color images in a paper file need to be scanned using a color scanning option. Depending on the placement of images and scanning strategy, all images may be scanned using a color option. Although more convenient, scanning in color generates much larger files even when the document may not contain any color. For example, a black and white scanned image may take up as little as 10,000 characters for a page. However, a color image could consume 1,000 times as much space or even more.

Dividers—Dividers may help or hurt the scanning process depending on your scanning and organization strategy. If you decide to split out more recent records from older clinical information, dividers may increase prep time. If you plan to scan images into sections that are the same as your dividers, then the dividers will speed the scanning process.

Slides—Slides that are contained in the paper chart can be scanned into the EHR using a special scanning device. But slides and other diagnostic images may add additional steps and time to your scanning effort.

Initially, the chart contents must be prepared for scanning. Depending on the chart order and the scanning strategy, the preparation effort can vary widely. At a minimum, you have to remove staples and paperclips as well as straighten the papers to feed the scanner. Other preparation strategies may be determined by the equipment you buy, and your scanning strategy. For example,

- One-sided scanners may require copying the back page of patient records to prepare the chart for scanning.

- Paper charts that are not kept in any specific order may require organizing the chart before scanning.
- Paper charts with significant amounts of useless materials may be edited before scanning.
- Some practices used family charts that mix patient information. Such information would have to be separated by patient before scanning.

Whatever your situation or problems, make sure you survey the paper charts to uncover the issues that you will have to deal with and test various paper handling and scanning strategies to determine the best one for you practice. Preparing the paper chart for scanning can easily exceed the time it takes to scan the document. Chart preparation can average 5–30 minutes per chart, depending on the size of the document, and your prep time. Large "phone book" charts could take an hour or more to prepare for scanning.

> **TIP**: Make sure your strategy balances the effort to scan and process the paper record with the resulting benefits of the scanned medical record. **ALERT:** Scanning a chart will not make the paper record look better or resolve the paper chart problems of the last 10 years. The resulting scanned images may be kept in a single group of the entire contents of the paper chart or split into various categories. For example, you may choose to have images organized by visit date or by type of document (e.g., office visit, radiology study, lab results, etc.)

Scanners and the target scanner software impact whether you can organize the patient chart before or after you scan the chart into the EHR. Some EHR scanning products only allow you to scan a one page document, while other products allow you to scan an entire chart and use the imaging software to organize the chart. In some cases, scanning software will help you organize the scanned images into groups of images that can be saved in separate folders. For example, you could pick out office notes from the past two years. The recent office notes could be put in one image folder and the rest of the paper chart could be stored in another image folder.

If you cannot organize the scanned images using the scanning software, then you may have to separate a single chart into several individual documents that must be separately scanned into the EHR. **TIP:** In general, scanning individual stacks into separate image folders is more time consuming than scanning the entire chart and using the scanning software to organize the various scanned image folders. Some scanning products use bar coded separator pages to allow you to scan stacks of paper at a time. Without the separators, you may have to use several scanning jobs to separate a single chart into the EHR pieces. These separate jobs will take more scanning time.

Some practices abstract information from the paper record in addition to or as a replacement for scanning. Key information—such as prior medical history, previous procedures, allergies, diagnoses—is entered into the EHR prior to the patient's first visit. In some cases, pulling information from the paper chart is difficult since many documents may be reviewed to gather information. **ALERT:** Entering information from the chart into the EHR will require a clinically experienced person to find the necessary information in the paper chart and follow-up on omissions in the paper chart. The information maybe entered as a dummy prior visit or as the start of the next patient visit. Practices that abstract without scanning frequently maintain a procedure to provide the paper chart on demand to the doctor. If the paper chart is not scanned, you must maintain a paper chart delivery process to insure that doctors can access pre-EHR information for continuity of care issues.

Indeed, some practices do not scan or abstract existing paper records. They merely start using the EHR. The paper records become obsolete for operational purposes, but the practice still keeps the paper chart according to medical record retention laws. The practice is also obligated to maintain the designated record set under the HIPAA privacy standards. In reality, the doctor may still need to go back to the paper chart to review continuity of care issues or a previous problem.

Given all of these issues and difficulties, the average practice would be scared away from doing anything with the current paper records. However, the practice must balance the desire to eliminate paper with the current condition of the paper medical record, and the effort involved with scanning the document. In the final analysis, your scanning strategy or lack thereof will depend on the utility of the final product and the value in the paper record balanced off with the costs of continuing to maintain the paper record after EHR activation. The general scanning options are reviewed in Table 10.8.

In the final analysis, there are no good solutions to the challenge of scanning paper charts into the EHR. If you don't scan anything, you will have to return to the paper chart whenever the doctor needs to research patient issues. If you selectively scan information, you may have to return to the same chart to scan incrementally additional information. If you scan everything, you can expect an intensive scanning process for 6 to 12 months after you start using the medical record.

Any analysis of your scanning strategy will have to consider the cost of scanning. Using an outside resource, scanned records cost .10 to .30 per image. Depending on the size of your charts the costs could significantly vary for each practice. However, your need to balance the cost of scanning with your continued maintenance and delivery costs for the paper record. If you expect to pull your charts more than 3 times after you switch over to the EHR, you should closely compare the true cost of pulling, handling, and returning the paper chart with the cost of scanning that same chart.

A number of strategies are available to ease the scanning and record abstraction burden on your practice. Your specific options will depend on your EHR activation strategy (see Chapter 11—Activating an EHR).

CONVERTING DATA FROM A PREVIOUS EHR

Moving from one EHR product to another is a challenging process. In order to appreciate the challenges, let's look at Practice Management System conversion.

Most PMS vendors will only provide limited demographic information from your PMS system. Typically, we cannot convert appointments, financial transactions, patient notes

TABLE 10.8

Option	Strengths	Limitations
No Scanning – Paper records are delivered until they are no longer needed.	No scanning requirements.	• Difficult to manage paper record and tablet. • Information could be written in the paper chart and not into the EHR. For example, a doctor may enter a note in the paper chart to highlight a trend or analyze a result. • Paper charts will never disappear since the paper chart will always be a part of the designated record set. • Managing the designated record set split among the EHR and paper record could be complicated. For example, paper chart information could be used in an encounter documented in the EHR. However, information used in medical decision-making from the paper record would not be in the EHR.
Abstract Paper Records – Important information is entered into the EHR, but the paper record is maintained and delivered to the physician until the paper chart is no longer needed.	Cuts down on accessing the paper chart.	• Consumes doctor or clinician time to prepare the patient record for the first visit. • Information could be missed when abstracted. • Doctor and clinicians would need to see the paper chart for selected patients. For example, the paper chart would contain important trend information for patients with a continuing problem. • Probably requires demand chart delivery in a stat mode for a long period of time. Even after the doctors generally decide the paper charts are no longer needed, the charts will be required on a demand basis. • Any time paper charts are delivered to the doctor or clinician, the practice runs the risk that new information will be recorded in the paper chart. • Difficult maintaining designated record set for each patient since information for EHR based decision-making will be in the patient chart. Paper charts will never disappear since the paper chart will always be a part of the designated record set.
Scan Selected/Current Information – Based on specific criteria, selected pages are scanned into the EHR. Criteria could include last visit information, all information after a certain date or all office notes. Each time the patient is seen, the doctor could request scanning of additional items from the paper chart.	Fewer EHR images to leaf through when the doctor is scanning the patient chart. Minimizes scanning of information.	• Longer time to select information, scan pages and rebuild the chart. One of the most difficult parts of scanning a paper chart is the preparation of the scanned images. Scanning selected information requires analyzing each document to select the items to be scanned. The selection process could be difficult and open to errors. Putting the chart back together in the order found could be time consuming. • Contextual issues may not be properly reflected in the EHR. Since selected items are scanned, the paper chart may include additional information, interim information or other results that may be needed to fully understand the scanned documents. • Information may not be scanned and could be missed by the doctor looking at only the EHR. • Physicians and medical record staff may need to constantly revisit previously processed charts to scan additional images for a problem already documented in the EHR or to get relevant paper chart information on a problem that is new to the EHR. • Difficult to maintain designated record set. • Paper charts will never disappear.
Limited Medical Record Scanning – Scan some medical records and not others based on some criteria (e.g., size).		• Requires electronic and paper medical record structures and costs. • Any time paper charts are delivered to the doctor or clinician, the practice runs the risk that new information will be recorded in the paper chart. • Requires maintaining paper medical records indefinitely.

Option	Strengths	Limitations
	Patients with smaller charts are scanned into the system, while larger charts can still be reviewed by flipping through the pages of the chart. Alternatively, the practice could establish a selection criteria for patients that trigger the scanning of the entire chart for patients that fit a problem or demographic profile.	• Requires maintaining paper medical records indefinitely. • Difficult to maintain designated record set for patients without scanned charts.
Scan Entire Record – The entire paper medical record is scanned into the EHR based on triggers to insure that the paper record is available when the doctors, clinicians or staff need access to the patient medical record. Note that charts could be scanned using different strategies. For example, a small-to-medium chart could be scanned as a single set of images, while large charts could be separately scanned by section, or current documents could be put in a special section of images.	Maintains designated record set. Once scanned, the paper chart will not have to be accessed again.	• Massive effort needed to scan the records into the EHR. • A variety of problems with scanning productivity since the paper records were not designed for scanning. • Large paper records could be organized into sections at an additional cost and effort.

and other PMS information. The information that we can convert must be translated from the current PMS to the new PMS. The translated data may be transposed, presented differently, or be limited in the new PMS. For example, when a practice transfers balances to a new PMS, the detailed information on the charges for management reporting, billing and claim submission is lost. As a practical matter, most practices run out the pre-new PMS charges on the old PMS. For management reporting, most practices must combine the information from the old and new PMS systems by hand.

You may be tempted to leave the old data in the old EHR and just pick up with the new EHR. However, there are a number of problems with that approach. First and foremost, you would have to continue paying support for the old EHR system and deal with maintaining the old EHR for an unknown period of time. This additional cost would not produce any benefits and could leave you with a number of go forward problems as the old EHR goes through the end of its product lifecycle. Secondly, you would have to provide continuing access to the old EHR to allow access to significant patient information. Finally, you have to properly introduce appropriate patient information into the new EHR in any case. For example, pediatricians may need immunization information, and surgeons may need information on procedures brought forward to the new EHR.

Unfortunately, we do not have the luxury of abandoning our EHR information from your old EHR system if you use the EHR to store any component of your patient's medical record. For example,

> Some practices have split their patient medical records between the EHR and the original paper record. In several cases, patient messages are maintained in the EHR, while all other patient information is in the patient's paper chart. From the practice's perspective the patient's medical record consists of the contents of the paper chart AND the messages in the EHR.

> A number of practices have replaced their paper charts with the scanned images of the chart contents in a document management system. Their doctors reference the document management system since there are no paper charts. The contents of the document management system contain the patient charts that must be preserved to meet patient chart retention requirements.

> Some practices use a particular EHR module to record information. For example, some practices implemented electronic prescriptions only. Those records are a defacto part of the patient's medical record. In order to produce the patient record, the practice must combine information from the paper chart with information from the electronic prescription module.

Indeed, some practices have patient charts split between several different pieces of software and still have a paper chart. For example, one practice used a separate document imaging system to maintain scanned images of selected patient documents, a transcription system to store dictated notes, and a third party electronic prescription service as well as a paper chart for items that were not elsewhere, administrative paperwork, and "key" documents from the electronic systems.

The actual trigger to move the practice from one EHR to another EHR may be due to a change in the practice, or the vendor. Acquisitions, change in services and growth are potential triggers to move to a different EHR. Vendor acquisitions and discontinued products can also necessitate the move to a different EHR product. CAUTION: If you have any information that your EHR product will be replaced or no longer supported, make sure that your move to a new or supported product as quickly as possible. Practices who are using unsupported EHR products may incur excessive expenses and significant challenges finding the technical expertise to pull the information from the old EHR to support conversion efforts. For example, one practice could not retrieve key clinical information from their EHR since the programming staff has dissolved after the company announced the discontinuation of the EHR product.

Unfortunately, moving from one EHR to another is not easy. Indeed, there are a number of key challenges facing a practice that is trying to move among EHRs:

> EHR activation is intense since you may have to move to the new EHR with few or no transition steps. As a practical matter, you cannot move over to a new EHR in stages. Splitting data, users, patients, functions or any other segmentation strategy may simply not be viable. For example, data conversion may not be split up due to the large number of connections between information in an EHR. Therefore, you may have to deal with a dramatic and sudden move to a completely new product. The only practical way to survive such an upheaval is to fully train, prepare and support you users with an adequate level of resources, Even then, you will encounter issues and challenges that will stress every doctor and staff person.

> EHR information may be stored in different structures. EHR products dramatically differ in the way they store information and the information that they store. In Chapter 6, four different EHR types were presented: document management, build a note, forms, and knowledgebase. If you are moving from one type of EHR to another, how will you be able to load information from the old EHR structure into the new structure? For example, if you are moving from a build a note or document management based EHR to a knowledgebase product, how will anyone be able to interpret the text from the notes or documents to trigger the correct knowledgebase selections. Similarly, a forms based EHR may have three or four different pieces of information that determine which knowledgebase finding is relevant.

> EHR information includes audit and source information that may not be available for conversion or be accommodated by the new EHR. For example, some EHRs store the audit trail in a separate log file that has to be viewed outside of the standard EHR functionality, while other EHR products attach the audit file to the EHR information.

> EHR products may differ in what images are accommodated and how they are stored. For example, BMP, JPG, and TIF are different image file types. Some EHRs only work with one type of image file. You may have to convert all of the images from the type used by the current EHR to a different image type supported by the new EHR.

EHR Conversion Challenges—As noted earlier, the key issue is that you cannot abandon the old EHR data, run it out and start using the new EHR. So, your practice will need to come up with strategies to move information from the old EHR to the new EHR. Unfortunately, the move is not a simple or standard process. For example,

Patient Identification—Many older EHR products were interfaced with the practice management systems. In some cases, practices actually entered patient demographic information into an EHR separately since the PMS didn't interface with the EHR. In these situations, the matching of patient clinical information with the patient demographics from the PMS could be a significant issue. Using a standard name, date or birth, gender and SSN can still be challenging. For example, some practices maintain multiple patient accounts, and, in some cases, separate patient clinical records in the EHR.

Medications and Prescriptions—Older EHR products may use a user maintained file of drugs instead of a drug database such as MediSpan or MULTUM. For example, one older EHR allows the practice to maintain a coded table of prescription drugs. The drug name library may only include the name, and not the various strengths and prescription options. Strengths and prescription options may be stored elsewhere or entered with the prescription. In many of these older products, the National Drug Code (NDC) is not stored. Therefore, it would be difficult or, in some cases, impossible to map the old drugs to a new EHR that uses the NDC codes. For example, separate tables of drug codes strengths and forms from the old EHR would have to be combined to create the NDC code.

Clinical Note Structure—Translating information from one medical record to another can be expensive and difficult. For example, different EHR structures (See above), codes, and storage techniques can undermine your ability to convert clinical information. For example, some EHRs store information that is processed through a document generator to create a clinical note. One would have to reverse engineer the EHR data and note generation program to produce the data that could be converted to the new EHR. In the final analysis, many EHR conversions will bring over old medical information as text in the new EHR. However, text conversion does not populate key patient information such as allergies, medications and orders. Indeed, you may encounter a situation where the patient has not been properly identified to the new EHR during the conversion process. For example, if the surgery note is brought over as text, the new EHR may not have surgical history information that triggers periodic check-ups (Ex. Annual checkups for total joint replacement.) You may have to manually enter key information into the new EHR to properly introduce the patient to the new EHR.

Data Stored in the New EHR that is Missing in the Old EHR—Newer EHRs may have information that is not available for conversion from the old EHR. For example, the new EHR may have a complete patient history that is not part of the old EHR record. In order to properly set up the patient in the new EHR may require manual backloading of information in the new EHR (See Chapter 10 on Implementation.)

Data Stored in the Old EHR that is not Accommodated in the New EHR—In some cases, the old EHR information is not maintained in the new EHR. For example, one EHR has screens of information on the patient that did not map to the new EHR. Similarly, one EHR did not have a place to store long text fragments that were an important part of the old EHR.

Mapping Different EHR Structures—EHR products have a variety of ways that information is connected and related. For example, some EHRs include tasks as part of the patient medical record, while other EHRs do not include tasks as part of the patient record. In some cases, EHR messages are directly connected to specific patient chart information such as lab results or an ER report. Other products merely associate the message with the patient. If you are moving from EHRs that handle messages differently, what will you do with the pointers from the old EHR when the new EHR does not have message pointers to the patient record? In such cases, you may append an informational message at the end of the converted information. However, that information will not be as obvious and notable as the linked messages in the old system.

Image File Formats—Images are stored in an EHR under one or more of a variety of image formats. JPG, BMP, and TIF are a few of the image formats that are available to store and manage scanned imaged of documents, and even images from diagnostic equipment. However, not all EHRs support all image formats. Even more frustrating is that some EHRs use proprietary image structures that are variations on the standard image structures. For example, some EHR products use a special version of an image file to store additional information, notations and amendments. The conversion of the image formats from one type to another can be a technical challenge and difficult. For example, some EHRs use proprietary "layering" within an image to accommodate notations on an image. If the new EHR does not accommodate layering in their standard images, how will you store the base image and the proprietary notes that are part of the historical image from the current EHR?

Dating Issues—As a matter of design, most EHR products have dating information that document the entry of information and all activities. The dating information may include the date of entry, completion, start and stop dates, verification dates and a wide range of information that not only documents activities, but determines presentation. For example, many products will display chart contents in reverse chronological order. When information from the previous EHR is loaded into the new EHR, the various dates associated with items in the old system may not be completely accommodated in the new EHR. Conversely, the new EHR may require more detailed dating information that was not tracked in the old EHR. Either problem could affect how your information is presented and accessed.

Audit Trails—EHRs significantly differ in how they support and maintain audit trails. The connection between you audit trail and the actual data may be built into the product or maintained as a list of activities associated with the patient record. In many cases, EHR data conversion does not allow for posting the old audit trails within the new EHR audit trails. The new audit trails may lack the specificity of the source, timing and sequence of information that was converted from the legacy EHR.

EHR Data Conversion Timing—EHR data conversion timing is particularly tricky due to the amount of data and time constraints. When you are converting data, typically, you must dump information from the old system, convert the information and then load the information into the new system. After the new information is loaded, you should verify that the conversion was successful before using your data in the new system. Due to the volume of information and conversion processes, such processes could take several days or even longer. For example, the conversion of a large number of images from an old EHR format to a new EHR format took over 2 weeks due to the large number of images and complex conversion necessitated by the significant differences between the two systems. Typically, during the conversion process, you cannot record information in the old EHR, and would have to undertake a catchup process to post information collected during the conversion process into the new EHR.

Conversion Strategy—In the final analysis, you will need to find a place in the new EHR for your information from the old EHR. In many cases, we will need to work around the limitations of the new EHR to find a place for the old EHR data and we will have to work around the limitations of the old EHR to properly load information into the new EHR.

The conversion of data from your current EHR to a new EHR is a daunting task that requires a substantial amount of analysis, testing, planning and verification efforts. In order to mitigate the challenges that you face, consider the following strategies:

Verify Feasibility of EHR Conversion Before Your Commit to a New EHR—As part of your EHR selection process, discuss the conversion options and strategies with the new EHR vendor. Make sure that you discuss the specific information in the old EHR and fully understand what the new EHR vendor plans to do with your information. Separate discussions will be needed about notes, messages, orders and other classes of information in the old EHR. The new EHR vendor should show you where the old information will be stored and you should verify that the strategy is viable and useful. For example, if the new EHR vendor suggests converting patient orders as a miscellaneous note, then you may not be able to manage outstanding old EHR orders in the new EHR. The key issue is to verify that the new EHR properly displays the old information and that the strategy to set up the old information in the new EHR does not distort the old EHR information or undermine the new EHR. **CAUTION:** Make sure that the conversion strategy works and is appropriate before you commit to any EHR product.

Detail the EHR Conversion in the Contract—Based on the feasibility analysis, include the conversion strategy in your contract. Be especially careful to list the classes of old EHR information to be converted and the conversion plan. The plan should include the process that will be used, define the conversion strategy, allow for a full test conversion and a final conversion as well as the acceptance process and a resolution strategy. CAUTION: You may need to defer some of the analysis and specifics until after the contract is signed and the project starts, but such a process and completion of a signed conversion plan should be inserted into the implementation plan included in the contract.

Include a Test Conversion—A full test conversion should be included in the implementation effort. Some vendors will only want to do a sample conversion. However, a limited conversion will not allow you to verify the convertability of all you data. Additionally, the full test conversion will allow you to get a good idea of the conversion process and the time needed for the live conversion.

Allow Extra Implementation Time—The conversion of data from an old EHR requires additional time for the EHR implementation effort. As a practical matter, you will not be able to attempt a test conversion until you have set up you EHR master files and trained staff on the use of the EHR. Additionally, you need to allow for complete verification of the testing process and sufficient practice time to accommodate the more compressed transition.

Prepare for Potential Break in EHR Use—During the conversion of the old EHR data to the new EHR, you may have to stop entering data into the EHR for a week or more while the new EHR is being loaded with your patient information. After the conversion has been verified, you will need to update the new EHR with the patient activity during the break. Note: The exact process and break will depend on the new EHR and your data conversion strategy.

Verify Test and Final Conversions—The conversion of the old EHR data to the new EHR will have to be vigorously tested and verified. You need to check the conversion of each class of information (Ex. Notes, images, prescriptions) as well as patient types. The proper access, use and setup of information in the new system will have to be verified. For example, previous procedure information should properly trigger health maintenance items (Ex. Proper immunization notification.)

There are many challenges and options for the disposition and handling of data from an old EHR. However, you will need to fully analyze the situation and options to insure that you have a practical and effective strategy to preserve the integrity of your patient charts that have been built in the old EHR.

TRAINING

EHR training strategies will be impacted by the contract and how you intend to support and train your users. In most practices, a designated group of EHR pioneers is established to champion the EHR implementation effort. These pioneers may be known as key users, super users, champions or a similar term.

Typically, the super users are trained by the vendor. The super users are responsible for setting up the EHR for use, and training the rest of the practice staff. This strategy is quite demanding since the super users must make key decisions on system setup and use as well as train others before they are fully familiar with the EHR.

In some cases, the vendor trains everyone. Most vendor training programs cover all staff on all aspects of the EHR. However, not all users may need to know how to manage and use all EHR features. Training all staff on all features does not let staff concentrate on the specific capabilities that they need to know. Indeed, you may end up training staff on certain capabilities that you may not even want them to know about. For example, setting up security and user access should be limited to a select group of users.

Your EHR training plan should address a number of distinct requirements:

General computer training—Frequently, practice doctors and employees lack the computer skills to use an EHR. Employees may not be comfortable with navigating around the system, using the Windows environment or operating a mouse. You can save money by providing general computer training from a local community college or a training service. Don't use EHR vendors to train your staff on general computer operations. Team staff familiar with the new systems with staff that do not have good computer skills. General computer training will help your staff feel more confident about exploring and using the EHR.

Device Training—Even users who may comfortable using a Windows environment may have problems with some of the new devices that you will be using. For instance, use of a tablet stylus in place of a mouse could pose some issues for various staff members. The best strategy is to give staff time using the various devices. On tablet devices, the user needs to know how to use the stylus, as well as how to change batteries and maintain contact through the wireless network. Other users may need to know how to operate a scanner or work new printers. Device training is best provided by practice staff. Device computer training may help you avoid problems, from connections between devices to turning on and off a device.

Setup Training—Setup training focuses on maintenance of security files, code tables, formularies and charges, as well as system administration. System setup also includes customizing EHR templates, screens, user preferences and practice standards. For example, your practice may design a custom screen to track a certain service that you provide. Setup training is provided by EHR vendors. However, you should limit setup training to a designated group of super users. In most cases, setup options should be driven by the EHR implementation team and management. EHR setup changes should not be made without the approval of your EHR implementation team. For example, the practice would not want a user to change a set of drug preferences unless the doctors had changed their list. Similarly, an EHR template should not be changed unless the doctors have agreed to the change in clinical documentation and have approved the cost of the change as well as identified tangible benefits from the change.

Application Training—Application training covers using the EHR features and functions. Note that vendor application training will not necessarily address your specific customizations, your workflow strategies or your setup standards. For example, the vendor trainer would cover how to access a clinical template, but the trainer may not understand the clinical details of your template or setups. **TIP:** Make sure your trainer understands the EHR features that will be relevant to your practice and services. For example, a trainer that does not have experience with orthopaedic practices may not have an effective strategy for managing the exchange of patients among orthopedic techs, PAs, and PT staff. Vendors do not typically set up training sessions to focus on specific areas that may be needed by practice employees. For example, you may want to train the phone center staff on messages and tasks but exclude other EHR features. Customized training sessions usually are the responsibility of the practice. **TIP:** Consider using a core team of clinical staff to develop the key training areas and train your staff on the specific items they need for their jobs.

Practice Procedures—EHR users should be trained on the EHR in light of the practice setups, templates and procedures. Practice procedures may include the various policies and workflows that have been designed by the practice to capitalize on the EHR. Practice procedure training may be built around practice-focused training on how to use the EHR. Indeed, practice procedures are the product of your workflow design and the various decisions that drive the EHR setup.

The actual training process may be staged to support the various stages of your EHR implementation. The following steps should be considered in developing your own training strategy:

Train super users—Super users training will be conducted by the vendor and cover all system features and capabilities. Super users are expected to serve the role of subject matter experts on the use and management of the EHR. Ideally, all users should have easy access to a super user. You may identify a super user for each location and/or department.

Develop practice training materials—Practice training materials allow you to focus on the specific strategies and setups of the EHR for your practice. This also allows you to integrate the training on the system with training staff on your own procedures, templates and setups. Training on practice procedures and practice training materials also support several HIPAA standards.

Train test and setup support staff—Additional staff can be used to support the system setup and testing process. For example, medical records staff can be used to test scanning options and clinical staff can be used to test templates and clinical documentation screens.

Identify training packages by role—Training all users on all aspects of the EHR will take a long time and provide many users with information that they will never use. Using the role definitions that drive the security setup, end users should be scheduled for training packages. The training packages should address the specific needs of each role.

Develop training plan—The end user training plan should train users for the work to be done in the current implementation step. The training should take place as close to the Go Live date for that particular function. For example, medical record training on scanning should be done immediately before scanning of medical records begins.

Train end users—End user training should take place as close to Go Live for the user as possible. For example, phone staff may train on messages immediately before they start using the EHR to log calls. End user training should include use of the workstation or tablet that will be used by the trainee. Note that end users may go through several training sequences as you expand the use of the system. For example, you may start off with imaging, move to workflow, proceed with charting and complete with order management. **TIP:** Remember that training classes should immediately precede actual use of the EHR. Otherwise the training effort will be a waste of time since most people will not remember how to use the system after a few weeks of inactivity. **TIP:** After a user is trained, make sure that they practice using the EHR in a test environment daily until Go Live. Ideally, you super users should check with each user each day on any problems they may have. You can encourage practicing with the EHR by broadcasting a problem of the day or finding information about a specific situation. **CAUTION:** Training of end users requires a different strategy for those practices moving from an old EHR to a new EHR. The end user training effort will have to allow a significant amount of time to allow users to practice with the new EHR and become more comfortable with the new EHR since the transition to a new EHR is more dramatic than the staged approach that can be taken with the transition from paper charts to an EHR.

Training practice staff on the EHR is an ongoing effort that will continue past EHR activation. Also, new employees will need to be fully trained on using the system. Current employees will need supplemental training on features that they have not used as well as changes to how the practice is making adjustments to EHR use. The EHR implementation effort allows the practice to set up the training materials and programs that will insure that the EHR usage is maintained according to the practice design as well as allow for evolving changes to meet practice needs and challenges (see Table 10.9).

TABLE 10.9

SMALL PRACTICE IMPLEMENTATION TASK	STATUS	ASSIGNED TO	START	END	COMMENT
ADMINSTRATIVE					
1. Develop an implementation strategy.					Develop an implementation strategy for implementing various aspects of the EHR and how the doctors will transition to the EHR. Smaller practices need the physician to lead the effort.
2. Establish supporting policies for the EHR project.					Define the policies to empower and support the implementation process including: Deployment Phases, EHR Policies/Strategies, and Vetting Workflow Changes.
3. Complete EHR Implementation, Project and Support Teams.					Select staff to support the EHR rollout.
POLICY AND PROCEDURE					
4. Develop EHR Medical Record Workflow Flow Charts.					Practice will develop a workflow model to support patient service, office flow, clinical charting,
5. Establish a retention policy for scanned charts and originals that are scanned into the EHR.					Need to consult legal counsel and risk manager.
6. Inventory Effect of EHR Procedure Changes on the Following Areas.					Practice will be establishing standard procedures based on services offered and specialty areas.
a. Staffing Responsibilities and Levels.					Smaller practices may have few changes since staff members may perform a wide range of functions.
b. Patient Service Procedures.					Tracking patient service item and office flow in the office.
c. Hardware Placement.					
d. Software Setup.					
7. Develop Detailed EHR Procedures.					
a. Clinical Content Changes					Small practices should be careful to limit modifications that may be difficult to support or manage. Smaller offices may rely more on the vendor for day to day support.

Continued

Continued from previous page

SMALL PRACTICE IMPLEMENTATION TASK	STATUS	ASSIGNED TO	START	END	COMMENT
b. Medical Records (Initial Use).					
c. Workflow					
d. Audit Procedures					
HARDWARE					
COMMUNICATIONS					
8. Analyze the effect of EHR traffic on practice communications. If necessary order more communication capacity.					The EHR will increase the number of active users and the amount of data exchanged on behalf of each user.
9. If necessary, install Wireless Network Equipment in the office.					Wireless networks will depend on the use of workstations and/or tablets.
10. Test Connectivity between Tablets and Wireless Network at from all appropriate areas in the office.					The wireless connection will be secured from outside access.
SERVERS					
11. Install EHR Server and infrastructure.					Smaller offices may use an ASP instead of an in-house server.
12. If interfacing with a PMS, verify working interface between PMS and EHR.					The smaller practice should limit interfaces which may be expensive to maintain. Ideally, the small practice should buy the EHR and PMS from the same vendor.
13. If interfacing with diagnostic equipment or lab devices, verify working EHR interface between diagnostic equipment, and lab service.					
WORKSTATIONS/TABLETS					
14. Order workstations and/or tablets to access the EHR.					
15. Identify, order, and install new Workstations needed in the office.					An EHR may increase the need for additional workstations. For example, shared workstations may not be practical with an EHR.
16. Order and install tablet devices, batteries, and charges as needed for EHR.					

Continued

Continued from previous page

SMALL PRACTICE IMPLEMENTATION TASK	STATUS	ASSIGNED TO	START	END	COMMENT
SCANNERS					
17. Determine the need for Medium and Heavy Duty EHR Scanners.					High speed scanners are needed for paper chart scanning. Smaller scanners will be used for daily scanning needs.
18. Order and install scanners.					
PRINTERS					
19. Identify, order and install new printers needed for EHR.					The practice will have to determine if additional printers are needed. Printers may be used to print documents that are currently generated by hand including prescriptions, office notes, and patient education documents.
CLINICAL CONTENT SETUP					
20. Compile Samples of Existing Clinical Forms, Letters, and Reports from All Offices.					The practice's forms and notes will be used to verify clinical content and use of the EHR.
21. Analyze EHR clinical content with the existing forms and documents.					The clinical content analysis will be completed for each area, disease and/or process.
22. Review results of analysis to determine work-around strategies and implementation issues.					Unresolved issues will be reviewed for significance and optional methods. The smaller practice should rely on the vendor to address items.
MASTER FILES					
23. Compile List of EHR Master File Analysis Guidelines and Information Requirements.					
24. Analyze Key Master Files Issues and Strategies.					The Master File setup strategy will be driven by the analysis of the workflow design and practice issues.
25. Compile EHR Master File Information.					Information to be collected could include lists of preferred treatments, pharmacies and other healthcare organizations that the practice may refer patients to.
26. Conduct EHR training on Master File Entry and Setup.					The EHR Setup team will need training to enter the setup information that will be the basis for training of other users.
27. Enter EHR Master File Information into EHR.					

Continued

Continued from previous page

SMALL PRACTICE IMPLEMENTATION TASK	STATUS	ASSIGNED TO	START	END	COMMENT
DATA CONVERSION					
28. Test scanning strategies and procedures with existing paper charts. Testing should include time and motion reviews.					The scope of scanning testing will depend on the data conversion and training strategies to fulfill data retention and patient service needs. The test is needed to verify the procedure and the setup of the EHR.
29. Develop scanning procedures, triggers, and strategies for the paper charts.					A detailed scanning plan and procedure will be developed for the selected training strategy. The triggers to process a paper chart may evolve as the EHR implementation effort proceeds. Alternatively, some practices do not scan any paper records into their EHR.
30. Load electronic clinical data from other sources.					Some small practices have previously collected data and clinical information that can be loaded into the EHR. For example, lab results, and transcription may be available.
31. Develop procedures for incoming faxes, and mail that is added to the EHR.					A scanning procedure will be needed for incoming documents.
TRAINING					
32. Identify Training Team for EHR System Administration, Operations and Production.					Training may include selected Super Users to help train other users, as well as, Computer Based Training and formal classes.
33. Identify EHR Training Packages.					The practice should develop training packages to focus training and support for classes of users (Ex. Physicians, MAs, Nurses, and Lab Techs.)
34. Develop Training Materials for EHR and Procedures.					A smaller practice may make more extensive use of the vendor materials in the practice's training manual.
35. Train Staff on appropriate functions and areas in focused training sessions.					Smaller practices should make more extensive use of the vendor's training program, since small practices typically have fewer in-house resources.
ACTIVATION					
36. Verify procedures for chartless patients.					The practice should verify the procedures for the dramatic change in workflow without a patient chart.

Continued

Continued from previous page

SMALL PRACTICE IMPLEMENTATION TASK	STATUS	ASSIGNED TO	START	END	COMMENT
37. If appropriate, set up production for chart scanning and clinical data backloading to support the EHR roll-out strategy.					The transition to an EHR for a particular patient may involve scanning paper chart items, and loading historic information into the EHR.
38. Initiate EHR Use.					The EHR may be rolled out on a staged basis defined in the implementation strategy. The stages will depend on the current practice situation, type of practice and practice strategy.
CONTINUING SUPPORT					
39. Conduct EHR Monthly Status Meetings.					

TABLE 10.10

LARGE PRACTICE IMPLEMENTATION TASK	STATUS	ASSIGNED TO	START	END	COMMENT
ADMINSTRATIVE					

1. Develop an implementation strategy.					Develop an implementation strategy including:
					
					    Rollout Order
					    Transition Strategy

2. Establish supporting policies for the EHR project.					Define the policies to empower and support the implementation process including:
					
					    Adoption Policies,
					    Deployment Phases,
					    Data Policies/Strategies,
					    Vetting Workflow Changes, and
					    Accepting Clinical Templates.

3. Complete EHR Implementation, Project and Support Teams.					Determine staffing to support EHR rollout. Factors include:
					
					    Implementation Team Composition
					    Office and Team Responsibilities

4. Develop interim staffing model and strategy for EHR Go Live.					Depends on the adoption and deployment strategy, Practice may use additional staff to support the transition to the EHR.
POLICY AND PROCEDURE					
5. Develop EHR Medical Record Workflow Flow Charts.					Practice will develop a workflow model to support patient service, office flow, and clinical charting,
6. Establish a retention policy for scanned charts and originals that are scanned into the EHR.					Need to consult legal counsel and risk manager.
7. Establish policies and procedures for audit and quality improvement activities using the EHR.					
8. Inventory Effect of EHR Procedure Changes on the Following Areas.					Practice will be establishing standard procedures and variations for offices based on office size, services offered and specialty areas.
a. Staffing Responsibilities and Levels.					

Continued

Continued from previous page

LARGE PRACTICE IMPLEMENTATION TASK	STATUS	ASSIGNED TO	START	END	COMMENT
b. Patient Service Procedures.					Tracking patient service item and office flow in each office.
c. Hardware Placement.					
d. Software Setup.					
9. Develop Detailed EHR Procedures.					
a. Security Access					
b. Clinical Content Changes					
c. Medical Records (Initial Use).					
d. Workflow					
e. Audit Procedures					
f. Office and Management					
HARDWARE					
COMMUNICATIONS					
10. Analyze the effect of EHR traffic on the communications with Offices.					The EHR will increase the number of active users and the amount of data exchanged on behalf of each user. Communication capacity between the offices and the EHR Server or ASP should be carefully analyzed.
11. Order additional communication lines and bandwidth.					Practice may need to increase the communications bandwidth as the EHR is rolled out.
12. Test and verify upgraded communications at each office.					
13. If necessary, install Wireless Network Equipment in all Offices.					Wireless networks will depend on the use of workstations and/or tablets.
14. Test Connectivity between Tablets and Wireless Network at from all appropriate areas at All Offices.					The wireless connection will be secured from outside access.
SERVERS					
15. Install EHR Server and infrastructure.					

Continued

Continued from previous page

LARGE PRACTICE IMPLEMENTATION TASK	STATUS	ASSIGNED TO	START	END	COMMENT
16. If interfacing with a PMS, verify working interface between PMS and EHR.					
17. If interfacing with diagnostic equipment or lab devices, verify working EHR interface between diagnostic equipment, and lab service.					
WORKSTATIONS/TABLETS					
18. Order workstations and tablets to support EHR efforts.					
19. Identify, order, and install new Workstations needed on an office by office basis.					An EHR may increase the need for additional workstations. For example, shared workstations may not be practical with an EHR.
20. Order and install tablet devices, batteries, and charges as needed for EHR.					
SCANNERS					
21. Complete Inventory of All Offices Requiring Medium and Heavy Duty EHR Scanner Service.					High speed scanners are needed for paper chart scanning. Smaller scanners will be put in each office for daily scanning needs. Some larger practices establish scanning centers at selected locations.
22. Order and install scanners.					
PRINTERS					
23. Identify, order and install new printers needed for EHR.					Each office will have to determine if additional printers are needed. Printers may be used to print a variety of documents that are currently generated by hand including prescriptions, office notes, and patient education documents.
CLINICAL CONTENT SETUP					
24. Compile Samples of Existing Clinical Forms, Letters, and Reports from All Offices.					Practice should collect a set of forms and notes from each Office. The forms and notes will be used to verify clinical content and use of the EHR.
25. Analyze EHR clinical content with the existing forms and documents.					The clinical content analysis will be completed for each area, disease and/or process. Offices may offer different services and/or expertise.

Continued

Continued from previous page

LARGE PRACTICE IMPLEMENTATION TASK	STATUS	ASSIGNED TO	START	END	COMMENT
26. Review results of analysis to determine work-around strategies and implementation issues.					Unresolved issues will be reviewed for significance and optional methods. Some items will be referred back to the vendor.
OTHER ISSUES					
27. Establish EHR Report and Production Schedule.					
MASTER FILES					
28. Compile List of EHR Master File Analysis Guidelines and Information Requirements.					The practice will consider the setup requirements for all of the offices. Larger practices should seek to limit the differences between locations. Make sure differences are substantiated by clinical issues, and needs.
29. Analyze Key Master Files Issues and Strategies.					The Master File setup strategy will be driven by the analysis of the workflow design and office specific issues.
30. Compile EHR Master File Information.					Information to be collected could include lists of preferred treatments, pharmacies and other healthcare organizations that the practice may refer patients to. Some master file information may be used by specific offices.
31. Conduct EHR training on Master File Entry and Setup.					The EHR Setup team will need training to enter the setup information that will be the basis for training of other users.
32. Enter EHR Master File Information into EHR.					
DATA CONVERSION					
33. Test scanning strategies and procedures with existing paper charts. Testing should include time and motion reviews.					The scope of scanning testing will depend on the data conversion and training strategies to fulfill data retention and patient service needs. The test is needed to verify the procedure and the setup of the EHR. Separate testing may be needed for each office.
34. Develop scanning procedures, triggers, and strategies for the paper charts.					A detailed scanning plan and procedure will be developed for the selected training strategy. The triggers to process a paper chart may evolve as the EHR implementation effort proceeds.
35. Load electronic clinical data from other sources.					The practice may have previously collected data and clinical information that can be loaded into the EHR. For example, lab results, transcription and information from a previous EHR may be available.

Continued

Continued from previous page

LARGE PRACTICE IMPLEMENTATION TASK	STATUS	ASSIGNED TO	START	END	COMMENT
36. Develop procedures for incoming faxes, and mail that is added to the EHR.					Faxes will be directed to a Fax Server for immediate loading into the EHR. A scanning procedure will be needed for incoming documents.
TRAINING					
37. Identify Training Team for EHR System Administration, Operations and Production.					Training may include selected Super Users to help train other users, as well as, Computer Based Training and formal classes.
38. Identify EHR Training Packages.					The practice should develop training packages to focus training and support for classes of users (Ex. Physicians, MAs, Nurses, and Lab Techs.)
39. Develop Training Materials for EHR and Procedures.					Training materials will focus on the way the EHR is used in the Practice by user class.
40. Train Staff on appropriate functions and areas in focused training sessions.					Several training classes will be held to focus on different classes of users and functions. For example, separate programs may be designed for scanning, charting, patient service, and workflow. Training versions may be office specific issues and services.
ACTIVATION					
41. Verify procedures for chartless patients.					The practice should verify the procedures for the dramatic change in workflow without a patient chart.
42. Set up production for chart scanning and clinical data backloading to support the EHR roll-out strategy.					The transition to an EHR for a particular patient may involve scanning paper chart items, and loading historic information into the EHR.
43. Initiate EHR Use.					The EHR may be rolled out on a staged basis defined in the implementation strategy. The stages will depend on the current practice situation, type of practice and practice strategy.
CONTINUING SUPPORT					
44. Establish EHR Super User and Support Team Structure.					Super users will be used to monitor EHR use and guide future activities.
45. Conduct EHR Monthly Status Meetings.					

Continued

Continued from previous page

MULTI-OFFICE PRACTICE IMPLE-MENTATION TASK	STATUS	ASSIGNED TO	START	END	COMMENT
ADMINSTRATIVE					
1. Identify Key Office EHR Implementation Staff.					Need to identify office staff that will be main contact and support for the EHR implementation.
2. Determine the readiness of the facilities at the office to support the EHR.					
POLICY AND PROCEDURE					
3. Present EHR Strategies and Procedures to the Office Staff.					
4. Verify applicability of policies and procedures for audit and quality assurance for the Office.					Office specific changes may be made to the policies and procedures. Such changes could also impact setup, clinical content, training and other activities.
5. Validate Office EHR Procedure Changes on the Following Areas.					
a. Staffing Responsibilities and Levels.					
b. Patient Service Procedures.					
c. Hardware Placement.					
d. Software Setup.					Software setup should only be affected in cases where the Office differs from the standard office procedures due to a business or care issue.
e. Data Conversion					Data conversion issues could significantly differ due to chart structure, information that must be loaded into the EHR, and office specific workflow and services.
HARDWARE					
COMMUNICATIONS					
6. If necessary, install Wireless Network Equipment at the Office.					
7. Test Connectivity between Tablets and Wireless Network at from all appropriate areas at the Office.					The wireless connection will be secured from outside access. Access to the EHR should be available from all locations in each office.

Continued

Continued from previous page

MULTI-OFFICE PRACTICE IMPLEMENTATION TASK	STATUS	ASSIGNED TO	START	END	COMMENT
8. Verify current communication facilities for use by EHR users from the Office.					The practice needs to insure that the incremental traffic from the Office will be accommodated by the practice's communication facilities.
WORKSTATIONS/TABLETS					
9. Order Tablets to support the Office.					
10. Identify Office Workstations that will need access to the EHR.					
11. Identify, order, and install new Workstations that will be needed to support the EHR at the Office.					
12. Order Tablet devices, batteries, and charges as needed for the Office.					
13. Install New Workstations.					
SCANNERS					
14. Verify scanning needs at the Office.					
15. Order Scanners for Office.					
16. Install EHR Scanners.					
PRINTERS					
17. Complete Inventory of New Printers Needed at the Office.					
18. Order Printers.					
19. Install Printers.					
OTHER ISSUES					
20. Inventory equipment that produces information for the EHR. Note that the equipment may be interfaced with the EHR or output may be scanned into the EHR.					The office needs a data collection or interface strategy for all of the equipment used. Options include scanning, generating a file, and interfacing with the EHR.

Continued

Continued from previous page

MULTI-OFFICE PRACTICE IMPLE-MENTATION TASK	STATUS	ASSIGNED TO	START	END	COMMENT
21. Order interfaces between Equipment, and EHR.					If appropriate and the equipment supports the interface, the practice could order and install the interface to diagnostic equipment.
22. Test and Activate the Interfaces between the equipment, and the EHR.					
OFFICE SPECIFIC CUSTOMIZATION					
23. Make office specific changes to the workflow model.					
24. Make office specific changes to clinical templates.					There may be situations where an office specific accommodation is necessary. For example, an office may need changes for a doctor who specializes in a precise area of medicine that has not been encountered in other offices.
25. Make office specific changes to the implementation plan.					
26. Enhance the EHR Setups for the office.					Office setups could include room configurations and provider clinical preferences.
27. Determine any facility changes needed to accommodate the EHR.					Facility issues can include a place to scan, availability of workstations, and places to store tablets.
TRAINING					
28. Identify Office EHR Super Users.					
29. After First office Go Live, doctors and staff will make site visits to operational offices to review and observe the use of the EHR as part of the training process.					
30. Schedule Staff for EHR Training.					
31. Train Staff on EHR in Coordination with Activation Activities.					Training will include use of the EHR, as well as workflow and patient service. Training packages were designed for the practice.
32. Test scanning of paper charts for the office.					Offices may have chart differences that necessitate test scanning.

Continued

Continued from previous page

MULTI-OFFICE PRACTICE IMPLEMENTATION TASK	STATUS	ASSIGNED TO	START	END	COMMENT
ACTIVATION					
33. Start up appropriate chart scanning and backloading of data into the EHR.					
34. Verify scanned documents with the appropriate doctors.					
35. Load electronic clinical data from other sources.					
36. Initiate Use of the EHR for scanning, workflow, and patient service.					The EHR may be rolled out on a staged basis defined in the implementation strategy. The stages will depend on the current office situation and experience with other offices.

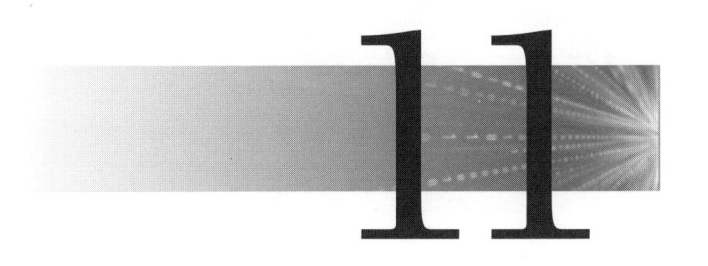

Activating an EHR

Once your practice starts moving to activate your EHR, expect some personnel and logistic issues. In some cases, staff and even doctors will leave a practice, protesting they "do not want to be computer operators." Some practices have experienced passive-aggressive behavior and sabotage. For example, doctors and employees may note that the EHR is slower that their paper-based process before they even fully use the system. You may even start questioning the value of the entire process.

The EHR will challenge employees who just do not like change. Some staff members will be afraid that they will lose their jobs or their influence. Other staff members may have years of time working with the paper record and be skeptical of the new EHR. Concern with job loss can be particularly acute in the most affected departments, such as medical records and transcription. Changes in staffing levels may be handled through normal attrition. In any case, don't expect to see job savings until several months after the EHR is activated. Indeed, most practices will experience greater expenses in the first transition year than the last non-EHR year. After the transition, you will be able to gauge the full effect and reap the benefits of the EHR.

EHR activation requires a massive change to every process and procedure. Know that the transfer of years of data and experience from the current records to an EHR is not accomplished in a day or two. The activation of the EHR requires a clear plan, commitment to the project and ability to address issues, because unexpected problems will arise in the middle of this massive change. For example, if patient flow depends on the EHR, then lapses in recording patient status or not checking the workflow screen on a constant basis will disrupt operations and frustrate everyone. EHR activation also requires patience and a focus on working out these problems.

Your activation strategy must consider the various factors and dynamics of the project as well as the need to complete the project. Activate the EHR only when your practice is ready. However, you need to move the project along at an even pace to complete activation in a manageable timeframe. The transition period accompanied by partial EHR use is complex and expensive to manage. For example, you have to pay for the management of paper records as well as the EHR during the transition period. As significant, maintaining a complete medical record may require addition efforts depending on your activation strategy.

In many cases, EHR activation is not so much an event, but a process. Depending on a wide array of issues, you may have various staff members using the EHR for work that is still paper based in other practice areas. For example, physician champions may be charting patient visits using the EHR, but medical records may still maintain the paper medical chart. Surviving and completing such transitions is the key to the activation process. Your practice, doctors, and staff will have to manage a number of transitions to complete the activation of the EHR. Some of these transitions will increase the workload of the practice, require additional resources, and frustrate everyone. However, coping with the changes during the transition is the only way to successfully activate and deploy the EHR. If you have a plan that the organization is behind, and you have the right product, then the process needed to implement the EHR should be allowed to proceed with the understanding that implementation is a complex and disruptive process. The successful completion of the activation process requires good management and commitment to the EHR strategy—throughout your organization.

ACTIVATION STRATEGIES

The activation of an EHR challenges the most capable staff and physicians. To succeed, you need to insure that all relevant doctors and staff understand their role and how you will activate the EHR. EHR activation can be based on any one of several strategies. Some vendors are very committed to one strategy, while others defer to the practice for the strategy and process. All EHR strategies consist of various groupings and orders of the following EHR capabilities:

Paperless chart stage—Some practices go through a paperless chart phase before they commence charting patient visits into the EHR. The paperless chart phase involves scanning the paper chart and providing access to the patient chart through the scanned EHR images. New information is entered on a paper form and the paper form is scanned into the EHR. The practice must deal with the EHR to access information but use paper to record information. In some cases, the paperless chart is the final end point of the EHR effort. The physicians will nonetheless benefit from immediate access to the patient chart instead of waiting for the paper record.

Charge and limited clinical information entry—The physicians and staff will use the EHR workstations and/or personal digital assistants to enter charge and limited EHR information, such as prescriptions, allergies and other basic patient data. Charges are passed to the PMS for billing. In some cases, you can also dictate directly into a transcription tool that is part of the EHR. For some practices, these functions are the end of their EHR effort. Some EHR vendors sell this limited set of capabilities as a "starting point" to move to the full EHR at a later date.

Doctor charting—Practices may start use of the EHR with selected patients and doctors to chart patient visits at time of service. Selected doctors will use the EHR to collect discrete information to document a patient visit while the patient is being served. For example, the nurse may enter vitals into the EHR record, but the doctor may dictate the assessment and plan. Using charting at time of service, the doctor enters information into the EHR and uses the EHR to calculate the E&M code for the visit. If the practice is not paperless, the chart record is printed from the EHR and filed in the patient's paper chart. *Note* that all doctors will not start charting at the same time, and will not start charting for all patients at once. Typically, the doctor will start charting for patient visits that they feel comfortable with. For example, a doctor may start with a single patient each day for a specific type of visit (for instance, flu, simple problem) and proceed to increase their EHR charting for all patients with the selected problem and then adding additional problems and conditions. The physician should practice with a previous visit, role play with staff, and/or shadow a patient visit to insure that he is ready to chart at time of service. The early-adopter physicians may mentor other doctors and users as they start using the EHR to chart patient visits. **CAUTION:** Doctors should cautiously move into charting with the EHR. Otherwise, they are putting too much pressure on themselves and the practice which could increase the chance of failure.

Transcription into the EHR—Dictated notes are entered into the EHR by a transcriptionist. The notes are saved in the EHR and the EHR may be used to coordinate review and distribution. If the practice is not paperless, the transcription may be printed and filed in the patient chart. For many practices, using the EHR to manage transcription offers an easy way to build up patient information in anticipation of implementing the EHR. Indeed, you may start using the transcription module to build up patient clinical content long before you are charting patient visits in the EHR. Immediate access to patient dictation is a significant benefit for practices that use dictation. **TIP:** EHR based access to transcription files is more effective and secure than transcription files that are generally available on a network server or stored on the transcriptionist's workstation.

Order entry and management—Doctors and clinical staff record and manage testing and treatment orders through the EHR. Orders are entered and assigned to the appropriate department. The order is managed by the department and the status of the order may be entered into the EHR. Note that the actual results may be managed through the paper record or through the EHR. The EHR offers the added benefit of being able to identify incomplete or pending services or treatments. EHR Order tracking is far superior to having outstanding items buried in a paper record or on a supplemental log. This capability can help the practice serve patients and follow-up on the doctor's advice. For example, the appointment clerk could check for outstanding tests or services when scheduling a patient.

Prescription entry—Prescriptions are entered into the EHR and produced for the patient. Prescriptions may be printed, faxed and/or electronically submitted to a designated pharmacy. In some cases, prescription writing is a separate module that may be used outside of implementing a complete EHR. Note that many practices have been disappointed with the final results of only entering prescriptions and not implementing an EHR. Some practices believe that they are only doing the pharmacy's data entry and seeing few benefits for the practice. Indeed, stand alone prescription systems do not necessarily save any work or time, since the prescription is still recorded in the patient note, prescription log and other documents.

Workflow—Practice staff and doctors use the EHR to manage patient workflow and issues. Patient messages, office issues, prescription refills and other items are entered and tracked in the EHR. The doctors and clinical staff access their assigned items, but need access to the paper chart to address the issue or answer the question. The resolution of the item is noted in the EHR. If the paper chart is still in use, the workflow items may be printed out and filed in the paper chart. EHR-based workflow tools will help management track items and insure that patient issues are addressed in a timely basis.

In some cases, vendors will group various capabilities together based on the structure of their system, your practice situation or any number of factors. For example, some vendors insist on charge entry and prescription writing for their initial EHR functions.

The activation sequence and what is included in each activation group should be seriously reviewed and considered before you move forward. **TIP**: Be especially careful to manage the implementation process on your schedule and not necessarily the "sunny day" schedule proposed by other parties. You need to be realistic about the practical effect of your activation strategy and steps. The various transition phases that are determined by your strategy will not necessarily save you time or money from the first step of your transition process. Converting to an EHR requires a lot of flexibility, enthusiasm, and commitment. You also need to be patient through the transition steps to complete the implementation process and take advantage of your investment.

For example, you need to let your key users digest the training on the EHR before you commence end-user training. Some vendors propose schedules that assume your newly trained key users return from training as experts. They rarely are that quickly. Additionally, you must be certain that a reliable patient medical record is available throughout the process. Split medical records with some information in the paper record and other information in the EHR can expose the practice to HIPAA compliant issues as well as inhibit patient care.

Using some features and adding additional capabilities over time is an excellent way to transition to the EHR. However, the transition period should be as short as possible due to the complexity of managing both the paper and computerized patient records. For example, charting patient visits on the EHR and printing for a paper record could create medical record continuity problems. Too many practices fall into the trap of implementing a few capabilities and stopping. A partially implemented EHR could be very dangerous and expensive. Your staff and doctors can only go so long with having to deal with patient information split between the EHR and your paper records. Indeed, some practices get to a point where they give up and go back to their paper records. The key to success is moving quickly through the implementation process and avoid sitting in transition for too long. For example, a scanned medical record may be more difficult for many doctors than the original paper record. However, order entry, charting and prescriptions will ultimately make things easier. If the practice is stuck in the scanned record mode for too long, the physicians and staff may get frustrated.

ACTIVATION READINESS

Now you're just about ready to use the EHR in your practice. To manage and control the process, you need to insure that you have the resources and support structure in place to deal with this dramatic and challenging step. This includes:

Physician champions—The biggest barrier to charting at time of service is clinical content. The verification and testing of clinical content is one challenge, but reaching a comfort level with the clinical content will make the difference for physicians. Your practice needs at least one physician champion to start EHR use. Some practices have several physician champions to cover various practice areas. The physician(s) must be willing to put up with the inevitable start up issues and adjustments. Of course, the more testing and training, the fewer problems. Physicians involved in the testing process should continue to use the charting tool to maintain training continuity and build experience. Physicians and staff need to practice documenting patient visits and using the EHR a number of times before they are ready to use the EHR for patient service. You may even consider generating the clinical record to be filed in your paper chart (to adequately control and maintain the designated record set). Physicians should be encouraged to use the charting tool to gain confidence and experience. These same physicians will become the mentors to the other doctors.

Employee readiness—The entire practice staff must be fully trained. Staff should be told to support new users of the EHR. Training materials, guides and workflow issues should be tested and ready for activation. A sufficient number of employees should have been involved in system setup and testing to provide a good base for activation. Immediately before activation, all of the remaining users will be trained on the EHR. As previously noted, such training should occur immediately before the user starts using the EHR—so the training is fresh in their minds. **TIP:** Make sure you take advantage of operational offices and doctors as part of your training process. For example, doctors who are using the EHR already could be mentors for doctors who are still training on EHR use. Clinical staff could be rotated into the locations that are already using the EHR prior to their EHR Go Live.

Activation meetings—As the activation date approaches, you need to monitor progress across a wide range of activities. Hold meetings with key staff across these activities. These allow you to allocate resources and make decisions to address issues as well as monitor their activities in preparing for EHR activation. These meetings should focus on practice readiness and critical path items to support the activation process. For example, the activation process may require the contemporaneous completion of user training and patient demographic loading from the PMS. Note that delays in the activation process will become more costly and disruptive as the project proceeds. For example, delay of the entire project is less disruptive than a delay between the start of scanning of medical records and the charting of patient visits.

Onsite support—Dedicated support staff should be positioned at each site in your practice as the EHR is activated. Support resources include vendor trainers, super users, managers and supervisors. Respond to user needs and issues quickly to get users over the initial startup challenges. For example, users may not be familiar with how to document a side issue that is outside the standard clinical data supported by the EHR. Make sure that each user has immediate access to a support person to help him through problems or issues. Additional support may be available by having software and hardware vendor staff onsite, as well as pulling other resources from various practice units. For example, you may place your computer support and billing office staff to provide additional support during the initial startup phase.

Key contacts—Keep a list of key contacts for hardware, software and support on call to immediately address any last minute challenges and items. You also need management ready to address procedural issues that may crop up during the initial system startup. For example, you may fall behind in scanning patient records for appointments.

Mentoring—In addition to training staff, the doctors and clinicians should be supported by mentors. The mentoring program should pair key users and computer savvy staff with less confident users. The mentoring process is critical to allow users to be served and not overwhelm the practice support staff during the activation and first few weeks of EHR use.

Your activation steps may follow several strategies. Some practices gradually adopt various EHR components on the way to full EHR use. Other practices implement several pieces at a time leading up to full EHR activation. After you have chosen your activation sequence, your activation plan should generally include the following tasks:

Verify policies and procedures—This insures that written training materials and procedures are properly documented. Be sure to check that users have current versions of your documents and *not* draft copies used during testing and setup.

Complete staff training—By the time you are ready to activate the EHR, a number of staff members should be fairly comfortable with the EHR. However, you may want to do some focused training on the use of the EHR in production mode that may differ from the training and testing to date. New user training should occur as close as possible to the date the user starts EHR use. Delays could result in lost knowledge and continuity problems.

Verify hardware operations—All hardware devices should be verified and staged for use by employees and doctors. Before activation, the various devices should be checked for access to the EHR and system facilities. For example, you need to verify that each tablet can correctly communicate with the wireless network. In some cases, hardware and software setups to back up training will not support the active system. For example, some EHRs have a test database that is actually maintained through a system initialization file. You should also verify that you can quickly and effectively respond to specific hardware problems and even failures. For example, you should have a person at each location that can swap out a problem piece of equipment and/or resolve a problem connecting to the EHR.

Complete EHR setup—The EHR setup should be completed. The physician super-users should verify that they have completed the setup of the clinical content. For example, some EHR setups that were staged in the test database must be transferred or entered in the production database. Note that the transferred clinical setups should be checked and verified to insure that the production database works. **CAUTION:** Some EHR products do not allow you to copy setup information from the test system to the production system: you have to reenter the setup information in the production system. Other EHR products do not even have test systems.

Initial load of demographic data—Prior to using the EHR, you need to load the demographic information that will be associated with the clinical data. Ideally, you should load these data electronically from your PMS. You need to activate the interface between the PMS and EHR systems and verify that the entire demographic database is available through the EHR. **TIP**: Verify the total number of demographic records and test search patient appointments for the first day. Do a test to verify that demographic changes are being passed from the PMS to the EHR. The verification process is needed to check that the production database (and not the test system) contains the appropriate information.

Initial load of appointment information—As noted with the demographic information, the appointment information must be initially loaded into the production database. You should also verify that the PMS is sending appointment updates to the production database and not the test database. **CAUTION:** Make sure to check the interface for patient checkin in the PMS (where applicable) to make sure the EHR workflow indicates the patients are available to be seen on a real time basis.

Initial load of electronic clinical data—A variety of clinical data may be loaded into the EHR before activation. Electronic clinical date may be available from diagnostic equipment and lab information systems that are interfaced with the EHR. Additional information sources include transcription files and information from the PMS. The electronic information should be loaded into the EHR according to the interface plan. Note that you may only download data based on a trigger (e.g., patient appointment) or all data from a selected period. **CAUTION:** Be sure to check the implications of information that is electronically loaded into the EHR with the same information that may be scanned from the patient's paper record into the EHR. **ALERT:** The loading of data from a legacy EHR is a complex issue that is addressed in Chapter 10 - Implementing an EHR.

Initial load of paper clinical data—To activate an EHR in place of a paper record, you need to provide the information needed from the paper medical record. Some practices continue use of the paper record during the transition period. Others practices scan the paper record into the EHR and use the EHR as the sole access point and repository of clinical information. The scanning process should be structured to work ahead of the appointment schedule in much the same way that you may pull charts three days before the appointment. Additional charts will be processed to support phone calls, hospital procedures and other clinical services. Depending on your activation strategy (see Chapter 10—Implementing an EHR), the initial load of paper clinical data may include a summarization of the paper record and/or the entry of key patient information into the EHR.

A timeline for two stage EHR activation is presented at the end of this chapter (see Figure 11.1). The timeline initially implements a paperless chart and workflow features. During the initial stage, physicians would document patient visits on paper or use dictation that would be saved in the EHR. A few weeks are allowed for adjusting to the scanning and workflow use as well as allowing for final testing of the clinical charting capability. The second phase activates clinical charting by physicians in two groups. Note that in both cases, the practice is counting on staff involved in setup and testing to provide a basic level of experience and support for new users. The other benefit of this strategy is that the setup and testing team understands the strategy and rational for the EHR setups used.

Only after the completion of the EHR rollout and its complete use will you be in a position to work towards the Meaningful Use standard. Therefore, attaining Meaningful Use requires the rollout of the EHR and the use of the EHR for a significant number of your patients. For example, one Meaningful Use measure is the use of electronic prescriptions for 80% of your patients. However, it would be difficult to attain that level of use without having a significant number of patients in the EHR system. Similarly, use of the patient portal by 10% of your patients requires virtually complete use of the EHR for those patients.

CHAPTER 11: Activating an EHR 257

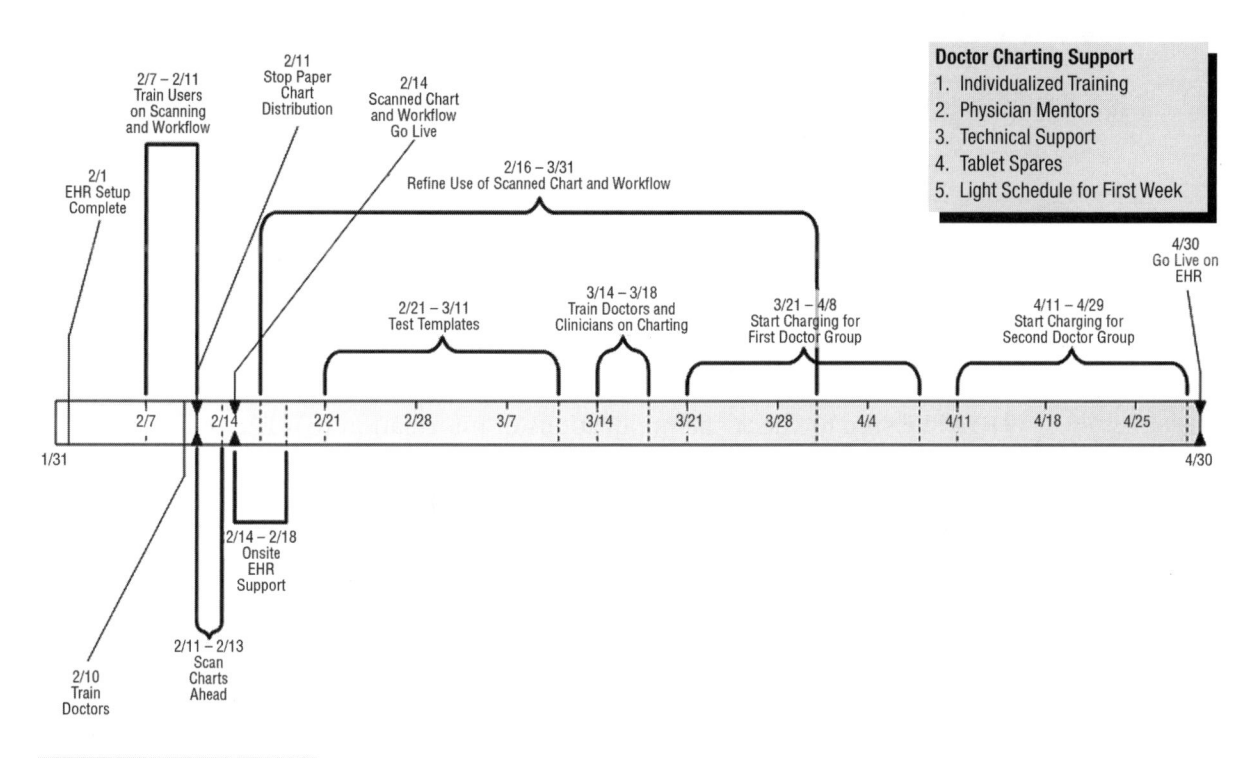

Doctor Charting Support
1. Individualized Training
2. Physician Mentors
3. Technical Support
4. Tablet Spares
5. Light Schedule for First Week

- 2/1 EHR Setup Complete
- 2/7 – 2/11 Train Users on Scanning and Workflow
- 2/10 Train Doctors
- 2/11 Stop Paper Chart Distribution
- 2/11 – 2/13 Scan Charts Ahead
- 2/14 Scanned Chart and Workflow Go Live
- 2/14 – 2/18 Onsite EHR Support
- 2/16 – 3/31 Refine Use of Scanned Chart and Workflow
- 2/21 – 3/11 Test Templates
- 3/14 – 3/18 Train Doctors and Clinicians on Charting
- 3/21 – 4/8 Start Charging for First Doctor Group
- 4/11 – 4/29 Start Charging for Second Doctor Group
- 4/30 Go Live on EHR

Timeline dates: 1/31, 2/7, 2/14, 2/21, 2/28, 3/7, 3/14, 3/21, 3/28, 4/4, 4/11, 4/18, 4/25, 4/30

Scanning Priorities
1. Current Day Contacts (Ex. Messages, Refills)
2. Appointments in Three Days
3. Current Therapy Patients
4. Procedures in Last 3 Months
5. Minor Charts

Chart Note Issues
1. Testing of Templates and Setups
2. Patient Information Sheet Entry
3. Entry of History for Current Patients
4. Charge Posting at Check-Out

FIGURE 11.1—*Sample Activation Timeline*

Supporting an EHR

Your practice has gone through a process that included reworking your operations, making policies and staging the EHR. The EHR implementation effort involved everyone in your practice and affected every patient. To preserve the value of your EHR investment, and avoid the painful process of recovery or, even worse, moving to another EHR, you need a multifaceted approach to control and monitor use. Protecting the EHR requires technical, organizational and management strategies. As an added bonus, some of these strategies will help you comply with various HIPAA security and privacy standards.

VENDOR/EHR PRODUCT MONITORING

One of the most important support strategies for your practice is monitoring the health and well being of your EHR vendor and product. Due to the reliance of your practice on the EHR, any significant problems or business issues with the vendor could significantly and dramatically affect your practice.

Part of your support strategy should be to maintain contact and monitor your vendor's activities. The key issue is to verify that the vendor is making progress in product development and maintains a relevant product. If the product does not attract new users or fails to meet ARRA HITECH Certification, then your practice may have to pursue another EHR strategy. Therefore, you should monitor vendor performance for your practice as well as how other users of your product are being treated and served. Similarly, you can maintain contact with new users to make sure that the vendor is competitive and responsive. When possible, you can review the financial statements or monitor press releases from the company.

As important, make sure that you share your concerns and issues with vendor management so that you maintain current information on the product that you depend on and can respond to any risks that could threaten the continued well being of the product and thereby affect your practice.

SUPPORT POLICIES

Your support program should be guided and empowered by practice policies designed to enforce procedures and training standards as well as structure changes. Unilateral decisions to change processes, use of system setups undermine your clinical documentation and management of the practice. For example, failure to follow initial intake information templates could lead to additional work for the doctor and a lower E&M code, costing you entitled reimbursement. The support policies should guide doctors as well as staff. Basic policies include:

Employee standards—The practice may choose to develop a general guideline for new employees. The guideline may include the level of computer competency as well as a pre-employment test on basic computer skills. Current employees should meet an escalating level of knowledge based on the needs of the practice and their position. For example, a phone operator will need additional training on demographics to staff the check-in desk. Employee standards should reflect these new needs. For example, suspended employees should not have access to the EHR.

Clinical charting standards—To support the clinical standards developed in the EHR implementation process, your chief medical officer should establish a clinical practices committee. The clinical practices committee will monitor use of charting standards as well as guide enhancements to the documentation standards. The committee will review, approve, design and test changes to templates and EHR setups. The clinical charting standards committee may also review compliance with the clinical standards by doctors and clinical staff. Some practices establish documentation standards that doctors must use to insure consistency and mitigate clinical and treatment risks. For example, a clinical treatment standard that included a certain test on a periodic basis would be used by all doctors.

Training standards—Establish training standards for doctors and staff. The training standards will specify the functional requirements for each role in the practice. For example, billing staff may be trained on accessing and printing medical record portions. You should also consider incentives to encourage employees to raise their knowledge and skills. **TIP**: Establish a bonus plan for employees who reach a certain level of EHR proficiency.

EHR access and use—Practice management should establish the access and use standards for the practice. These standards should meet the HIPAA privacy and security guidelines. EHR access should be clearly defined for each employee role. The policy should specify the penalties for violations. The EHR access and use policies may include audit requirements and rules for reporting compliance issues to management. For example, an audit procedure may verify the "need-to-know" standard for selected patients and employees on a periodic basis. Violations may be reported to management, perhaps, on a monthly basis.

Performance monitoring and problem resolution—The practice should establish a mechanism to monitor EHR performance and problems. The policy may require reporting on interruptions, problems and issues on a monthly basis. The management oversight will insure that key issues are addressed at the executive level and appropriate communications are maintained with vendors and staff on use issues. This mechanism will assure management oversight of this increasingly important function.

TRAINING PROGRAM

Training and retraining users insures they are fully informed and adequately knowledgeable on how to use the EHR. The practice should schedule training programs to introduce new users and update current users on EHR use. You training program is part of your HIPAA privacy and security compliance efforts. The training program will insure that the system is used consistently throughout the practice according to the established policies and procedures.

Be sure the training program has written documentation and/or manuals. The written materials can include screen shots and instructions to guide use of the system. The documentation should reflect your specific procedures as well as how you set up the EHR. For example, you may establish new department breakdowns and roles to capitalize on instantaneous access to the patient chart. The training materials should focus on your practice. Don't delve into non-relevant topics. For example, a urology practice may exclude training on the use of the EHR growth charts.

You can undertake an elaborate document or piece together information from copies of manual pages. In any case, the training manual should focus on how the system is used in the practice and your expectations. For example, you may include lists of your document types and what documents are classified for each of your document types. The document could include routing and priority standards for each document type. Such priority standards could be used by practice managers to focus resources on an operational basis as well as monitor average response times for management tracking.

New employees should be trained on the features that are relevant to their job according to user roles. Train new employees as soon as they come on board. Ideally, each new employee should be assigned a mentor to insure that the new employee adapts to the practice's EHR methods using your own procedures. **TIP**: Use the audit records to monitor new employee performance and double-check their work. Note that new employees can be an excellent source of ideas and suggestions.

Retrain current employees on a periodic basis. The retraining effort should include a review of the EHR features and procedures used in their areas. Such training could be conducted by employees who have demonstrated a superior command of the product. Retraining insures that all employees are using the same processes on a consistent basis. Employees who have difficulty using the EHR within the established procedure framework should receive supplemental training. For example, a user who documents phone messages in a patient note instead of a patient task would receive supplemental training in both areas.

On occasion, you will need to train all current users on a change to the system or a new software release. The training program should be designed to cover all employees in a compressed timeframe. The updated process should be supported by appropriate training materials and procedure documentation. **TIP**: Conduct the training in a room that includes the equipment used in the practice.

HARDWARE AND SOFTWARE SUPPORT

Supporting an EHR requires an ongoing hardware and software maintenance effort. The entire technology base should be continually reviewed to insure it meets your needs, and that your system evolves to meet the changes to your practice. In too many cases, the completion of EHR implementation leads to complacency. Lack of attention to your system can cause troubles.

Your system is subject to changes due to business, industry, management and clinical issues. For example, new diagnostic equipment may speed the intake of patients requiring a frequently administered test. A new office, new service offering, changes in your patient base, and/or additional doctors could affect your technology needs. Additional clinical services may require more clinical content that the EHR doesn't have.

Even if the EHR contains appropriate clinical content, the clinical content has to be tested by the practice. Additional offices and users could exceed the communication capacity that was designed for the system. Additional users and increased volume could exceed the designed capacity of the system or consume disk space at a more rapid rate. Although growth and changes are not a problem, the EHR must be enhanced and expanded to meet the changes in your practice. Otherwise, the EHR could fall into disuse and risk failure. For example, the new doctors may use another system because the practice's EHR lacks support for their subspecialty. Multiple EHRs in a single practice is costly and harms coordination.

Any strategic decision should include an analysis of the technology impact. The existing technology should be reviewed in light of the projected change. For example, new diagnostic equipment may be able to directly interface with the EHR to speed patient services. Yet, introduction of mid-level providers enabled by the EHR may increase the user count and the load on the system.

The projected changes should be analyzed to insure that the servers, communications and software setups will be able to support the changes. For example, new services may require a new department setup instead of crowding patient flow and messages into an existing department. Additional services may necessitate the review of classifications and management structures to avoid the growth of "miscellaneous" classifications throughout the system. Note that system enhancements should be completed before you need them and *not* in the middle of a performance crisis.

Regardless of the expense and effort, you cannot cost effectively eliminate the possibility that the EHR may fail. You can invest in redundant hardware, uninterruptible power supplies and a host of options and still experience a failure. On the other hand, some practices go for years without a disruption. As a matter of prudence, assume that you will lose access to the EHR for 1–2 days/year. The loss may be due to a communication problem, power failure, hardware failure and/or a software issue, but you should be prepared to get by for a day or two without the EHR. **TIP**: Design your system to tolerate problems, monitor your system to catch issues before you experience a system failure, have a plan for operating in the event of a failure and be prepared to quickly address failures.

Effective hardware support begins with good system design. We have previously discussed a number of strategies and options to consider in your initial purchase. However, your hardware base will change over time due to expansion of the practice, new offices and services, device replacements and hardware capacity. Manage your hardware situation by reviewing each change for:

Strategic hardware and software support—Changes to the hardware and software should be completed within the structure of a strategic plan. For example, piecemeal workstation upgrades could lead to continuing disruptions to the entire system. If you need more powerful workstations, you should plan ahead to insure new workstations are based on the evolving requirements and not the baseline needs of the current software. And you can avoid separate virus protection purchases for each workstation by employing a virus-detection system on a server. Backup device planning should be based on strategic needs and not the minimum requirements. A number of practices have had to suddenly contend with the inability to back up their systems overnight. Switching to a weekly backup leaves the practice seriously exposed to a tragic loss of information.

EHRs will consume substantially more space in a much shorter time than anything the practice has previously encountered. Diagnostic images and scanned medical charts can consume more space in a day than your may need for a year of financial transactions. A number of practices have had to suddenly contend with the inability to back up their system overnight. The backup equipment and strategy should accommodate complete backups of the entire database on a periodic basis as well as interim partial backups. For example, some EHRs ask you to backup every 30–60 minutes.

Security Issues and Enhancements—Monitoring security issues and challenges is a continuing process. Any new hardware and software should be reviewed in light of your security and privacy standards. New hardware should be set up to support the existing security standards including communications, virus protection, access codes and automatic logging off. New software should be reviewed to insure that the appropriate security features and options are used. For example, you may need to review your security access strategy by user role. Be especially careful to check that intermediate files containing patient information are kept on unsecured devices. For example, print images, intermediate image files from diagnostic devices and workstation-based documents require cleanup and maintenance to assure confidentiality. On a periodic basis, you should review compliance with your security standards as well as any security problems. For example, firewall logs and software audit records should be reviewed on a periodic basis for security violations and intrusion attempts. In some cases, practices use a third-party systems' integrator to review the system logs and stability of the database on a periodic basis.

System access—An increasing number of healthcare organizations and vendors will seek to exchange data with your systems. You need to be extremely vigilant and skeptical to insure that you maintain the security of your systems. For example, a software vendor requested opening the firewall for easier access. The easier access for the vendor would have exposed the practice to computer attacks from other parties. In some cases, practices are giving access to EHR data for related providers and physicians. Note that such access may not be supported by your EHR product and could open your practice to security and privacy problems.

In some cases, you may get early warning of impending system problems. Intermittent interruptions, slow performance and other problems may be early signs of a larger system problem. To avoid these issues, the practice should monitor performance and check hardware components on a periodic basis. For example, some systems require maintenance tasks to recapture disk space. You should also monitor hardware for problems that may indicate the end of the useful life of system components. System components should be replaced before and not because of catastrophic failures.

If your EHR is at a secured hosting site or you use an Application Service Provider (ASP), you should conduct periodic reviews of any changes at the site as well as examine any interruptions that required the use of backup systems and communication links. A periodic meeting with the ASP representative and appropriate reports will allow you to make sure you are protected.

On a periodic basis, you will need to upgrade your software. For example, your EHR vendor may release a new upgrade to support additional features and address problems. In many cases, vendors will only support a previous version or two of the product. Ideally, you should wait to install the upgrade until you have verified that other practices are successfully using the new version. You should insure that the system includes all of the functionality and modules that you are currently using. For example, you may have to wait until the vendor includes a module you use in the next product upgrade.

You should also verify that your hardware and system software will support the new version of your EHR. For example, a new version may require additional disk space for a new access and audit log. In other cases, the vendor may have changed the minimum hardware requirements. If you are sure that the update is stable, then you should perform a test conversion or installation and verify the update works. Having completed testing, you need to coordinate training on the new update with its planned installation of live data. Note that some system upgrades are easily installed with your current data, while others may require conversion of your current data. In any event, make sure you always maintain a backup of the pre-update system to allow you to fall back to the working system in the event of a problem.

You should also be careful to validate the amount of time needed for the conversion to the upgrade. In some cases, upgrades require a weekend conversion. The actual conversion time will depend on the complexity of the upgrade, the speed of your hardware and the size of your database.

Disaster Recovery

In the unlikely event of a failure, you should have a remediation and recovery plan for various potential problems. The plan should have specific instructions to address various system failures, including the full or partial loss of the EHR and localized loss of system access. For example, you may lose the ability to print anything from the EHR. The plan documentation should include a detailed explanation of the current system components and software. The plan should allow for continuing operations while you work on the problem.

In many cases, you may encounter a problem that increases the risk of a serious problem, but does not noticeably affect operations. For example, the failure of a communication line to an office that is closed for the day may go immediately unnoticed but is a sign of a serious problem. Address such issues with urgency. Practices often fail to fix the little problems until a big failure occurs. By proactively going after problems and monitoring system issues and performance, you may be able to resolve them before they cause disruptions.

Your remediation plan should include:

Notification protocols—Depending on the type of loss, your plan should indicate the various parties that should be notified. Practice management, key vendors and supervisors should be informed of the problem and status. Note the vendor response and monitor it. Throughout the crisis, practice staff and management should be updated on status and expected recovery.

Operational protocols—The operational strategy during the system loss should be documented and available to all employees. Employees should be periodically trained on the fall-back procedures. For example, paper flowsheets may be used during the loss to continue patient services. In cases where the hardware features fall-back options, you may need to scale back EHR use. For example, you may need to stop scanning from remote locations when you use a slower backup communications link to a remote office. Similarly, you may need to limit the number of users if a key server fails.

EHR recovery—Once the EHR is operational, the plan should specify how the information accumulated during the outage will be added to the EHR system. Verify that full operations are restored. Some outages may require staged activation of EHR components. For example, it may take longer to reestablish interfaces with diagnostic equipment than to restart the EHR.

Post-recovery review—After the problem has been resolved and the system has been restored, the problem and recovery activities should be reviewed to determine potential improvements to the plan and changes to avoid future problems. Such a review should be undertaken for unexpected situations and failures. For example, frequent disk failures could target what needs to be corrected to avoid future problems.

USER SUPPORT

To protect your EHR investment, you need to set up a structure that avoids "creeping disability." Creeping disability results from changes to meet evolving issues without fully evaluating the effects on the practice. Creeping disability also is caused by users abandoning the EHR for other solutions. For example, a doctor may start documenting patient visits using typed notes instead of templates and clinical content. Quality assurance reports and patient selection reports based on template information may not include patient notes. Employees who use their own task classification codes and priority flags will not be included in management reports and performance tracking.

In reality, your practice staff will know more about the EHR in your practice than your vendor after 3–6 months. Vendor support staff may not be familiar with the various setups and templates you use. You need to establish a process that insures that you control user support and maintain the value of your EHR investment. The support mechanism insures that you keep using the system as you designed and that the EHR evolves in a way that better serves your practice.

User support addresses user issues on a day-to-day basis. The best support structures provide immediate feedback to users who have a question or issue. Informal support structures may not produce resolutions. Indeed, the support structure helps the user but also enforces the practice's standards. User support requires a hierarchical approach that provides front-line support on a continuing basis that is backed by management strategies:

Front-line support—Each department and working area should have a "go to" person for daily support issues. The front-line support person should be knowledgeable in the EHR functions and practice procedures that are relevant to the department. The front-line support person should be able to perform basic troubleshooting on local hardware issues and to answer software questions. User issues and needs should get to super users or computer support through the front-line support person. The front-line support person insures that you make the best use of each level of staff to identify, address and resolve computer issues.

Super-user support—If a problem requires a change to the way you use the EHR or one of your procedures, the problem must be passed on to a super user. The practice managers or super users will be able to make decision on changes to the EHR use or practice procedures that can be applied to the entire practice. The super users should be able to look at the issue from a practice level. This helps to make sure changes that are helpful to one department will not create problems in another area. For example, scanning incoming clinical documents may complicate operations at the front desk but significantly eases clinical workflow.

Computer support—If the front-line support staff is unable to resolve a technical computer hardware or software issue, get the designated computer support person/staff involved. The computer support person/staff serves as the resident technical expert on the computer system as well as the point of contact with vendors on technical issues. In some cases, the practice staff includes a basic technical support person that is supplemented with an outside consultant or network support group. In other cases, practices employ a complete technical support team to administer the computer network and address technical issues. The practice computer support staff coordinates EHR server or application issues with the EHR vendor. Frequently, the application and procedure issues are managed by super users.

Regardless of how well you implemented the EHR, new issues and situations will evolve that will require adjustments and changes. The practice needs a mechanism to identify, analyze and resolve these issues. Your solution to evolving issues rests in the same structure you used to implement the system: your implementation team and super users.

Key EHR users should meet on a monthly basis to review EHR use and evolving issues. The purpose of the monthly EHR review meetings is to maintain the momentum of adaptation, and identify problems to fix. The meeting should identify the go-forward strategy for each problem. Issues may be solved through changes to procedures, adjustments to the system setups and/or changes to templates. In some cases, changes will require vendor enhancements. The monthly review meetings should consider a list of all outstanding issues. Report these issues to the practice management team.

Due to the number of users and the critical nature of the EHR, the practice should consider the use of automated support tools to log problems and provide assistance. The computer support software should allow designated users to log problems, as well as facilitate management and tracking of support issues by managers and designated IT staff. For example, you may want to know EHR problems by type and resolution. A number of products can support your practice computer support needs. DataTrack (www.magnosoft.biz) and Track-It (www.itsolutions.intuit.com) are examples of products that manage computer user support issues.

SYSTEM AUDIT PROCEDURES

In many systems, a variety of information is maintained behind the scenes to track user activities and system performance. Based on the information maintained by the EHR, you should conduct periodic audits of various system activities. System audit procedures will help you maintain practice performance and support users. System audit areas can include user activities, unauthorized activities by users and attempts to access the system by unauthorized users. Other audit procedures may track open clinical notes, incomplete tasks and overdue patient procedures. Hardware and network audits may analyze attacks on the firewall, virus attacks and events, quarantined files and failed exchanges among practice systems.

The system audit should include tracking of monthly activities and trend analysis. The system audit results should be reported to management.

APPENDIX

CCHIT (www.cchit.org) provides certification based on an analysis of electronic health records. CCHIT measures products under a defined and published standard. The CCHIT status has been added to our vendor chart to identify those products that have met the CCHIT certification standard.

EHR Product	Company, Phone, Website	CCHIT Certification
ABELMed EHR-EMR/PM 9	ABELSoft Corporation 800-267-2235 x3 www.abelmedicalsoftware.com	2008 Certified 01/28/09
ABELMed EHR—EMR / PM 11 Pre-Market	ABELSoft Corporation 800-267-2235 x3 www.abelmedicalsoftware.com	2011 Certified 11/23/09
ABELMed PM—EMR Version 8	ABELSoft Corporation 800-267-2235 x3 www.abelmedicalsoftware.com	2007 Certified 06/17/08
Abraxas EMR 4.1.	Abraxas Medical Solutions 877-777-6500 / 949-502-7776 www.abraxasmedical.com	2008 Certified 04/17/09
Accelerator Graphical Health Record 4.4	Catalis, Inc. 888-241-1325 www.TheCatalis.com	2006 Certified 01/29/07
Acumen EHR 5	HIT Services Group 877-535-5566 www.acumenehr.com	2007 Certified 12/11/07
Advance EMR MD 2.1 Pre-Market	Medical Software Technology, Inc. 888-367-4110 www.advanceemrmd.com	2008 Certified 05/14/09
Advantage/EHR 10 Pre-Market	Compulink 800-456-4522 www.compulinkadvantage.com	2011 Certified 12/16/09
Agastha Enterprise Healthcare Software v 1.2	Agastha, Inc. 704-544-6504 www.agastha.com	2008 Certified 05/21/09
AllMeds EMR Version 7	AllMeds, Inc. 888-343-MEDS www.allmeds.com	2006 Certified 04/30/07
AllMeds EMR Version 8	AllMeds, Inc. 888-343-MEDS www.allmeds.com	2008 Certified 06/17/09
Allscripts MyWay 2008	AllscriptsMisys, LLC 800-654-0889 www.allscripts.com	2007 Certified 02/22/08
Allscripts Professional EHR 8.2, 8.3, 9.0	AllscriptsMisys, LLC 800-654-0889 www.allscripts.com	2008 Certified 01/08/09
Allscripts Professional EHR 8.1	AllscriptsMisys, LLC 800-654-0889 www.allscripts.com	2007 Certified 01/23/08

Continued

Continued from previous page

EHR Product	Company, Phone, Website	CCHIT Certification
Amazing Charts 5	AmazingCharts.com, Inc. 866-382-5932 www.amazingcharts.com	2008 Certified 05/29/09
Aprima 2009 (formerly called iMedica PRM2008) Build 8.1	Aprima Medical Software, Inc. 866-960-6890 Option 7 www.aprimaEHR.com	2007 Certified 02/22/08
Aprima 2010 2010 Pre-Market	Aprima Medical Software, Inc. 866-960-6890 Option 7 www.aprimaEHR.com	2008 Certified 06/04/09
ASG-Medappz iSuite v4.0	Allen Systems Group, Inc. (ASG) 800-932-5536 www.asg.com	2008 Certified 03/20/09
AssistMed EHR 1.2.0.0	AssistMed, Inc. 888-774-7717 www.assistmed.com	2008 Certified 09/30/08
athenaClinicals™ 0.27	athenahealth, Inc. 800-981-5084 www.athenahealth.com	2006 Certified 4/30/07
athenaClinicals™ 9.15.1	athenahealth, Inc. 800-981-5084 www.athenahealth.com	2008 Certified 06/02/09
Avatar PM 2006 Release 02	Netsmart Technologies 800-421-7503 / 631-968-2000 www.ntst.com	2006 Certified 10/23/06
Axolotl's Elysium 9	Axolotl Corporation 888-296 5685 / 408-920-0800 www.axolotl.com	2008 Certified 05/19/09
CareRevolution 5.2a	EHS 205-871-1031 / 888-879-7302 www.ehsmed.com	2007 Certified 06/20/08
CattailsMD Version 5	Marshfield Clinic 800-782-8581 x 1-8164 www.cattailsmd.com / www.marshfieldclinic.org	2006 Certified 1/29/07
CattailsMD Version 5.9	Marshfield Clinic 800-782-8581 x 1-8164 www.cattailsmd.com / www.marshfieldclinic.org	2008 Certified 06/04/09
Centricity Electronic Medical Record 9.2	GE Medical Systems 888-436-8491 www.gemedical.com	2008 Certified 06/11/09
Centricity EMR 9.0	GE Medical Systems 888-436-8491 www.gemedical.com	2007 Certified 06/24/08
Centricity Enterprise 6.7	GE Medical Systems 888-436-8491 www.gemedical.com	2007 Certified 06/24/08

Continued

Continued from previous page

EHR Product	Company, Phone, Website	CCHIT Certification
Centricity Practice Solution 9.0	GE Medical Systems 888-436-8491 www.gemedical.com	2007 Certified 06/24/08
CentriHealth Individual Health Record (IHR) Release 2009.1.17 *eRx Conditional*	CentriHealth, Inc. 615-345-0318 www.centrihealth.com	2008 Certified 07/01/09
Cerner Millennium PowerChart/PowerWorks EMR 2007	Cerner Corporation 816-201-1024 www.cerner.com	2007 Certified 04/24/08
Cerner Millennium Powerchart/PowerWorks EMR 2007.19	Cerner Corporation 816-201-1024 www.cerner.com	2008 Certified 04/22/09
ChartMaker 3.0.5	STI Computer Services Inc. 610-650-9700 www.sticomputer.com	2007 Certified 04/22/08
ChartMaker Clinical Version 3.2	STI Computer Services Inc. 610-650-9700 www.sticomputer.com	2008 Certified 03/23/09
ClinixMD 7.1	Clinix Medical Information Services LLC 866.CLINIXMIS (866.254.6496) www.clinixmis.com	2006 Certified 01/29/07
Criterions 1.0.0	Criterions, LLC 516-466-1942 www.criterions.com	2008 Certified 05/29/09
CureMD 9.0	CureMD Corporation 212-509-6200 www.curemd.com	2006 Certified 4/30/2007
CureMD EHR 10 *(eRx Conditional)*	CureMD Corporation 212-509-6202 www.curemd.com	2008 Certified 4/29/09
dChart EMR 4.5	NCG Medical Systems, Inc. 800-959-1906 www.ncgmedical.com	2006 Certified 2/9/07
digiChart OBGYN 7.0	digiChart, Inc. 615-777-2727 www.digichart.com	2007 Certified 03/20/08
Doctations v1.0106062008	Doctations, Inc. 516-536-7841 www.doctations.com	2007 Certified 06/24/08
DocuTAP EMR and Practice Management Solution 2.8.2	Integrity On Site LLC, dba DocuTAP 877-697-4696 www.urgentcareemr.com	2007 Certified 06/06/08
e-MDs Solution Series 6.3	e-MDs 888-344-9836 / 512-257-5200 www.e-MDs.com	2008 Certified 02/03/09

Continued

Continued from previous page

EHR Product	Company, Phone, Website	CCHIT Certification
e-Medsys—Electronic Health Record (EHR) 5.2	PracticeOne 877-363-3797 x 2922 www.practiceone.com	2008 Certified 04/17/09
e-Medsys—Electronic Health Record 5.0	PracticeOne 877-363-3797 x 2922 www.practiceone.com	2007 Certified 11/30/07
eCast EMR 7.0	eCast Corporation 919-334-6300 www.ecastsoftware.com	2007 Certified 09/21/07
eClinicalWorks 8.0	eClinicalWorks 508-836-2700 / 866-888-6929 www.eclinicalworks.com	2008 Certified 09/30/08
Eclipsys PeakPractice 1093	Eclipsys Corporation 800-869-8300 www.eclipsys.com	2008 Certified 01/22/09
EdgeEHR 2.4	Edge Health Solutions, Inc. 888-542-8522 www.edgehealthsolutions.com www.edgeehr.com	2007 Certified 02/22/08
EHS CareRevolution 5.3 *Pre-Market*	EHS, Inc. 888-879-7302 / 205-871-1031 www.ehsmed.com	2011 Certified 12/17/09
Electronic Patient Charts 20	American Medical Software 800.423.8836 www.americanmedical.com	2008 Certified 11/12/08
emr4MD Version 6.0.2	MedNet System 877-MEDNET-4 www.mednetsystem.com	2008 Certified 06/22/09
EMRge 7.0 Release 1.0	SSIMED 800-276-6992 www.ssimed.com	2007 Certified 06/20/08
EncounterPRO EHR 5	EncounterPRO Healthcare Resources, Inc. 800-677-5653 / 770-91997220 www.jmjtech.com	2006 Certified 07/18/06
EncounterPRO EHR 5.0	JMJ Technologies, Inc. 2000 RiverEdge Parkway Suite GL 100A Atlanta, GA 30328 770-919-7220/800-677-5653 www.jmjtech.com	2006 Certified 7/18/06
Endosoft	Utech Products, Inc. EndoSoft (A Division of Utech Products, Inc.) 518-831-8000 www.endosoft.com	2006 Certified 4/30/07
Enterprise 11.1.6	AllscriptsMisys, LLC 800-334-8534 www.allscripts.com	2008 Certified 03/26/09

Continued

Continued from previous page

EHR Product	Company, Phone, Website	CCHIT Certification
E-Paperless EMR V2.01	BMD Services 281-208-5403 www.bmdservices.net	2006 Certified 4/30/07
EpicCare Ambulatory EMR Spring 2008	Epic Systems Corporation 608-271-9000 www.epic.com	2008 Certified 09/30/08
EpicCare Ambulatory EMR Summer 2009	Epic Systems Corporation 608-271-9000 www.epic.com	2008 Certified 09/30/08
EpiChart 5.2	Polaris Medical Management, Inc. 401-781-7810 www.PolarisMedical.com	2006 Certified 4/30/07
ezEMRxPrivate 7.00	Total OutSource, Inc. 630-872-5000 www.ezemrx.com	2008 Certified 05/21/09
gCare 4.0 Release 6.3	gMed, Inc. 888-577-8801 www.gmed.com	2007 Certified 06/17/08
GEMMS ONE G1.07	Gateway Electronic Medical Management Systems (GEMMS) 800-773-3111 / 317-819-5060 www.gemmsnet.com	2008 Certified 10/28/08
GenesysMD EHR 2.0	Physician Advantage 866-935-8069 / 314-993-4378 www.genesysmd.com	2007 Certified 07/27/07
GlaceEMR 2.0	Glenwood Systems, LLC 888-Glace-MD www.glaceemr.com	2006 Certified 4/30/07
GlaceEMR 3.0	Glenwood Systems, LLC 888-Glace-MD www.glaceemr.com	2008 Certified 05/11/09
gloEMR 5.0	gloStream, Inc. 877-gloEMR1 www.glostream.com	2008 Certified 04/10/09
gloEMR 4.0	gloStream, Inc. 877-gloEMR1 www.glostream.com	2007 Certified 06/17/08
HealthMatics EHR 2007.1	AllscriptsMisys, LLC 800-334-8534 www.allscripts.com	2007 Certified 01/23/08
HealthPort EHR v9.0	HealthPort 800 999-0788 x 1173 www.healthport.com	2007 Certified 05/01/08
HealthTec Fusion 4.4	HealthTec Software, Inc. 210.545.1010 www.healthtec-software.com	2006 Certified 01/29/07

Continued

Continued from previous page

EHR Product	Company, Phone, Website	CCHIT Certification
HemOncPro 4.2	MedSym Inc. 866-339-8463 www.medsyminc.com	2006 Certified 01/29/07
Horizon Ambulatory Care™ Version 9.4	McKesson Provider Technologies 404-338-6000 www.mckesson.com	2006 Certified 7/18/06
iAchieve EHR Version 2008	ChartLogic 800-686-9651 www.chartlogic.com	2006 Certified 04/30/07
IC-Chart Release 6.0	InteGreat Concepts, Inc. 800-676-1360 www.igreat.com	2006 Certified 1/29/07
Ingenix CareTracker 6.2	Ingenix 866-427-6802 www.ingenix.com	2007 Certified 06/11/08
InSync 4.1	Intivia, Inc. 877-246-4848 www.intivia.com	2007 Certified 06/26/08
Intelligent Medical Software (IMS) 2007	Meditab Software, Inc. 510-632-8021 / 866-994-6367 www.meditab.com	2006 Certified 1/29/07
Intelligent Medical Software (IMS) 12	Meditab Software, Inc. 510-632-8021 / 866-994-6367 www.meditab.com	2008 Certified 05/07/09
Intergy EHR by Sage	Sage Software Healthcare, Inc. 877-932-6301 www.sagehealth.com	2007 Certified 01/17/08
iSuite 4.0	Medappz, LLC 877-633-2779 www.medappz.com	2008 Certified 03/20/09
KeyChart 4.0.0.0	KeyMedical Software, Inc. 765-482-7964 / 888-953-9633 www.keymedicalsoftware.net	2011 Certified 12/21/09
Longitudinal Medical Record (LMR) 5.1.1	Partners HealthCare System, Inc. 978-741-1200 www.partners.org	2006 Certified 04/30/07
Lytec MD 2009	McKesson Provider Technologies 800-333-4747, Option 5 www.lytec.com	2008 Certified 09/30/08
MD-REPORTS 9i	INFINITE SOFTWARE SOLUTIONS INC. [D/B/A: MD-REPORTS] 718-982-1315 www.md-reports.com	2008 Certified 07/08/09

Continued

Continued from previous page

EHR Product	Company, Phone, Website	CCHIT Certification
MDLAND Electronic Health Record and Practice Management Systems 8.0	MDLAND 212-684-9038 www.mdland.com	2006 Certified 4/30/07
MD-Navigator Clinical 5.0	Benchmark Systems 800-779-0902 www.benchmark-systems.com	2007 Certified 12/11/07
MDTABLET 2.6.7	MDTablet 888-989-1965 www.mdtablet.com	2006 Certified 4/30/07
mdTablet 4.0.0	MDTablet 888-989-1965 www.mdtablet.com	2008 Certified 07/02/09
MEDAZ 60720.001	MedAZ.Net, LLC (wholly owned subsidiary of Koni Ameri Tech Services, Inc) 888-633 2972 www.MedAZ.net	2006 Certified 1/29/07
MedcomSoft Record UE (V 4.5)	Electronic Claims Processing Inc. d/b/a PBF Online 800-699-5533 www.pbfonline.com www.medcomsoft.com	2007 Certified 05/15/08
MedConnect EHR 1.0	MedConnect 334-215-3568 www.medconnect-inc.com	2008 Certified 06/30/09
MEDENT 18.1	Community Computer Service, Inc. 315-255-1751 www.medent.com	2008 Certified 09/30/08
Medical and Practice Management (MPM) Suite Client/Server Version 5.6 *eRx Conditional*	LSS Data Systems (Lake Superior Software) 952-941-1000 www.lssdata.com	2008 Certified 05/21/09
Medical and Practice Management (MPM) Suite MAGIC Version 5.6	LSS Data Systems (Lake Superior Software) 952-941-1000 www.lssdata.com	2006 Certified 1/29/2007
Medical and Practice Management (MPM) Suite MAGIC Version 5.64	LSS Data Systems (Lake Superior Software) 952-941-1000 www.lssdata.com	2008 Certified 05/21/09
Medical Messenger Astral Jet EMR 3.7.1	Medical Messenger 800-965-9959 www.mymedicalmessenger.com	2006 Certified 4/30/07
Medical Practice EMR 14	CPSI 800-711-2774 www.cpsinet.com	2006 Certified 10/23/06
Medicat 8.8	Medicat, LLC 866-633-4053 www.medicat.com	2006 Certified 01/29/07

Continued

Continued from previous page

EHR Product	Company, Phone, Website	CCHIT Certification
MedicsDocAssistant 3.0	AdvancedMD Software, Inc 801-984-9500 www.advancedmd.com	2006 Certified 01/29/07
MedicsDocAssistant 4.0.1	AdvancedMD Software, Inc 801-984-9500 www.advancedmd.com	2008 Certified 02/09/09
MedicWare EMR 7	MedicWare, Inc 626-334-5678 www.medicware.com	Certified 1/29/07
MedInformatix V 6.0	MedInformatix, Inc 310-348-7367 www.medinformatix.com	2006 Certified 01/29/07
MedInformatix V 7.0	MedInformatix, Inc 310-348-7367 www.medinformatix.com	2008 Certified 10/28/08
MediNotes "e" 5.2	Eclipsys Corporation 800-869-8300 www.eclipsys.com	2007 Certified 01/24/08
Medisoft Clinical 15	McKesson Provider Technologies 800-333-4747 www.medisoft.com www.mckesson.com/practicepartner	2008 Certified 09/30/08
MediSYS EHR 1.0	MediSYS for Physicians, Inc. 205-631-5969 www.medisysinc.com	2008 Certified 06/30/09
MedLink TotalOffice 3.1	MedLink International, Inc. 631-342-8800 www.medlinkus.com	2008 Certified 09/30/08
MedPlexus EHR 9.2.0.0	MedPlexus, Inc. 408-990-9080 www.medplexus.com	2008 Certified 09/30/08
MedPointe 9	Health Systems Technology, Inc. 800-398-6170 / 585-271-6170 www.HSTcentral.com	2008 Certified 05/07/09
meridianEMR 3.6.1	meridianEMR, Inc. 877 411-4367 www.meridianEMR.com	2006 Certified 4/30/07
MicroMD EMR 7.0	Henry Schein Medical Systems 800-624-8832 www.micromd.com	2008 Certified 12/19/08
MicroMD EMR 4.5	Henry Schein Medical Systems 800-624-8832 www.micromd.com	2006 Certified 01/29/07

Continued

Continued from previous page

EHR Product	Company, Phone, Website	CCHIT Certification
Misys EMR 9.10	AllscriptsMisys, LLC 800-334-8534 www.allscripts.com	2007 Certified 02/22/08
mMD.Net EHR 9.0.9	Health Communication Systems, LLC 800-741-0981 www.healthcomsys.com	2006 Certified 7/18/06
mMD.Net EHR 10.8 eRx Conditional	Health Communication Systems, LLC 800-741-0981 www.healthcomsys.com	2011 Certified 12/21/09
MTBC EMR 4.0	MTBC (Medical Transcription Billing Corporation) 866-266-MTBC (6822) www.mtbc.com	2008 Certified 05/11/09
MyEMR 2.0 Pre-Market	Secure Infosys, LLC 859-578-3815 www.secureinfosys.com	2008 Certified 06/24/09
MyWinmed EMR 1.2 (Pre-Market)	Complete Medical Solutions, LLC 800-256-2803 www.doctornetwork.com	2008 Certified 06/25/09
NetPractice EHR 6.0	Noteworthy Medical Systems, Inc. 877-891-8777 www.noteworthymedical.com	2007 Certified 01/17/08
NetPracticeEHRweb 7.0 Pre-Market	Noteworthy Medical Systems, Inc. 877-891-8777 www.noteworthymedical.com/netpractice_EHRweb.shtml	2008 Certified 04/02/09
NexTech Practice 2010 9.3	NexTech Systems Inc. 866) 856-0784 www.nextech.com	2008 Certified 06/24/09
NexTech Practice 2011 9.5 Pre-Market	NexTech Systems Inc. 866) 856-0784 www.nextech.com	2011 Certified 01/26/10
NextGen EMR 5.5	NextGen Healthcare Info. Sys. 215-657-7010 www.nextgen.com	2007 Certified 06/25/07
NextGen EMR 5.5.27	NextGen Healthcare Info. Sys. 215-657-7010 www.nextgen.com	2008 Certified 09/30/08
NextGen EMR 5.6 Pre-Market	NextGen Healthcare Info. Sys. 215-657-7010 www.nextgen.com	2011 Certified 12/08/09
Nightingale On-Demand V8.2	Nightingale Informatix Corporation 877-852-3663 www.nightingale.md	2007 Certified 02/22/08

Continued

Continued from previous page

EHR Product	Company, Phone, Website	CCHIT Certification
NueMD EHR 5.2	Nuesoft Technologies, Inc. 800-401-7422 www.nuesoft.com	2007 Certified 05/05/08
Nuevita EHR 5.2	Nuesoft Technologies, Inc. 800-401-7422 www.nuesoft.com	2007 Certified 05/05/08
Office Practicum 8.1 *eRx Conditional*	Connexin Software Inc. 800-218-9916 / 212-366-6987 www.officepracticum.com	2008 Certified 04/10/09
OfficeEMR 2008	iSALUS Healthcare 888-280-6678 iSALUShealthcare.com	2006 Certified 04/30/07
OIS EMR 4.1	OIS 800-338-8436 www.oisi.com	2008 Certified 04/17/09
OmniMD EMR 6.0.5	Integrated Systems 914-332-5590 www.omnimd.com	2006 Certified 04/30/07
OpenChart 8.0	Point and Click Solutions, Inc 781-272-9800 www.pointnclick.com	2006 Certified 04/30/07
Patient Chart Manager 5.3	Prime Clinical Systems, Inc. 800-523-5977 / 626-449-1705 www.primeclinical.com	2006 Certified 04/30/07
Patient Chart Manager 5.5 *eRx Conditional*	Prime Clinical Systems, Inc. 800-523-5977 / 626-449-1705 www.primeclinical.com	2008 Certified 06/24/09
PEARL EMR 6.0	Business Computer Applications, Inc. 800-648-1555 www.bca.us	2006 Certified 4/30/07
Physician Practice Documentation (PPD) 9.0.0	Healthland, Inc. 800-323-6987 www.healthland.com	2007 Certified 06/13/08
Physician's Solution 3.0	Universal EMR Solutions 516-869-4535 www.uniemr.com	2006 Certified 04/30/2007
Practice Partner 9.3	McKesson Provider Technologies 800-594-9145 www.mckesson.com/practicepartner	2008 Certified 09/30/08
Praxis V4.0	Praxis EMR, Inc 800-985-6016 www.praxisemr.com	2006 Certified 07/31/06
PrimeSuite PrimeSuite 2008	Greenway Medical Technologies 866-242-3805 www.greenwaymedical.com	2008 Certified 09/30/08

Continued

Continued from previous page

EHR Product	Company, Phone, Website	CCHIT Certification
PrimeSuite 2011	Greenway Medical Technologies 866-242-3805 www.greenwaymedical.com	2011 Certified 12/08/09
Pro-Filer 2007.0.0	UNI/CARE Systems, Inc. 941-954-3403 www.unicaresys.com	2006 Certified 04/30/07
PrognoCIS 1.81	BizMatics, Inc. 866-873-3030 www.bizmaticsinc.com	2006 Certified 04/30/07
Pulse Patient Relationship Management 4.1.02	Pulse Systems, Inc. 800-444-0882 www.pulseinc.com	2011 Certified 12/11/09
Resource and Patient Management System 2008 *Pre-Market*	Indian Health Service 505-248-4191 www.ihs.gov	2007 Certified 06/30/08
Sage Intergy EHR v5.5	Sage 877-932-6301 www.sage.com	2008 Certified 04/09/09
SequelMed EMR V7.50	Sequel Systems, Inc. 800-965-2728 www.sequelsys.com	2006 Certified 04/30/07
Sevocity 5.2	Conceptual MindWorks, Inc. 877-777-2298 www.Sevocity.com	2007 Certified 05/05/08
Sevocity Version 08	Conceptual MindWorks, Inc. 877-777-2298 www.Sevocity.com	2008 Certified 05/26/09
SmartClinic 16	VIP Medicine, LLC 201-675-1507 www.vipmedicine.com/smartclinic	2008 Certified 09/30/08
SOAPware 2008	SOAPware, Inc. 800-455-7627 www.soapware.com	2007 Certified 06/12/09
SOAPware 2010	SOAPware, Inc. 800-455-7627 www.soapware.com	2007 Certified 06/12/09
SpringCharts EHR 9.0	Spring Medical Systems 888-767-4827 / 281-537-0186 www.springmedical.com	2006 Certified 01/29/07
STIX EHR Release 9.1	Integritas, Inc. 800-458-2486 www.integritas.com	2008 Certified 04/09/09
Streamline EHR 10.8 *eRx Conditional*	StreamlineMD, LLC 866.406.2224 www.streamlineMD.com	2011 Certified 12/21/090

Continued

Continued from previous page

EHR Product	Company, Phone, Website	CCHIT Certification
SuiteMed Intelligent Medical Software 12	SuiteMed 877-682-7482 www.suitemed.com	2008 Certified 05/07/09
Sunrise Ambulatory Care 5.0 SP1, Eclipsys Auditing Services 1.0 XA and Eclipsys Security Services 1.0 XA 5.0 SP1 *Pre-Market*	Eclipsys Corporation 800-869-8300 www.eclipsys.com	2007 Certified 06/27/08
Sunrise Ambulatory Care 4.5C SP5 *Pre-Market*	Eclipsys Corporation 800-869-8300 www.eclipsys.com	2007 Certified 04/22/09
Symphony Plus EMRx 1.00 *Pre-Market*	Symphony Corporation 888-338-0010 www.symphony.cc/healthcare_emr.html	2008 Certified 05/21/09
SynaMed EMR 5.487	SynaMed 866-SYNAMED / 866-796-2633 www.synamed.com	2006 Certified 04/30/07
The CareData Solutions 2.7	CareData 800-775-6709 www.caredata.med.pro	2007 Certified 02/18/08
TouchChart 3.3	Encite 800-714-7199 www.encite.us	2006 Certified 01/29/07
TouchWorks V11.1	AllscriptsMisys, LLC 800-334-8534 www.allscripts.com	2007 Certified 04/30/08
TransMed CS 3.0	TransMed Network, Inc 877-999-TMED (8633) www.transmed.net	2007 Certified 06/20/08
UroChart EHR 3.0	Intuitive Medical Software 877.570.8721 www.intuitivemedical.com	2008 Certified 03/13/09
VersaSuite 7.5	Universal Software Solutions, Inc. VersaSuite US 866-395-8774 www.versasuite.com	2006 Certified 01/29/07
Visionary Dream EHR 7.1	Visionary Medical Systems, Inc. 813-594-1026 / 888-895-2466 www.visionarymed.com	2006 Certified 01/29/07
vxVisitA V1.0	Document Storage Systems, Inc. 561-227-0207 www.dssinc.com	2006 Certified 04/30/07
Waiting Room Solutions Practice Management System 3	Waiting Room Solutions 866-977-4367 www.waitingroomsolutions.com	2006 Certified 04/30/07

Continued

Continued from previous page

EHR Product	Company, Phone, Website	CCHIT Certification
Wellogic Consult and GBA MEDfx Release X and MEDfx v3.0	Wellogic and GBA Health Network Systems 617-621-9775 www.wellogic.com	2007 Certified 03/26/08
workflow EHR 2.1	Workflow.com, LLC 877-438-9332 / 440-808-2700 www.workflow.com	2006 Certified 04/30/07
WorldVistA EHR™	WorldVistA—(System was originally developed by the U.S. Department of Veterans Affairs (VA)) 416-232.-206 www.worldvista.org www.worldvista.org/World_VistA_EHR	2006 Certified 04/30/07
XUMIX VERSION 1.0 *eRx Conditional*	Medicmatics Inc www.medicmatics.com	2008 Certified 07/18/09

A

access restrictions, 159
activation
   initial load of data, 255–256
   meetings, 254
   readiness
      complete EHR setup, 255
      onsite support, 254
      policies and procedures, 255
      verifying hardware, 255
   staff training, 255
      employees, 253–254
      key contacts, 167, 254
      mentoring, 254
      physician champions, 253
   strategies
      charge and limited clinical information, 250–251
      order entry and management, 251–252
      paperless chart stage, 250
      physician charting, 251
      prescription entry, 252
      transcription, 251
   timeline, 257
   workflow, 252
active directory server (ADS), 136–137
America Recovery and Reinvestment Act (ARRA), 6–7
   certification and support, 56, 156
   electronic interfaces, 8–9
   Meaningful Use standard, 6, 21
application services provider (ASP), 137
appointments
   documenting, 95–96
   document management, 218–219
   initial load of data, 255–256
   recall triggers, 42
   tracking, 213
   workflow management, 51
   see also patients
ARRA *see* America Recovery and Reinvestment Act
ASP *see* application services provider
auditing, 61
   converting from old EHR, 242–243
   policies, 184

B

Bridges to Excellence, 8
Bright Futures, 8
Business Associate Agreement, 160

C

CCR (*see* Continuity of Care Record)
Certification Commission for Healthcare Information Technology (CCHIT), 269
charge capture, 21–22
charge information, 43
clinical charting, 67–73, 158
clinical content, 160–161
   malpractice issues, 90
clinical orders, 42
clinical reporting, 76
coding levels, 20, 49
collections, 22–23
computers (*see* hardware)
confidential information, 161–162
content management, 183
Continuity of Care Record (CCR), 9
contracts
   final agreement, 172–174
   malpractice issues, 92–93
   negotiating
      business points, 150–154
      final agreement, 172–174
      terms, 154–172
   price, 151–152
   support, technical, 153–154
   vendors, 150–151
   warranties, 152–153
   see also vendors
copyrights, 168
costs
   budget, comprehensive, 25
      cost basis, 141–142
   comparing, 138–144
   estimate
      basic, 25–26, 107–108
      working, 26
   functionality, 142
   hard, 24–26
      hardware, 139
      implementation, 142, 180
      interfaces, 139

locations, 139
missing items, 141
price, final, 151–152
  discounts, 143
quotes, 141–142
return on investment (ROI), 24, 140
scope, 140
soft, 26, 28–29 (*see also* evaluation)
  clinical content development, 143–144
  connecting with PMS, 49–50
  entities (corporate), 138
  support, technical, 143, 181
  training, 139–140
  upgrades, 143
  users, number of, 138–139
vendor contracts, negotiating, 155–156
customer service (*see* service, customer)
customization services, 162

D

data conversion, 216–219
  and changing systems, 4
  initial load of data, 255
  malpractice issues, 94–95
data exchanges, 161
diagnostic studies
  and EHR evaluation, 72
disaster recovery, 265–266
  see also software
disease management, 8
documentation, limitations on, 162
document management
  America Recovery and Reinvestment Act (ARRA) incentives, 6–7, 8
  certainty, 217
  current procedures, 197
  diagnostic equipment, 217–218
  EHR types, 109–112
  improving, 17
    lost files, 18
  lab information system (LIS), 217
  malpractice issues, 89–90
  master files, 41, 218
  organization, 217
  paper records, 219–223
    color images, 221
    conversion, 216

different sizes, 220
eliminating, 5, 6–7
file folder, 220
loose documents/forms, 221
physical defects, 221
preparations, 11
retention, 185–186
two-sided, 220
and patients
  appointments, 218–219
  demographics, 217
  identification, 217
production, 215–216
retrospective records, 215
scanning options, 222–223
slides, 221
unnecessary information, 220

E

EHR (*see* electronic health records)
electronic data interchange (EDI), 163
electronic healthcare records (EHR), 21
electronic health records (EHR)
  activation, 249–257
  clinical content development, 143–144
  converting from previous, 223–231
    negotiating help from vendor, 156
  difficulties, 2–3
  effects on private practice, 4
  hardware provisioning, 134–137
  and the healthcare industry, 4–9
  implementation, 177–257
  information
    exchanges of, 10
    improved access, 17–18
  interfaces (electronic), 45
    costs, 139
    evaluation, 62–64
    screen samples, 116–121
  malpractice risk, 85–98
  open EHR options, 39
  and paper records, 219–223
  and PMS, 37–51
    clinical focus, 49
    features, 49
    information exchange, 40–44

interfaces, 39–40
relationships with, 44–45
technology, 49
products
changes, 3–4
list of, 269–281
review, 113–132
selection, 99–112
types, 109–112
reporting, 75, 76
selection, 1–14 (*see also* activation; evaluation; implementation; support; training)
checklist, 13–14
contracts, negotiating, 149–176
deciding against, 11–12
final, 133–147
review, 99–112
support, technical, 259–260
workflow evaluation, 73–75
strategic and tactical effect, 4
electronic transactions and clearinghouses, 157
employees (*see* staff)
EMR (Electronic Medical Record), replacement of term, viii–ix
error definition, 164–165
evaluation
analysis tools, 75–76
benefits, 17–23
clinical charting, 67–73, 118–119
evaluation list, 53–83
final decision, 144–145
financial
Basic EHR Estimate, 25–26
Comprehensive Working Budget, 26
Quick Working Estimate, 26
hardware provisioning, 134–137
less-than-complete product, 16
overview, 15–35
purchasing the wrong product, 15–16
with respect to PMS, 47–48
scenario list, 114–115
size of practice, 9–10
summarizing, 133–134
vendor demonstration, 114–115
see also costs; evaluation list

evaluation and management (E&M), 20
evaluation list
comments, 79–80
creating, 76–80
example, 81–83
factors, 54–76
features, 76–78
significant, 56–80
trivial items, 78
importance, 79
needs of the practice, 78
required components, 78
scoring, 78–79
specific criteria, 77
standards
common, 78
and the vendor, 114
see also evaluation
exit strategy, 165

F

facilities
clinical office, 206
computer room, 204–205
department areas and locations, 212
front desk, 206
management, 204–207
reception, 206
training room, 205–206
forms, 109–110

G

glossary, 291
Go Live, 26, 170, 291
government stimulus program, vi–vii, ix
see also America Recovery and Reinvestment Act (ARRA)

H

hardware
costs, 139
and EHR activation, 255
environment, 164
improved, 141
insufficient, 16
issues, learning from client, 157

personal digital assistant (PDA), 61
provisioning, 134–137
reliability, 54
scanners, 208
servers
  backup, 58, 98, 137
  cluster, 291
  high-availability, 136–137
  hosting, 137, 205
  hot swap disk drive, 291
support, technical, 165–166, 262–266
  enhancements, 263–264
  security, 263–264
  strategic, 263
system access, 264
tablet devices, 54, 205–206, 208
upgrades
  PMS, 48
  unexpected, 28
warranties, 153
workstations, 205–206, 208
  upgrades, 24–25
see also software
healthcare industry
  common care standards, 8
  and EHR, 4–9
Healthcare Information Technology (HITECH) Stimulus Program, vi–vii, ix
Health Information Exchange (HIE), 157
Health Insurance Portability and Accountability Act (HIPAA), 3
  Business Associate Agreement, 160
  compliance, 166
  electronic transactions and clearinghouses, 157
  operational standards, 197
  PMS and EHR information sharing, 51
  privacy standards, 65, 182–185
  security standards, 65, 183–184, 204
  Transactions, 65
  Transaction Set, 8–9
Health Level 7 (HL7), 11
Highmark BCBS, 7
HIPAA (*see* Health Insurance Portability and Accountability Act)

I

image files
  converting, 218
  malpractice issues, 90
implementation
  clinical issues
    content, 214
    standards, 178–182
  costs, 180
    productivity losses, 26
    services, 142
    startup, 28
  documentation, 180
  facilities management, 204–207
  Go Live, 26, 170, 291
  less-than-complete product, 16
  malpractice issues, 93–94
  overview, 177–178
  policies, 182–186
  procedures, 195–203
  project management, 186–195
  reporting, 180–181
  software
    data conversion, 216–219
  strategy, 125–126
  technology
    base, 207–209
    strategy, 12
  testing, 215–216
  training, 231–248
    provider time, 26
  upgrades
    design changes, 214
    frequent releases, 57
    network, 25
    workflow,
      differences, 180
    workstation, 24–25
information exchange, 40–44
interfaces (electronic)
  America Recovery and Reinvestment Act (ARRA) incentives, 6
  diagnostic equipment, 11–12, 166–167
  lab orders, 167
  and PMS, 45
    supported, 45

investment
  analysis, 29–35
  insufficient, 12, 15

K

knowledgebase, 110–111

L

lab information systems (LIS), 217
lab orders
  and EHR evaluation, 71
  EHR interfaces, 167
  malpractice issues, 91
letter writing, 76
licenses, 46–49
  assignment of, 159–160
  costs, 142
  providers, 169
  users, 171
  vendors, 155, 168
  see also software

M

malpractice risk
  choosing EHR, 85–88
  contract issues, 92–93
  data conversion, 94–95
  implementation, 93–94
  product design issue examples, 88–92
  support issues, 97–98
  usage issues, 95–97
Meaningful Use standard, 6, 8, 56
Medcin, 109–110
Medicaid, 6, 21
medical records
  expenses, 19–20
  and project management, 191–192
  see also electronic health records
Medicare
  America Recovery and Reinvestment Act (ARRA) payment for EHR implementation, 6, 21
  Pay for Performance, 7

N

network (electronic)

application services provider (ASP), 137
backups
  communications, 205
  sites/servers, 137
communications, 205
Internet access, 54
security, 29
upgrades, 25
  communications, 28
  see also hardware; software
notes, clinical, 43, 111–112

P

P4P (*see* Pay for Performance)
paper (*see* document management)
patents, 168
patients
  appointments, 41
    documenting, 95–96
    initial load of data, 255–256
    recall triggers, 42
    tracking, 213
  classification, 51
  collaboration with, 17
  education, 72
  identification, 217
  information
    converting to new EHR, 228
    demographics, 41, 218
    evaluation, 65–67
    malpractice issues, 88–89
    presentation, 50–51
  services, improved, 18
payer information, 42
Pay for Performance (P4P), 7–8, 21
Physician Quality Reporting Institute (PQRI), 7, 21
practice management systems (PMS)
  converting information, 223–231
  and data conversion, 216
  defined, 291
  and EHR, 2, 37–51
    costs, 49–50
    features, 12
    information exchange, 40–44
    interfaces, 39–40, 45

joint marketing, 39
relationships with, 44–45
support, technical, 46
interfaces, 48, 167, 213
and EHR selection, 107–108
licenses, 46–49
products, 38–40
companion, 38
integrated, 38, 40
interfaced, 38–40
replacing, 50–51
review of, 44–49
satisfaction, 44
upgrades, 25, 46, 48
vendors, 45–46
see also private practice
prescriptions
and EHR activation, 252
EHR conversion, 228
and EHR evaluation, 71
reported, 91
screen samples, 119–120
price (*see* costs)
privacy, patient, 65
HIPAA, 182–185
see also security
private practice
closure and merging, 156
and EHR, 9–11
features to look for, 77
management, 2
organization, 2
procedures, 2
responsibilities for EHR implementation, 151
structure, 58–60
see also practice management systems
procedure orders
and EHR evaluation, 72
malpractice issues, 91
product review
checking references, 128–129
demonstration, 121–126
functionality, 142
modularization, 143
overview, 113–132

preparations, 113–115
request for proposal (RFP), 127–128
screen samples, 116–117
site visits, 129–132
see also screen samples
product selection
candidates
identifying, 99–112
manageable list, 112
paring down, 105–108
clinical areas, 106
complexity, 124
customization, 123
and EHR evaluation, 73
EHR status, 101–102
enhancements, 123
upcoming, 125
hospital support, 100–101
limited data, 123
list of commercial products, 269–281
outstanding issues, 125
overview, 99
patient service style, 106–107
PMS
deferring to, 124–125
interface, 107–108
practice size, 105–106
process, 101
recommendations, 100
situations to avoid, 102–105
starting point, 4
support strategy, 125
systems of interest, 100
systems supported by key partners, 101
vendors
comparable, 124
service coverage, 4
verbal explanations, 124
workarounds, 124
product types
document management, 109–112
forms, 109–110
knowledgebase, 110–111
list of commercial products, 269–281
notes, 111–112
project management

access, instantaneous, 196
ad-hoc discussions, 192
business office, 192
clinical content tracking, 189
clinical resources, 191
implementation, 186–195
information velocity, 196
internal project meetings, 193
issues to consider, 194–195
key EHR features, 199
key issues, 187
medical records, 191–192
personnel
    project manager, 190
    staff interaction and use, 196
project plan, 187
    critical path, 188–189
    timeline, 188
technical resources, 190–191
vendor project meetings, 192–193
workflow
    design, 198–200
    issues, 201–203

R

Recovery and Reinvestment Act *see* America Recovery and Reinvestment Act
references, 128–129
referrals, 43
regulation (government), 3
request for proposal (RFP), 127–128
    see also product review
return on investment (ROI), 24, 29, 140

S

screen samples
    clinical charting, 118–119
    diagnostic testing, 121
    image review, 119
    lab order, 121
    message/to-do, 118
    patient information, 117–118
    patient summary, 116
    prescriptions, 119–120
    workflow, 116–117
security

access
    clinical data, 185
    role-based, 185
    system, 264
backup sites/servers, 58, 98, 137
evaluation, 58
facilities, 204–207
HIPAA, 65, 183–184
network, 29
officers, 183–184
personal use, 185
remediation plan, 265–266
software, 211
support, technical, 264
see also network
selection (*see* product selection)
servers (*see* hardware)
service, customer
    continuing support, 29
    costs, negotiating, 155
    coverage, 4
    evaluation
        ARRA support, 56
        basic, 56–58
        system setup, 61–62
    implementation, 142
    provider time, 26
    quality, 10
    warranties, 153
    see also support, technical
site visits, 129–132
    see also product review
software
    appointment tracking, 213
    data conversion, 216–219
    imaging, 212
    interfaces
        diagnostic equipment, 213–214
        PMS, 213
    licensing costs, 24
    plan items, 213
    requirements, 170
    screen samples, 116–121
    security, 211
        disaster recovery, 265–266
        system access, 264

source code escrow, 170
support, technical, 262–266
  enhancements, 264–265
  strategic, 263
tasks, 212
upgrades
  network, 25
  PMS, 25, 46, 48
  unexpected, 28
warranties, 153
see also network

staff
  clinical, 138
  difficulties, 3
  and EHR activation, 253–254
  interaction and use, 196
  mentoring, 254
  super users, 233
  support staff
    continuing, 29
    standards, 260
    training, 233–234
  training, 255
  see also training

support, technical
  access and use, 260–261
  contract, negotiating, 163–164
  and contracts, 153–154
  costs, 143, 155–156, 181
  documentation, 126
  and EHR activation, 254
  evaluation, 61–62
  hardware and software, 262–266
    disaster recovery, 265–266
  malpractice issues, 97–98
  overview, 259–260
  performance monitoring, 261
  and PMS, 46
  policies, 260–261
    clinical charting, 260
    employee standards, 260
    training, 260
  remediation plan, 265–266
  strategy, 125
  system audits, 267–268
  training, 260

  users, 266–267
    front-line, 266
    super-users, 267
  warranties, 153
  see also service, customer
surgery, scheduling, 43, 73
system audits, 267–268

T

technical support (*see* support, technical)
technology
  issue list, 210
  reliance upon, 2–3
  verifying installation, 211
third party vendor exclusions, 91, 171
timeline, vendors', 157
training
  application-specific, 233
  costs, 139–140
  device-specific, 232
  and EHR
    activation, 255
    contract, 158
    implementation, 231–248
    product review, 126
  end users, 233, 234
  facilities, 205–206
  general, 232
  packages, 234
  plan, 234
  practice procedures, 233
  setup, 232–233
  support
    standards, 260
    technical, 260
  see also implementation; support, technical
transcription, 19
  capturing, 12
  and EHR activation, 251
  file conversion, 217

U

uninterruptible power supplies (UPS), 205
user access, 159
user licenses (*see* licenses)

V

vendors
  bill payment, 160
  comprehensive quotes, 141–142
  and contracts, 150–151
    discounts, 143
    negotiation issues, 155–172
    payment, 149
    termination clause, 149–150
  cost estimates, 24
  issues list, 173
  list of commercial products, 269–281
  and mentoring, 254
  payment schedule, 168
  PMS, 45–46
  project meetings, 192–193
  third party exclusions, 171
  see also contracts
volume, 22

W

warranties, 149, 152–153, 171–172
  see also contracts
worksheets
  Basic Implementation Plan, 235–248
  Clinical Content Tracking, 189
  Comprehensive Working Budget, 31–35
  Cost Reduction and Revenue Benefits, 23
  EHR Cost Comparison, 146–147
  EHR Return on Investment, 30
  Evaluation List, 81–83
  key Issues, 187
  Quick EHR Working Budget, 27–28
  Reference Check/Site Visit Questionnaire, 130–132

GLOSSARY

Cluster Server—A cluster server is actually two separate computers that maintain the EHR. One of the servers is the active server and the second mimics the first server. If the primary server fails, the second server becomes the primary server.

Hot Swap Disk Drive—Hot swap disks offer a fail-safe option for EHRs. Hot swap disks are typically used in redundant disk setups. Pairs of hot swap disks are used to store the same information. If one of the disks fails, you can remove it and replace it with a new disk. The system will automatically copy the contents of the working disk to the new disk.

Go Live—The point when your practice is using the EHR as the primary repository of clinical information in the practice.

PMS—Practice Management Systems (PMS) typically includes an appointment scheduler and allows for processing of charges and payments.